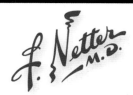
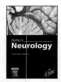

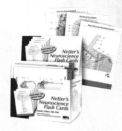

Netter's Concise Neuroanatomy

Michael Rubin, M.D., F.R.C.P.(C)
Professor of Clinical Neurology
Weill Cornell Medical College
New York, New York

Joseph E. Safdieh, MD
Assistant Professor of Neurology and Neuroscience
Weill Cornell Medical College
New York, New York

Illustrations by Frank H. Netter, MD

Contributing Illustrators
John A. Craig, MD
Carlos A.G. Machado, MD
James A. Perkins, MS, MFA

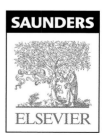

SAUNDERS

ELSEVIER

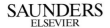

SAUNDERS
ELSEVIER

1600 John F. Kennedy Blvd.
Ste 1800
Philadelphia, PA 19103-2899

Netter's Concise Neuroanatomy

ISBN-13: 978-1-933247-22-9
ISBN-10: 1-933247-22-3

Library of Congress Cataloging-in-Publication Data

Rubin, Michael, 1957–
   Netter's concise neuroanatomy / Michael Rubin, Joseph E. Safdieh ; illustrations by Frank H. Netter ; contributing illustrators, John A. Craig, Carlos A.G. Machado, James A. Perkins. – 1st ed.
      p. ; cm.
   ISBN-13: 978-1-933247-22-9
   ISBN-10: 1-933247-22-3
      1. Neuroanatomy—Atlases.   I. Safdieh, Joseph E.   II. Netter, Frank H. (Frank Henry), 1906–1991.
III. Title.   IV. Title: Concise neuroanatomy.
      [DNLM: 1. Nervous System—anatomy & histology—Atlases.   2. Nervous System Diseases—
Atlases. WL 17 R8955n 2007]
   QM451.R83 2007
   611'.8—dc22

2006052204

Acquisitions Editor: Elyse O'Grady
Developmental Editor: Marybeth Thiel
Publishing Services Manager: Linda Van Pelt
Project Manager: Priscilla Crater
Design Direction: Lou Forgione

Printed in China
Last digit is the print number: 9 8 7 6 5

Working together to grow
libraries in developing countries

www.elsevier.com | www.bookaid.org | www.sabre.org

ELSEVIER   BOOK AID International   Sabre Foundation

To my wife, Annette.
Without you, little would be possible.
Even less would be worthwhile.
—M.R.

In honor of my wife, Esther, who is a source of unyielding support and devotion.
In memory of Mrs. Audrey Nasar, who served as a constant source of
inspiration for me.
—J.S.

Preface

Neuroanatomy is the key to neurology; a solid grounding in neuroanatomy goes a long way in solving any neurodiagnostic challenge. Many fine neuroanatomy textbooks are available, some large, some small. What makes this text unique is the unparalleled Netter series of diagrams, coupled with the relevant points that the student needs to master, all presented in a clear, simplified, straightforward, tabulated format. Easy to grasp and review at a glance, they offer the student what (s)he needs to know without being overburdened with the details needed primarily by the board-certifying neurologist.

Arranged, for the most part, using the standard anatomic approach found in most texts, this atlas is designed to be broadly applicable to medical, dental, allied health and undergraduate neuroanatomy courses. Netter's illustrations provide an illustrative venue for understanding neuroanatomy, a science that is nothing if not visual. Netter's rich illustrations say more than words, while the text, primarily in tabular and point form, supplements and highlights the important aspects of the figures which you, the student, must master.

Acknowledgments

We would like to thank the reviewers who, anonymously, have helped us improve this text to the best of our ability. Any errors that remain are, of course, our own. Our developmental editor, Marybeth Thiel, has patiently worked with us in getting this atlas completed in a timely fashion, and has demonstrated that writing a book can be an enjoyable pastime. Michael Rubin would like to thank his father, a retired cardiologist and outstanding clinician in his own right, for being his guiding light, teacher, and exemplar of what it means to be a teacher and physician. Joseph Safdieh would like to thank his parents for their perpetual support. Finally, we both owe our thanks to Paul Kelly who, though unable to see this to completion, was the initiator of the project and to him we owe our gratitude.

Michael Rubin
Joseph Safdieh

About the Authors

Michael Rubin, M.D., F.R.C.P.(C), is Professor of Clinical Neurology at the Joan and Sanford I. Weill Medical College of Cornell University and Director of the Neuromuscular Service and Electromyography Laboratory at New York Presbyterian Hospital-Cornell Medical Center. Dr. Rubin has been Director of the Neurology Clerkship at Weill-Cornell since 1996 and has received several teaching awards from medical students and neurology residents. In 2002, he was awarded the Teacher Recognition Certificate of the AB Baker Section on Education from the American Academy of Neurology, given to nationally recognized neurologic educators, and he has served as an Associate Examiner for the American Board of Psychiatry and Neurology. In addition to his clinical neurology practice and medical education focus at the student and resident level, Dr. Rubin directs the EMG Fellowship for post-residency trainees. His research interests encompass therapeutic clinical trials in the area of diabetic and HIV-associated peripheral neuropathy. Dr. Rubin is an assistant editor of Neurology Alert, a monthly survey of developments in neurologic medicine. A nonpracticing ordained orthodox rabbi, he enjoys giving a nightly Talmud class at his synagogue.

Joseph E. Safdieh, MD, is Assistant Professor of Neurology and Neuroscience at Joan and Sanford I. Weill Medical College of Cornell University and Assistant Attending Neurologist at New York Presbyterian Hospital. He serves as Associate Director of the Neurology Clerkship at Weill Medical College of Cornell University and Director of Outpatient Training for the Neurology Residency Program at New York Presbyterian Hospital. He has received numerous awards for his academic and teaching achievements, including being selected as the 2005 Academic Neurology Teaching Fellow by the American Neurological Association. He is a member of Phi Beta Kappa and Alpha Omega Alpha. Dr. Safdieh received his bachelor's degree in neuroscience and his medical degree from New York University. He completed his neurology residency training at the Weill Cornell Campus of New York Presbyterian Hospital, where he also served as chief resident in neurology.

Frank H. Netter was born in 1906, in New York City. He studied art at the Art Student's League and the National Academy of Design before entering medical school at New York University, where he received his MD degree in 1931. During his student years, Dr. Netter's notebook sketches attracted the attention of the medical faculty and other physicians, allowing him to augment his income by illustrating articles and textbooks. He continued illustrating as a sideline after establishing a surgical practice in 1933, but he ultimately opted to give up his practice in favor of a full-time commitment to art. After service in the United States Army during World War II, Dr. Netter began his long collaboration with the CIBA Pharmaceutical Company (now Novartis Pharmaceuticals). This 45-year partnership resulted in the production of the extraordinary collection of medical art so familiar to physicians and other medical professionals worldwide.

Icon Learning Systems acquired the Netter Collection in July 2000 and continued to update Dr. Netter's original paintings and to add newly commissioned paintings by artists trained in the style of Dr. Netter. In 2005, Elsevier, Inc. purchased the Netter Collection and all publications from Icon Learning Systems. There are now over 50 publications featuring the art of Dr. Netter available through Elsevier, Inc.

Dr. Netter's works are among the finest examples of the use of illustration in the teaching of medical concepts. The 13-book *Netter Collection of Medical Illustrations,* which includes the greater part of the more than 20,000 paintings created by Dr. Netter, became and remains one of the most famous medical works ever published. *The Netter Atlas of Human Anatomy,* first published in 1989, presents the anatomical paintings from the Netter Collection. Now translated into 16 languages, it is the anatomy atlas of choice among medical and health professions students the world over.

The Netter illustrations are appreciated not only for their aesthetic qualities, but, more importantly, for their intellectual content. As Dr. Netter wrote in 1949 "... clarification of a subject is the aim and goal of illustration. No matter how beautifully painted, how delicately and subtly rendered a subject may be, it is of little value as a *medical illustration* if it does not serve to make clear some medical point." Dr. Netter's planning, conception, point of view, and approach are what inform his paintings and what makes them so intellectually valuable.

Frank H. Netter, MD, physician and artist, died in 1991.

Acknowledgments

The Netter collection of medical illustrations contains a rich assortment of art depicting the complexities of the structure and function of the nervous system. The success of these illustrations is because of close collaboration of content expert and artist. Dr. Frank Netter's most comprehensive collection of neuroanatomy artwork is found in Volume 1, Part 1 of *The Netter Collection of Medical Illustrations*. Since Dr. Netter's passing, several artists have continued in the Netter tradition, working with leaders in various specialties to update some of the Netter plates and to develop new ones that reflect current scientific thought and clinical practice. In preparing *Netter's Atlas of Human Neuroscience*, David Felten, M.D., Ph.D. worked with artists John Craig, M.D. and Jim Perkins to create 117 new illustrations and modify 35 others for the Netter collection of medical illustrations. The creation of these fine images owes much to Dr. Felten who was the content expert for these illustrations, many of which appear in this book. Elsevier thanks them for their contributions to the collection without which many of the illustrations contained in this book would not have been available for reuse and modification.

Netter's Concise Neuroanatomy

Table of Contents

CHAPTER 1

Bony Coverings of the Brain and Spinal Cord

SKULL: ANTERIOR VIEW

STRUCTURE	ANATOMIC NOTES	FUNCTIONAL SIGNIFICANCE
Supraorbital notch	Transmits supraorbital nerve	A useful pressure point for evaluation of arousability in a comatose patient
Infraorbital foramen	Transmits infraorbital nerve	Supplies the skin of lower eyelid, cheek, side of nose, and upper lip
Mental foramen	Transmits mental nerve	Mental neuropathy causes a numb chin and may be a symptom of underlying malignancy; requires aggressive evaluation

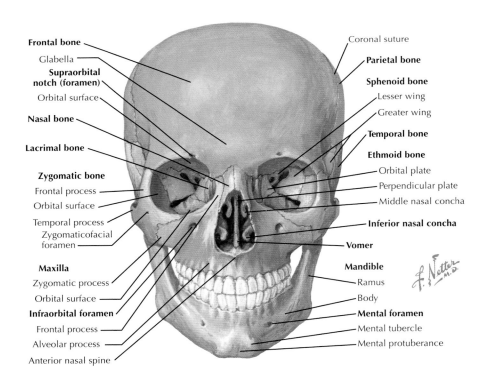

Frontal bone
Glabella
Supraorbital notch (foramen)
Orbital surface
Nasal bone
Lacrimal bone
Zygomatic bone
Frontal process
Orbital surface
Temporal process
Zygomaticofacial foramen
Maxilla
Zygomatic process
Orbital surface
Infraorbital foramen
Frontal process
Alveolar process
Anterior nasal spine

Coronal suture
Parietal bone
Sphenoid bone
Lesser wing
Greater wing
Temporal bone
Ethmoid bone
Orbital plate
Perpendicular plate
Middle nasal concha
Inferior nasal concha
Vomer
Mandible
Ramus
Body
Mental foramen
Mental tubercle
Mental protuberance

ORBIT: ANTERIOR VIEW

STRUCTURE	ANATOMIC NOTES	FUNCTIONAL SIGNIFICANCE
Optic foramen	Transmits optic nerve (CN-II) and ophthalmic artery	Compression of CN-II causes blindness
Superior orbital fissure	Transmits oculomotor nerve (CN-III), trochlear nerve (CN-IV), and nasociliarly branches of ophthalmic division of trigeminal nerve (V_1) and abducens nerve (CN-VI)	Tolosa-Hunt syndrome: idiopathic inflammatory process involving superior orbital fissure, causing eye pain and ophthalmoplegia from involvement of CN-III, -IV, and -VI
Inferior orbital fissure	Transmits maxillary nerve, venous plexus channels, fascicles from pterygopalatine ganglion	Trigeminal neuralgia (tic douloureux) usually involves maxillary and mandibular divisions of trigeminal nerve, rarely ophthalmic division

Right orbit: frontal and slightly lateral view

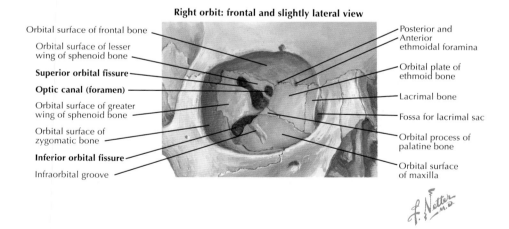

Orbital surface of frontal bone

Orbital surface of lesser wing of sphenoid bone

Superior orbital fissure

Optic canal (foramen)

Orbital surface of greater wing of sphenoid bone

Orbital surface of zygomatic bone

Inferior orbital fissure

Infraorbital groove

Posterior and Anterior ethmoidal foramina

Orbital plate of ethmoid bone

Lacrimal bone

Fossa for lacrimal sac

Orbital process of palatine bone

Orbital surface of maxilla

SKULL: LATERAL VIEW

STRUCTURE	ANATOMIC NOTES	FUNCTIONAL SIGNIFICANCE
Zygomatic bone	Yokes temporal (zygon), sphenoid (greater wing), frontal, and maxillary bones	Sphenoid wing is a common site of origin of meningioma
Pterion	Point where greater wing of sphenoid meets anteroinferior angle of parietal bone	Beneath the pterion lies the anterior branch of the middle meningeal artery, often injured from skull fracture
Nasion	Depression in midline at root of nose	Falx cerebri begins here and extends posteriorly to the inion
Inion	Identical to external occipital protuberance, junction of head and neck	Line joining nasion over skull to inion indicates the position of underlying falx cerebri, superior sagittal sinus, and longitudinal interhemispheric cerebral fissure

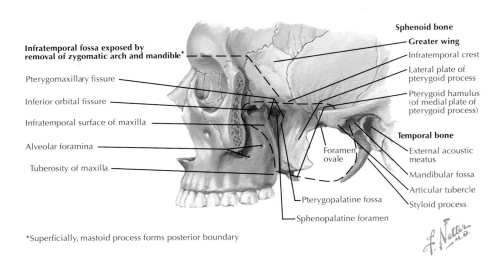

Infratemporal fossa exposed by removal of zygomatic arch and mandible*

Pterygomaxillary fissure

Inferior orbital fissure

Infratemporal surface of maxilla

Alveolar foramina

Tuberosity of maxilla

Sphenoid bone
Greater wing
Infratemporal crest
Lateral plate of pterygoid process
Pterygoid hamulus (of medial plate of pterygoid process)

Temporal bone
External acoustic meatus
Mandibular fossa
Articular tubercle
Styloid process

Foramen ovale

Pterygopalatine fossa

Sphenopalatine foramen

*Superficially, mastoid process forms posterior boundary

SKULL: LATERAL VIEW *continued*

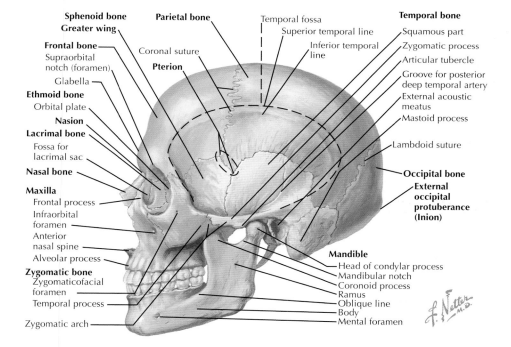

Sphenoid bone
Greater wing

Parietal bone

Temporal fossa
Superior temporal line
Inferior temporal line

Temporal bone
Squamous part

Frontal bone
Supraorbital notch (foramen)
Glabella

Coronal suture

Pterion

Zygomatic process
Articular tubercle
Groove for posterior deep temporal artery
External acoustic meatus
Mastoid process

Ethmoid bone
Orbital plate

Nasion

Lacrimal bone
Fossa for lacrimal sac

Nasal bone

Lambdoid suture

Occipital bone
External occipital protuberance (Inion)

Maxilla
Frontal process
Infraorbital foramen
Anterior nasal spine
Alveolar process

Zygomatic bone
Zygomaticofacial foramen
Temporal process

Zygomatic arch

Mandible
Head of condylar process
Mandibular notch
Coronoid process
Ramus
Oblique line
Body
Mental foramen

SKULL: LATERAL RADIOGRAPH

CLINICAL NOTE:
Enlargement of sella turcica on skull x-ray suggests pituitary tumor.

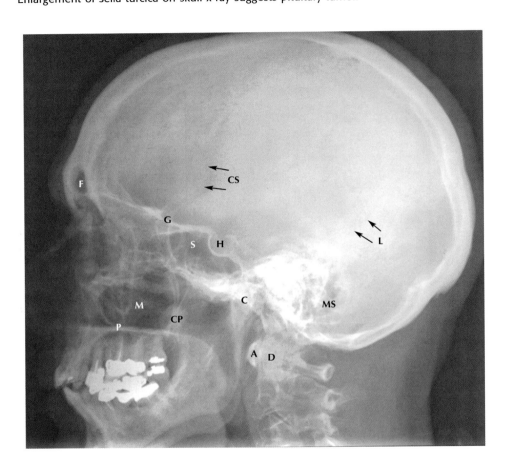

A	Anterior arch of atlas (CI vertebra)	**G**	**Greater wing of sphenoid**
C	Condyle of mandible	**H**	**Hypophyseal fossa (sella turcica)**
CP	Coronoid process of mandible	**L**	Lambdoid suture
CS	Coronal suture	**M**	Maxillary sinus
D	Dens of axis (C2 vertebra)	**MS**	Mastoid air cells
F	Frontal sinus	**P**	Palatine process of maxilla
		S	Sphenoid sinus

SKULL: MIDSAGITTAL VIEW

STRUCTURE	ANATOMIC NOTES	FUNCTIONAL SIGNIFICANCE
Internal acoustic (auditory) meatus	Transmits facial nerve (CN-VII), vestibulocochlear nerve (CN-VIII), and internal auditory artery	Internal acoustic meatus is near the cerebellopontine angle. Tumors in this region cause facial weakness (CN-VII nerve compression), deafness, tinnitus, and vertigo (CN-VIII nerve compression).
Jugular foramen	Lodges superior bulb of internal jugular vein and transmits glossopharyngeal nerve (CN-IX), vagus nerve (CN-X), and spinal accessory nerve (CN-XI)	Jugular foramen syndrome affects CN-IX, -X, -XI, causing hoarseness (vocal cord paralysis), dysphagia, deviation of soft palate to normal side, posterior pharyngeal wall anesthesia, trapezius and sternocleidomastoid weakness. May be due to posterior fossa tumor, vertebral artery aneurysm, or, on leaving the skull, internal carotid artery dissection.
Hypoglossal canal	Transmits hypoglossal nerve (CN-XII)	Hypoglossal nerve lesions (Lou Gehrig's disease, polio) cause tongue atrophy, weakness, and fasciculations.
Cribriform plate	Transmits olfactory nerves (CN-I) from nasal mucosa to olfactory bulb	Meningiomas of cribriform plate cause unilateral anosmia.

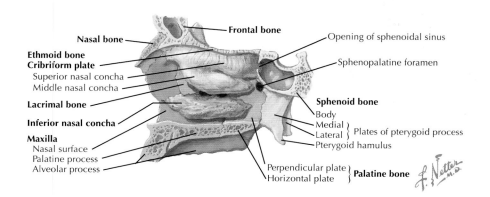

Nasal bone — Frontal bone — Opening of sphenoidal sinus

Ethmoid bone
Cribriform plate
Superior nasal concha
Middle nasal concha

Sphenopalatine foramen

Lacrimal bone

Sphenoid bone
Body
Medial } Plates of pterygoid process
Lateral }
Pterygoid hamulus

Inferior nasal concha

Maxilla
Nasal surface
Palatine process
Alveolar process

Perpendicular plate } Palatine bone
Horizontal plate }

SKULL: **MIDSAGITTAL VIEW** *continued*

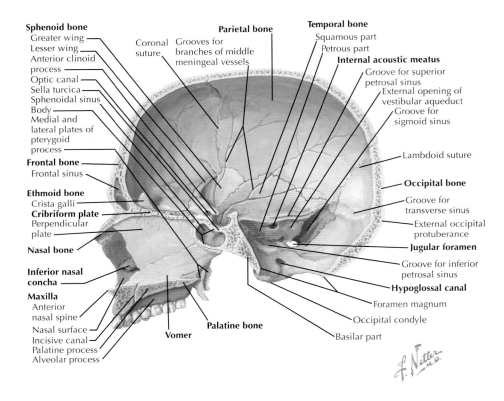

Sphenoid bone
Greater wing
Lesser wing
Anterior clinoid process
Optic canal
Sella turcica
Sphenoidal sinus
Body
Medial and lateral plates of pterygoid process

Frontal bone
Frontal sinus

Ethmoid bone
Crista galli
Cribriform plate
Perpendicular plate

Nasal bone

Inferior nasal concha

Maxilla
Anterior nasal spine
Nasal surface
Incisive canal
Palatine process
Alveolar process

Coronal suture

Grooves for branches of middle meningeal vessels

Parietal bone

Vomer

Palatine bone

Temporal bone
Squamous part
Petrous part
Internal acoustic meatus
Groove for superior petrosal sinus
External opening of vestibular aqueduct
Groove for sigmoid sinus

Lambdoid suture

Occipital bone
Groove for transverse sinus
External occipital protuberance
Jugular foramen
Groove for inferior petrosal sinus
Hypoglossal canal
Foramen magnum
Occipital condyle
Basilar part

CALVARIUM

STRUCTURE	ANATOMIC NOTES
Calvarium	Skullcap Roof of the cranium is formed by frontal, parietal, and occipital bones
Frontal bone	Meets parietal bones at coronal suture
Parietal bones	Meet each other at midline sagittal suture, meet occipital bones at lambdoid suture
Bregma	Meeting point of sagittal suture and coronal suture
Lambda	Meeting point of sagittal suture and lambdoid suture
Vertex of skull	Highest point, lies in midline of sagittal suture
Skull bones	Possess outer and inner lamellae separated by diploe: layer of cancellous bone

CALVARIUM *continued*

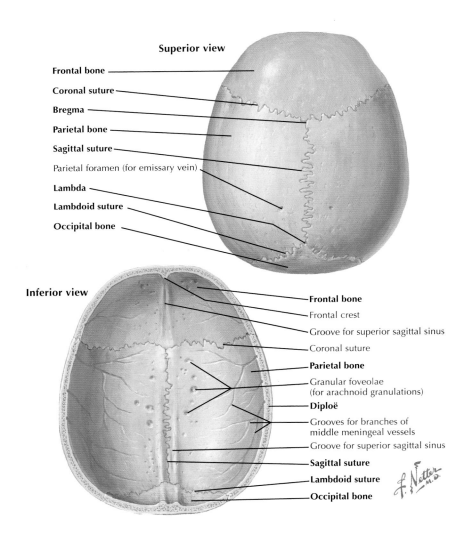

Superior view

Frontal bone

Coronal suture

Bregma

Parietal bone

Sagittal suture

Parietal foramen (for emissary vein)

Lambda

Lambdoid suture

Occipital bone

Inferior view

Frontal bone

Frontal crest

Groove for superior sagittal sinus

Coronal suture

Parietal bone

Granular foveolae
(for arachnoid granulations)

Diploë

Grooves for branches of
middle meningeal vessels

Groove for superior sagittal sinus

Sagittal suture

Lambdoid suture

Occipital bone

Bony Coverings of the Brain and Spinal Cord

BASE OF SKULL: FROM BELOW

STRUCTURE	ANATOMIC NOTES
Incisive foramen	Transmits nasopalatine nerve terminal branches
Greater and lesser palatine foramina	Transmit corresponding nerves and arteries
Stylomastoid foramen	Transmits CN-VII
Jugular fossa	Lodges superior bulb of internal jugular vein

CLINICAL NOTES:
- Paget's disease may cause basilar invagination of skull base, resulting in lower cranial nerve (CN-IX, -X, -XI, -XII) abnormalities, high spinal myelopathy, and cerebellar findings.
- Nasopharyngeal carcinoma can spread from the nasopharynx along the skull base, picking off individual cranial nerves along its course and causing multiple cranial mononeuropathies, usually the trigeminal nerve (CN-V) and CN-VI, with resulting facial numbness (CN-V) and horizontal diplopia (CN-VI).

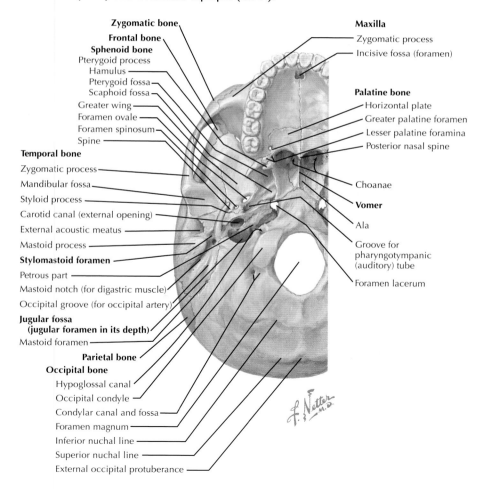

Bony Coverings of the Brain and Spinal Cord

BASE OF SKULL: FROM ABOVE

STRUCTURE	ANATOMIC NOTES
Anterior cranial fossa	Houses the frontal lobes
Middle cranial fossa	Houses the temporal lobes
Posterior cranial fossa	Houses the cerebellum, pons, and medulla
Sella turcica	Houses the pituitary gland

CLINICAL NOTES:
Lesser sphenoid wing meningiomas may expand medially to involve cavernous sinus (affecting CN-III, -IV, and -VI), anteriorly into orbit causing exophthalmos, or laterally into temporal bone, causing bulging of bone.

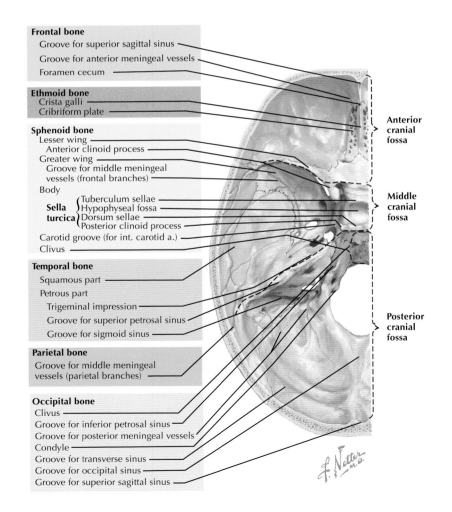

Frontal bone
Groove for superior sagittal sinus
Groove for anterior meningeal vessels
Foramen cecum

Ethmoid bone
Crista galli
Cribriform plate

Sphenoid bone
Lesser wing
Anterior clinoid process
Greater wing
Groove for middle meningeal
vessels (frontal branches)
Body
Sella turcica {Tuberculum sellae
Hypophyseal fossa
Dorsum sellae
Posterior clinoid process
Carotid groove (for int. carotid a.)
Clivus

Temporal bone
Squamous part
Petrous part
Trigeminal impression
Groove for superior petrosal sinus
Groove for sigmoid sinus

Parietal bone
Groove for middle meningeal
vessels (parietal branches)

Occipital bone
Clivus
Groove for inferior petrosal sinus
Groove for posterior meningeal vessels
Condyle
Groove for transverse sinus
Groove for occipital sinus
Groove for superior sagittal sinus

Anterior cranial fossa

Middle cranial fossa

Posterior cranial fossa

BASE OF SKULL: FROM ABOVE *continued*

CLINICAL NOTES:
- Chronic meningeal diseases often involve the skull base (internally).
- Multiple cranial mononeuropathies occur as a result of contiguous spread of process with involvement of cranial nerves.
- Differential diagnoses include infection, autoimmune, and neoplasms.
- Foramen lacerum: Internal carotid artery enters foramen through carotid canal and then turns upward and forward into cavernous sinus.

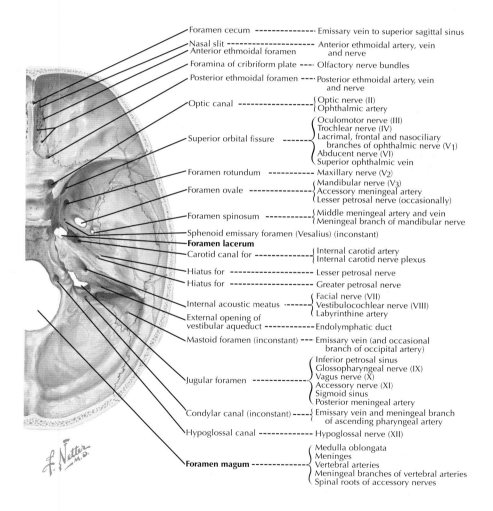

Foramen cecum — Emissary vein to superior sagittal sinus

Nasal slit — Anterior ethmoidal artery, vein and nerve
Anterior ethmoidal foramen

Foramina of cribriform plate — Olfactory nerve bundles

Posterior ethmoidal foramen — Posterior ethmoidal artery, vein and nerve

Optic canal — Optic nerve (II) / Ophthalmic artery

Superior orbital fissure — Oculomotor nerve (III) / Trochlear nerve (IV) / Lacrimal, frontal and nasociliary branches of ophthalmic nerve (V_1) / Abducent nerve (VI) / Superior ophthalmic vein

Foramen rotundum — Maxillary nerve (V_2)

Foramen ovale — Mandibular nerve (V_3) / Accessory meningeal artery / Lesser petrosal nerve (occasionally)

Foramen spinosum — Middle meningeal artery and vein / Meningeal branch of mandibular nerve

Sphenoid emissary foramen (Vesalius) (inconstant)

Foramen lacerum

Carotid canal for — Internal carotid artery / Internal carotid nerve plexus

Hiatus for — Lesser petrosal nerve

Hiatus for — Greater petrosal nerve

Internal acoustic meatus — Facial nerve (VII) / Vestibulocochlear nerve (VIII) / Labyrinthine artery

External opening of vestibular aqueduct — Endolymphatic duct

Mastoid foramen (inconstant) — Emissary vein (and occasional branch of occipital artery)

Jugular foramen — Inferior petrosal sinus / Glossopharyngeal nerve (IX) / Vagus nerve (X) / Accessory nerve (XI) / Sigmoid sinus / Posterior meningeal artery

Condylar canal (inconstant) — Emissary vein and meningeal branch of ascending pharyngeal artery

Hypoglossal canal — Hypoglossal nerve (XII)

Foramen magum — Medulla oblongata / Meninges / Vertebral arteries / Meningeal branches of vertebral arteries / Spinal roots of accessory nerves

BONY FRAMEWORK OF HEAD AND NECK

STRUCTURE	ANATOMIC NOTES	FUNCTIONAL SIGNIFICANCE
Pterygopalatine fossa	Small space behind and below the orbital cavity	Communicates: • Laterally with infratemporal fossa through pterygomaxillary fissure • Medially with nasal cavity through sphenopalatine foramen • Superiorly with skull through foramen rotundum • Anteriorly with orbit through inferior orbital fissure

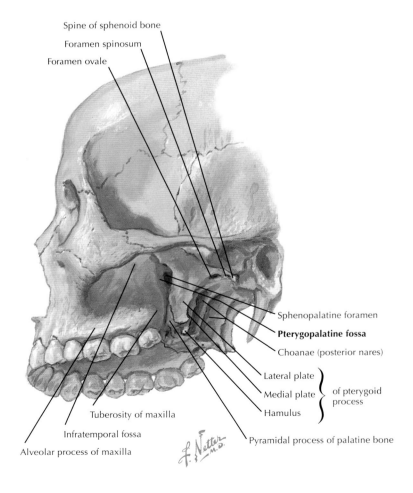

Spine of sphenoid bone

Foramen spinosum

Foramen ovale

Sphenopalatine foramen

Pterygopalatine fossa

Choanae (posterior nares)

Lateral plate ⎱
Medial plate ⎰ of pterygoid process

Hamulus

Tuberosity of maxilla

Infratemporal fossa

Alveolar process of maxilla

Pyramidal process of palatine bone

SURFACE ANATOMY BACK

STRUCTURE	ANATOMIC NOTES	FUNCTIONAL SIGNIFICANCE
Spinous process of C7 vertebra	Vertebra prominens	First spinous process to be felt; 1-6 are covered by ligamentum nuchae
Iliac crests	Horizontal line joining their highest point corresponds to L3-4 interspace	Landmark for lumbar puncture
Posterior superior iliac spines	Horizontal line joining them passes through S2 spinous process	Subarachnoid space with cerebrospinal fluid extends to this level

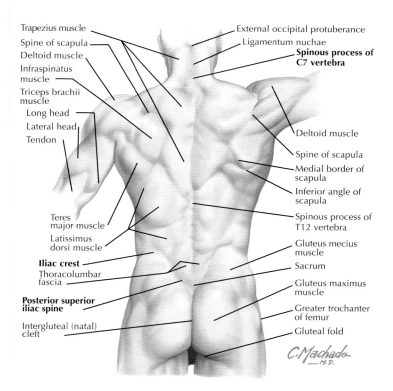

Trapezius muscle

Spine of scapula

Deltoid muscle

Infraspinatus muscle

Triceps brachii muscle

Long head

Lateral head

Tendon

Teres major muscle

Latissimus dorsi muscle

Iliac crest

Thoracolumbar fascia

Posterior superior iliac spine

Intergluteal (natal) cleft

External occipital protuberance

Ligamentum nuchae

Spinous process of C7 vertebra

Deltoid muscle

Spine of scapula

Medial border of scapula

Inferior angle of scapula

Spinous process of T12 vertebra

Gluteus mecius muscle

Sacrum

Gluteus maximus muscle

Greater trochanter of femur

Gluteal fold

C.Machado
—M.D.

VERTEBRAL COLUMN

STRUCTURE	ANATOMIC NOTES	FUNCTIONAL SIGNIFICANCE
33 Vertebral bodies	7 Cervical, 12 thoracic, 5 lumbar, 5 fused sacral, 4 fused coccygeal	Increase in size caudally due to increasing weight they bear
Intervertebral discs	Between each vertebrae but lacking between occiput and atlas and between atlas and axis	Act as shock absorbers for spinal column
C7	Called vertebra prominens because it is the longest cervical spinous process	Highest spinous process palpable is C7

LEVEL	CORRESPONDING STRUCTURE
C2-3	Mandible
C3	Hyoid bone
C4-5	Thyroid cartilage
C6	Cricoid cartilage
C7	Vertebra prominens
T3	Spine of scapula
T8	Point of inferior vena cava piercing diaphragm
T10	Xiphisternal junction
T10	Point of esophagus entering stomach
T12	Point of aorta entering abdomen
L1	End of spinal cord
L3	Subcostal plane
L3-4	Umbilicus
L4	Bifurcation of aorta
L4	Iliac crests
S2	End of dural sac

From Hansen, J.T., & Lambert, D.R. (2006). Netter's Clinical Anatomy. Philadelphia, Elsevier.

CLINICAL NOTES:
• Lumbar disc herniation is more frequent than cervical herniation.
• Disc between L5 and S1 vertebrae is the most common herniated disc.
• As one ascends, lumbar discs herniate with decreasing frequency in sequence (i.e., L4-5 more often than L3-4 > L2-3 > L1-2).
• Thoracic discs represent 0.5% of all surgically verified disc protrusions.
• Lower four thoracic interspaces are the most frequently involved.
• Lumbar puncture is done at L3-4 interspace, or the space above or below, to avoid puncturing the spinal cord that ends at L1-2 interspace.

VERTEBRAL COLUMN *continued*

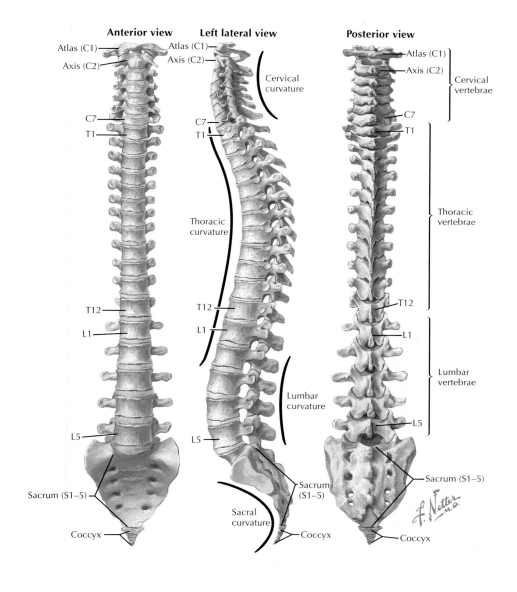

Anterior view

Atlas (C1)
Axis (C2)

C7
T1

T12
L1

L5

Sacrum (S1–5)

Coccyx

Left lateral view

Atlas (C1)
Axis (C2)

Cervical curvature

C7
T1

Thoracic curvature

T12
L1

Lumbar curvature

L5

Sacrum (S1–5)

Sacral curvature

Coccyx

Posterior view

Atlas (C1)
Axis (C2)

Cervical vertebrae

C7
T1

Thoracic vertebrae

T12

L1

Lumbar vertebrae

L5

Sacrum (S1–5)

Coccyx

CERVICAL VERTEBRAE: ATLAS AND AXIS

STRUCTURE	ANATOMIC NOTES	FUNCTIONAL SIGNIFICANCE
Atlas	First cervical vertebra Has no body Forms ring enclosing vertebral foramen Transverse processes pierced by transverse foramen for vertebral artery Occipital condyles of skull rest on superior articular facets of atlas	Paget's disease may cause basilar invagination (upward bulging of occipital condyles), causing neck shortening, cerebellar signs, and myelopathy
Axis	Second cervical vertebra	Hangman fracture, suffered in hanging death, involves fracture of C2, axis, with or without subluxation (slippage) of C2 on C3 and causes death by paralyzing breathing
Dens	Tooth-like process, projects upward from body A divorced portion of atlas that has united with axis	Forms a pivot around which atlas and skull can rotate

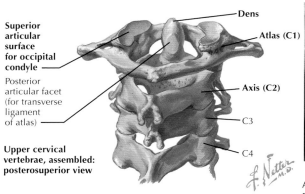

Dens

Atlas (C1)

Axis (C2)

C3

C4

Superior articular surface for occipital condyle

Posterior articular facet (for transverse ligament of atlas)

Upper cervical vertebrae, assembled: posterosuperior view

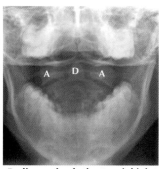

Radiograph of atlantoaxial joint

A   Lateral masses of atlas (CI vertebra)
D   Dens of axis (C2 vertebra)

CERVICAL VERTEBRAE: ATLAS AND AXIS *continued*

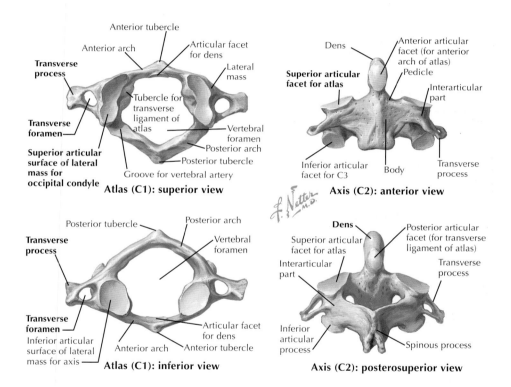

Anterior tubercle

Anterior arch

Articular facet for dens

Transverse process

Lateral mass

Tubercle for transverse ligament of atlas

Transverse foramen

Vertebral foramen

Posterior arch

Superior articular surface of lateral mass for occipital condyle

Posterior tubercle

Groove for vertebral artery

Atlas (C1): superior view

Dens

Anterior articular facet (for anterior arch of atlas)

Superior articular facet for atlas

Pedicle

Interarticular part

Inferior articular facet for C3

Body

Transverse process

Axis (C2): anterior view

Posterior tubercle

Posterior arch

Transverse process

Vertebral foramen

Transverse foramen

Articular facet for dens

Inferior articular surface of lateral mass for axis

Anterior arch

Anterior tubercle

Atlas (C1): inferior view

Dens

Superior articular facet for atlas

Posterior articular facet (for transverse ligament of atlas)

Interarticular part

Transverse process

Inferior articular process

Spinous process

Axis (C2): posterosuperior view

CERVICAL VERTEBRAE

STRUCTURE	ANATOMIC NOTES
Cervical vertebra C1-7	Foramen in transverse processes for vertebral artery, which passes anterior to transverse process of C7 and runs upward from C6 to C1
Pedicles	Project posterolaterally from body of vertebra
Laminae	Directed medially and fuse posteriorly as spinous process
Superior and inferior articular facets	Lie at the junction of pedicle and lamina
Intervertebral foramina	Bordered by pedicles above and below, by intervertebral discs anteriorly, and by facets and facet joints posteriorly

CLINICAL NOTES:
- Dorsal and ventral spinal nerve roots fuse in the intervertebral foramen to form spinal nerve.
- Most common cervical herniated disc is C6-7 (70%).
- Next most common is C5-6 disc (20%), followed by C4-5 and C7-T1 (10%).

4th cervical vertebra: anterior view

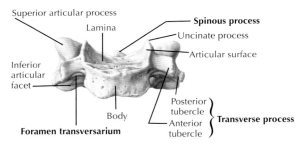

Superior articular process
Lamina
Spinous process
Uncinate process
Articular surface
Inferior articular facet
Body
Posterior tubercle
Anterior tubercle } Transverse process
Foramen transversarium

7th cervical vertebra: anterior view

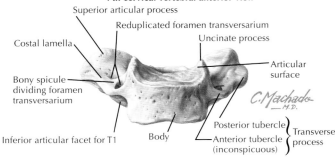

Superior articular process
Reduplicated foramen transversarium
Uncinate process
Costal lamella
Articular surface
Bony spicule dividing foramen transversarium
C.Machado
—M.D.
Posterior tubercle } Transverse process
Inferior articular facet for T1
Body
Anterior tubercle (inconspicuous) } process

CERVICAL VERTEBRAE *continued*

Inferior aspect of C3 and superior aspect of C4 showing the sites of the facet and uncovertebral articulations

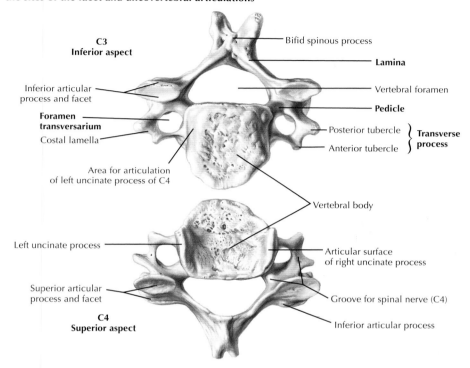

C3
Inferior aspect

Bifid spinous process

Lamina

Inferior articular process and facet

Vertebral foramen

Foramen transversarium

Pedicle

Costal lamella

Posterior tubercle } **Transverse**

Anterior tubercle } **process**

Area for articulation of left uncinate process of C4

Vertebral body

Left uncinate process

Articular surface of right uncinate process

Superior articular process and facet

Groove for spinal nerve (C4)

C4
Superior aspect

Inferior articular process

7th cervical vertebra (vertebra prominens): superior view

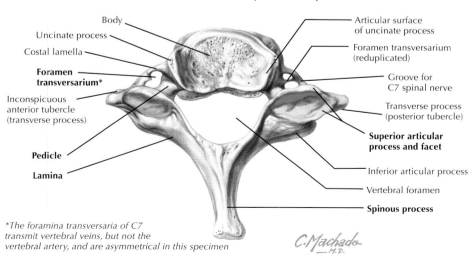

Body

Articular surface of uncinate process

Uncinate process

Foramen transversarium (reduplicated)

Costal lamella

Foramen transversarium*

Groove for C7 spinal nerve

Inconspicuous anterior tubercle (transverse process)

Transverse process (posterior tubercle)

Superior articular process and facet

Pedicle

Inferior articular process

Lamina

Vertebral foramen

Spinous process

*The foramina transversaria of C7 transmit vertebral veins, but not the vertebral artery, and are asymmetrical in this specimen

C.Machado
—M.D.

EXTERNAL CRANIOCERVICAL LIGAMENTS

STRUCTURE	ANATOMIC NOTES
Anterior longitudinal ligament	Runs anterior to vertebrae from base of skull to sacrum
Posterior longitudinal ligament	Runs within vertebral canal, posterior to vertebral body, from base of skull to sacrum (not shown)
Anterior atlanto-occipital membrane	Connects anterior margin of foramen magnum with anterior arch of atlas. It is the continuation of anterior longitudinal ligament
Posterior atlanto-occipital membrane	Connects posterior margin of foramen magnum with posterior arch of atlas
Ligamentum nuchae	Runs from external occipital protuberance to posterior tubercle of atlas and spinous processes of all cervical vertebrae
Ligamentum flavum	Connects laminae of adjacent vertebrae but is absent between skull and atlas

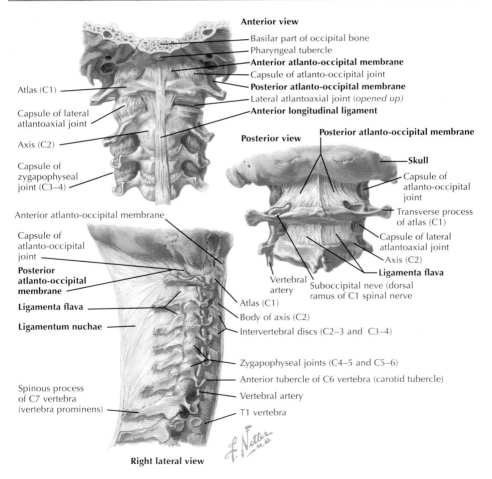

Anterior view

Basilar part of occipital bone
Pharyngeal tubercle
Anterior atlanto-occipital membrane
Capsule of atlanto-occipital joint
Posterior atlanto-occipital membrane
Lateral atlantoaxial joint (opened up)
Anterior longitudinal ligament

Atlas (C1)

Capsule of lateral atlantoaxial joint

Axis (C2)

Capsule of zygapophyseal joint (C3–4)

Posterior view

Posterior atlanto-occipital membrane

Skull

Capsule of atlanto-occipital joint

Transverse process of atlas (C1)

Capsule of lateral atlantoaxial joint

Axis (C2)

Ligamenta flava

Anterior atlanto-occipital membrane

Capsule of atlanto-occipital joint

Posterior atlanto-occipital membrane

Ligamenta flava

Ligamentum nuchae

Vertebral artery

Suboccipital neve (dorsal ramus of C1 spinal nerve)

Atlas (C1)

Body of axis (C2)

Intervertebral discs (C2–3 and C3–4)

Zygapophyseal joints (C4–5 and C5–6)

Anterior tubercle of C6 vertebra (carotid tubercle)

Vertebral artery

T1 vertebra

Spinous process of C7 vertebra (vertebra prominens)

Right lateral view

INTERNAL CRANIOCERVICAL LIGAMENTS

STRUCTURE	ANATOMIC NOTES
Posterior longitudinal ligament	Runs along posterior surface of vertebral bodies along anterior aspect of the vertebral canal
Tectorial membrane	Upward continuation of posterior longitudinal ligament; runs from posterior surface of dens to anterior/lateral margins of foramen magnum
Alar ligament	Connects dens (odontoid process) to the medial side of occipital condyles
Apical ligament	Connects apex of dens to the anterior margin of foramen magnum
Transverse ligament of atlas	Connects (right and left) lateral masses of atlas
Superior longitudinal fascicle	Runs from transverse ligament to basilar part of occipital bone
Inferior longitudinal fascicle	Runs from transverse ligament to posterior surface of body of axis
Cruciform (cruciate) ligament	Composed of transverse ligament of atlas and superior and inferior longitudinal fascicle

CLINICAL NOTE:
Alar ligament prevents excessive head rotation.

INTERNAL CRANIOCERVICAL LIGAMENTS *continued*

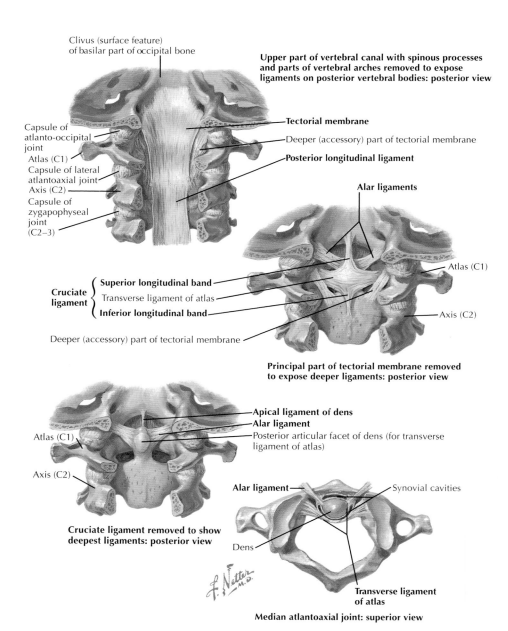

Clivus (surface feature) of basilar part of occipital bone

Upper part of vertebral canal with spinous processes and parts of vertebral arches removed to expose ligaments on posterior vertebral bodies: posterior view

Tectorial membrane

Capsule of atlanto-occipital joint

Deeper (accessory) part of tectorial membrane

Atlas (C1)

Posterior longitudinal ligament

Capsule of lateral atlantoaxial joint

Axis (C2)

Alar ligaments

Capsule of zygapophyseal joint (C2–3)

Atlas (C1)

Axis (C2)

Cruciate ligament { **Superior longitudinal band**
Transverse ligament of atlas
Inferior longitudinal band }

Deeper (accessory) part of tectorial membrane

Principal part of tectorial membrane removed to expose deeper ligaments: posterior view

Apical ligament of dens
Alar ligament
Posterior articular facet of dens (for transverse ligament of atlas)

Atlas (C1)

Axis (C2)

Alar ligament

Synovial cavities

Dens

Cruciate ligament removed to show deepest ligaments: posterior view

Transverse ligament of atlas

Median atlantoaxial joint: superior view

THORACIC VERTEBRAE

- Vertebral bodies of all thoracic vertebrae have superior and inferior costal facets for ribs.
- Transverse processes of thoracic vertebra T1-10 also have transverse costal facets for ribs.

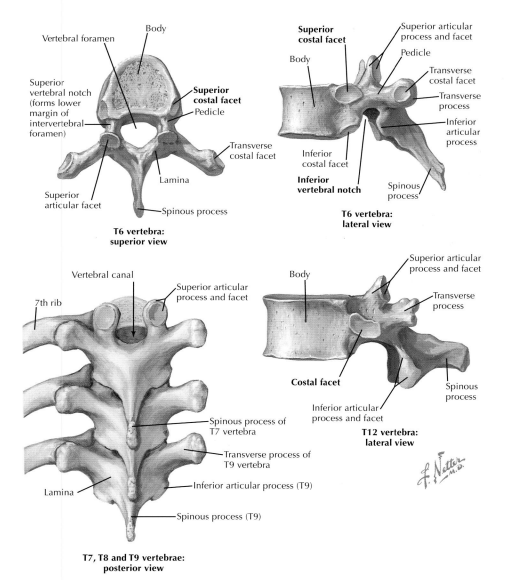

Body
Vertebral foramen
Superior vertebral notch (forms lower margin of intervertebral foramen)
Superior costal facet
Pedicle
Transverse costal facet
Lamina
Superior articular facet
Spinous process

T6 vertebra: superior view

Superior costal facet
Body
Superior costal facet
Pedicle
Superior articular process and facet
Pedicle
Transverse costal facet
Transverse process
Inferior articular process
Inferior costal facet
Inferior vertebral notch
Spinous process

T6 vertebra: lateral view

Vertebral canal
7th rib
Superior articular process and facet
Spinous process of T7 vertebra
Transverse process of T9 vertebra
Inferior articular process (T9)
Lamina
Spinous process (T9)

T7, T8 and T9 vertebrae: posterior view

Body
Superior articular process and facet
Transverse process
Costal facet
Inferior articular process and facet
Spinous process

T12 vertebra: lateral view

LUMBAR VERTEBRAE

STRUCTURE	ANATOMIC NOTES	FUNCTIONAL SIGNIFICANCE
Lumbar vertebrae	Largest individual vertebra L5 is largest lumbar vertebra	As one ascends, lumbar discs herniate with decreasing frequency in sequence (i.e., L4-5 more often than L3-4 > L2-3 > L1-2)
Intervertebral discs	Composed of annulus fibrosus and nucleus pulposus	Disc between L5-S1 vertebrae is most common herniated disc

CLINICAL NOTES:
- Intervertebral discs make up 25% of the length of the vertebral column.
- With aging, discs desiccate and lose height. Hence aging is associated with becoming shorter.
- Lumbar disc herniation is more frequent than cervical herniation.

LUMBAR VERTEBRAE *continued*

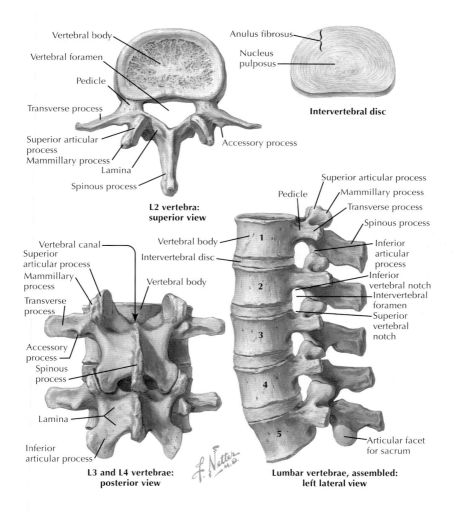

Vertebral body

Vertebral foramen

Pedicle

Transverse process

Superior articular process

Mammillary process

Lamina

Spinous process

Anulus fibrosus

Nucleus pulposus

Intervertebral disc

Accessory process

**L2 vertebra:
superior view**

Vertebral canal

Superior articular process

Mammillary process

Transverse process

Accessory process

Spinous process

Lamina

Inferior articular process

Vertebral body

Intervertebral disc

Vertebral body

Superior articular process

Mammillary process

Transverse process

Pedicle

Spinous process

Inferior articular process

Inferior vertebral notch

Intervertebral foramen

Superior vertebral notch

Articular facet for sacrum

**L3 and L4 vertebrae:
posterior view**

**Lumbar vertebrae, assembled:
left lateral view**

VERTEBRAL LIGAMENTS OF SPINAL COLUMN

STRUCTURE	ANATOMIC NOTES
Anterior longitudinal ligament	Runs anterior to vertebrae from base of skull to sacrum
Posterior longitudinal ligament	Runs within vertebral canal, posterior to vertebral body, from the base of the skull to the sacrum
Ligamentum flavum	Connects adjacent laminae
Supraspinous ligament	Connects the tips of the vertebral spines throughout the spinal column
Interspinous ligament	Runs between adjacent spines throughout the spinal column, anterior to the supraspinal ligament

CLINICAL NOTE:
• Ligamentum nuchae, present in the neck only, are greatly thickened supraspinous and interspinous ligament.

VERTEBRAL LIGAMENTS OF SPINAL COLUMN *continued*

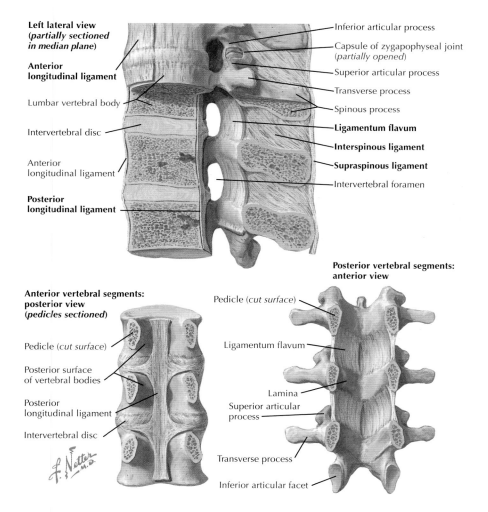

Left lateral view (*partially sectioned in median plane*)

Anterior longitudinal ligament

Lumbar vertebral body

Intervertebral disc

Anterior longitudinal ligament

Posterior longitudinal ligament

Inferior articular process

Capsule of zygapophyseal joint (*partially opened*)

Superior articular process

Transverse process

Spinous process

Ligamentum flavum

Interspinous ligament

Supraspinous ligament

Intervertebral foramen

Anterior vertebral segments: posterior view (*pedicles sectioned*)

Pedicle (*cut surface*)

Posterior surface of vertebral bodies

Posterior longitudinal ligament

Intervertebral disc

Posterior vertebral segments: anterior view

Pedicle (*cut surface*)

Ligamentum flavum

Lamina

Superior articular process

Transverse process

Inferior articular facet

SACRUM AND COCCYX

STRUCTURE	ANATOMIC NOTES
Sacrum	Consists of 5 fused vertebrae, wedge-shaped, narrow inferior apex articulates with coccyx
Coccyx	Formed by fusion of 4 rudimentary tail vertebrae

CLINICAL NOTES:
- First four sacral nerve root ventral rami exit through four ventral pelvic sacral foramina to join the sacral plexus.
- First four sacral nerve root dorsal rami exit through four dorsal sacral pelvic foramina to supply the lower paraspinal muscles and skin.

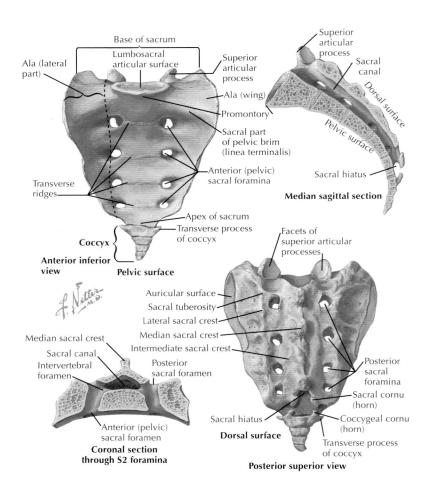

CHAPTER 2

ross Anatomy of the Brain and Spinal Cord

LATERAL SURFACE OF THE BRAIN

NOTABLE LATERAL SULCI	
Structure	**Anatomic Notes**
Lateral (Sylvian) fissure	Separates the temporal lobe from frontal and parietal lobes
Central (Rolandic) sulcus	Separates the frontal lobe from the parietal lobe

CORTICAL LOBES: LATERAL VIEW			
Lobe	**Notable Gyri**	**Notable Sulci**	**Notable Functions**
Frontal	Superior frontal gyrus Middle frontal gyrus Inferior frontal gyrus Precentral gyrus	Superior frontal sulcus Inferior frontal sulcus Precentral sulcus	Motor control, expressive speech, personality, drive
Parietal	Postcentral gyrus Superior parietal lobule Inferior parietal lobule: • Supramarginal gyrus • Angular gyrus	Postcentral sulcus Intraparietal sulcus	Sensory input and integration, receptive speech
Temporal	Superior temporal gyrus Middle temporal gyrus Inferior temporal gyrus	Superior temporal sulcus Inferior temporal sulcus	Auditory input and memory integration
Occipital		Transverse occipital sulcus Lunate sulcus	Visual input and processing

LATERAL SURFACE OF THE BRAIN *continued*

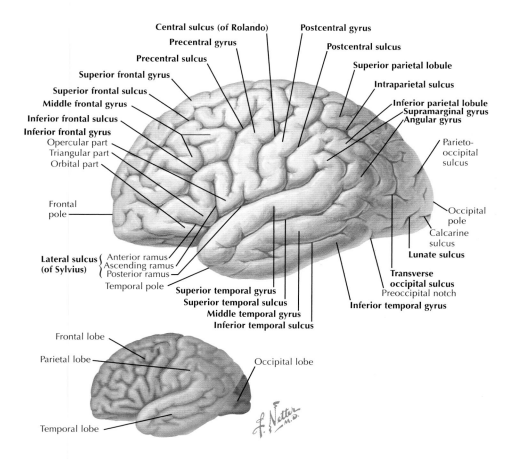

Central sulcus (of Rolando)
Precentral gyrus
Precentral sulcus
Superior frontal gyrus
Superior frontal sulcus
Middle frontal gyrus
Inferior frontal sulcus
Inferior frontal gyrus
Opercular part
Triangular part
Orbital part

Frontal pole

Lateral sulcus { Anterior ramus
(of Sylvius) { Ascending ramus
{ Posterior ramus
Temporal pole
Superior temporal gyrus
Superior temporal sulcus
Middle temporal gyrus
Inferior temporal sulcus

Postcentral gyrus
Postcentral sulcus
Superior parietal lobule
Intraparietal sulcus
Inferior parietal lobule
Supramarginal gyrus
Angular gyrus
Parieto-occipital sulcus

Occipital pole
Calcarine sulcus
Lunate sulcus
Transverse occipital sulcus
Preoccipital notch
Inferior temporal gyrus

Frontal lobe
Parietal lobe
Temporal lobe

Occipital lobe

INSULA *(INSULAR CORTEX)*

STRUCTURE	ANATOMIC NOTES
Circular sulcus of the insula	Surrounds and demarcates the insula
Central sulcus of the insula	Divides the insula into anterior and posterior parts
Limen	The apex of the insula at its inferior margin
Short gyri and long gyrus	Gyri of the insula

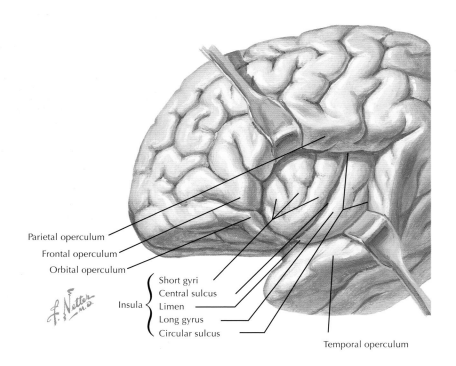

Parietal operculum
Frontal operculum
Orbital operculum
Insula {
Short gyri
Central sulcus
Limen
Long gyrus
Circular sulcus
}
Temporal operculum

MEDIAL SURFACE OF THE BRAIN

MEDIAL CORTICAL STRUCTURES		
Structure	Anatomic Notes	Functional Significance
Medial frontal gyrus	Medial portion of frontal lobe	Involved in motivation
Cingulate sulcus	Separates medial frontal gyrus from cingulate gyrus	
Cingulate gyrus	C-shaped gyrus, which loops around the corpus callosum	Involved in emotion as part of limbic system
Paracentral lobule	Medial extension of precentral and postcentral gyri	Controls motor and sensory function of legs
Precuneus	Part of the medial extension of parietal lobe	
Parieto-occipital sulcus	Prominent sulcus separating parietal and occipital lobes	
Cuneus	Superior portion of medial occipital lobe	Functions in visual processing
Calcarine sulcus	Separates occipital lobe into (upper) cuneus and (lower) lingua	Primary visual center lies on banks of this sulcus
Lingual gyrus	Inferior portion of medial occipital lobe	Functions in visual processing

INTERHEMISPHERIC CONNECTIONS (COMMISSURES)	
Commissure	Anatomic Notes
Anterior commissure	Contiguous and below the rostrum of corpus callosum
Corpus callosum	Large, C-shaped major conduit between 2 hemispheres
	Has following components:
	Rostrum—tapered extension from genu; forms part of the floor of the lateral ventricle
	Genu—curves anterior to the lateral ventricle
	Trunk (body)—largest portion; forms the roof of the lateral ventricle
	Splenium—the posterior-most portion
Posterior commissure	Crosses at the upper end of the cerebral aqueduct
Habenular commissure	Small commissure crossing superior to the pineal gland

MEDIAL SURFACE OF THE BRAIN *continued*

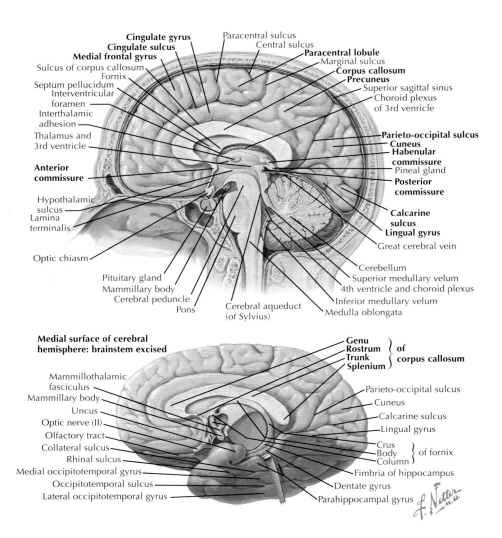

Cingulate gyrus
Cingulate sulcus
Medial frontal gyrus
Sulcus of corpus callosum
Fornix
Septum pellucidum
Interventricular foramen
Interthalamic adhesion
Thalamus and 3rd ventricle
Anterior commissure
Hypothalamic sulcus
Lamina terminalis
Optic chiasm
Pituitary gland
Mammillary body
Cerebral peduncle
Pons

Paracentral sulcus
Central sulcus
Paracentral lobule
Marginal sulcus
Corpus callosum
Precuneus
Superior sagittal sinus
Choroid plexus of 3rd venricle
Parieto-occipital sulcus
Cuneus
Habenular commissure
Pineal gland
Posterior commissure
Calcarine sulcus
Lingual gyrus
Great cerebral vein
Cerebellum
Superior medullary velum
4th ventricle and choroid plexus
Inferior medullary velum
Medulla oblongata

Cerebral aqueduct (of Sylvius)

Medial surface of cerebral hemisphere: brainstem excised

Mammillothalamic fasciculus
Mammillary body
Uncus
Optic nerve (II)
Olfactory tract
Collateral sulcus
Rhinal sulcus
Medial occipitotemporal gyrus
Occipitotemporal sulcus
Lateral occipitotemporal gyrus

Genu)
Rostrum } of
Trunk } corpus callosum
Splenium)

Parieto-occipital sulcus
Cuneus
Calcarine sulcus
Lingual gyrus
Crus)
Body } of fornix
Column)
Fimbria of hippocampus
Dentate gyrus
Parahippocampal gyrus

INFERIOR SURFACE OF THE BRAIN

CORTICAL STRUCTURES		
Structure	**Anatomic Notes**	**Functional Significance**
Frontal pole	Anterior-most portion of frontal lobe	Vulnerable to injury during head trauma
Straight gyrus (gyrus rectus)	Most medial and inferior gyrus of frontal lobe	
Olfactory sulcus	Separates straight gyrus from more lateral orbital gyri	Olfactory tract travels with this sulcus
Orbital gyri and sulci	Form the floor of frontal lobes; rest on the roof of orbits	
Temporal pole	Anterior-most portion of temporal lobe	Vulnerable to injury during head trauma
Uncus	Medial-most bulb-shaped projection of temporal lobe	If swollen may compress the ipsilateral midbrain, causing contralateral hemiparesis
Parahippocampal gyrus	Large inferomedial temporal lobe gyrus	Involved in emotion as part of the limbic system
Collateral sulcus	Separates parahippocampal gyrus from medial occipitotemporal gyrus	
Medial occipitotemporal gyrus	Lies lateral to parahippocampal gyrus	
Occipitotemporal sulcus	Separates medial and lateral occipitotemporal gyri	
Lateral occipitotemporal gyrus	Forms inferolateral border of temporal lobe; contiguous with inferior temporal gyrus	
Occipital pole	Posterior-most portion of the occipital lobe	Vulnerable to injury during head trauma

INFERIOR SURFACE OF THE BRAIN *continued*

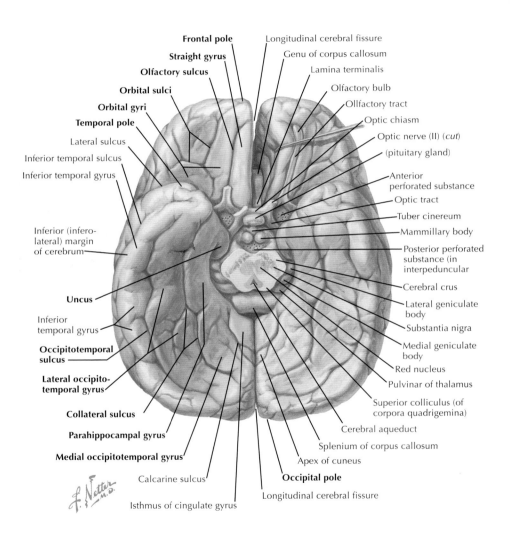

Frontal pole
Straight gyrus
Olfactory sulcus
Orbital sulci
Orbital gyri
Temporal pole
Lateral sulcus
Inferior temporal sulcus
Inferior temporal gyrus
Inferior (infero-lateral) margin of cerebrum
Uncus
Inferior temporal gyrus
Occipitotemporal sulcus
Lateral occipito-temporal gyrus
Collateral sulcus
Parahippocampal gyrus
Medial occipitotemporal gyrus
Calcarine sulcus
Isthmus of cingulate gyrus

Longitudinal cerebral fissure
Genu of corpus callosum
Lamina terminalis
Olfactory bulb
Olfactory tract
Optic chiasm
Optic nerve (II) (*cut*)
(pituitary gland)
Anterior perforated substance
Optic tract
Tuber cinereum
Mammillary body
Posterior perforated substance (in interpeduncular
Cerebral crus
Lateral geniculate body
Substantia nigra
Medial geniculate body
Red nucleus
Pulvinar of thalamus
Superior colliculus (of corpora quadrigemina)
Cerebral aqueduct
Splenium of corpus callosum
Apex of cuneus
Occipital pole
Longitudinal cerebral fissure

BRAINSTEM: MEDIAL VIEW

COMPONENT	ANATOMIC NOTES	FUNCTIONAL SIGNIFICANCE AND CLINICAL NOTES
Midbrain	Encircles the cerebral aqueduct Dorsal tectum composed of superior and inferior colliculi Ventral tegmentum contains nuclei of cranial nerve III (CN-III) and CN-IV, red nucleus, substantia nigra, and cerebral peduncles (which contain fibers of corticospinal tract)	Serves as the center for vertical gaze and the pupillary light reflex In Parinaud's syndrome of the dorsal midbrain compression, upgaze is impaired Degeneration of the substantia nigra is responsible for Parkinson's disease
Pons	Pontine tectum lies anterior to fourth ventricle Contains nuclei of CN-V, -VI, -VII, and -VIII Pontine tegmentum forms large, conspicuous bulge and contains fibers of corticospinal tract	Serves as the center for horizontal gaze Tegmental pontine lesions can cause weakness of all four extremities and the face, with preserved consciousness, known as the *locked-in syndrome,* and sometimes mistaken for a coma
Medulla oblongata	Lowest portion of brainstem, between pons and spinal cord Contains nuclei of CN-IX, -X, -XI, and -XII Corticospinal tract and dorsal column decussation occurs here	Controls visceral and autonomic functions in the body Large, compressive lesions can lead to respiratory arrest and death

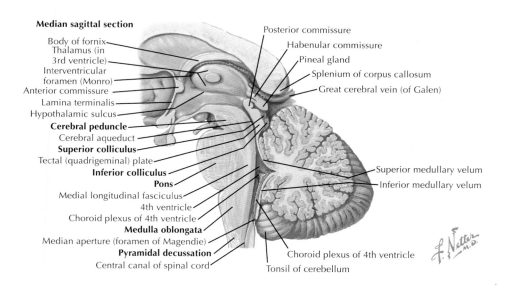

Median sagittal section

Body of fornix
Thalamus (in 3rd ventricle)
Interventricular foramen (Monro)
Anterior commissure
Lamina terminalis
Hypothalamic sulcus
Cerebral peduncle
Cerebral aqueduct
Superior colliculus
Tectal (quadrigeminal) plate
Inferior colliculus
Pons
Medial longitudinal fasciculus
4th ventricle
Choroid plexus of 4th ventricle
Medulla oblongata
Median aperture (foramen of Magendie)
Pyramidal decussation
Central canal of spinal cord

Posterior commissure
Habenular commissure
Pineal gland
Splenium of corpus callosum
Great cerebral vein (of Galen)
Superior medullary velum
Inferior medullary velum
Choroid plexus of 4th ventricle
Tonsil of cerebellum

BRAINSTEM: ANTERIOR AND VENTRAL VIEWS

STRUCTURE	ANATOMIC NOTES	FUNCTIONAL SIGNIFICANCE AND CLINICAL NOTES
Optic chiasm	Two optic nerves join at the optic chiasm, partly decussate, and become optic tracts	Upward pressure on chiasm from pituitary masses can cause specific visual-field deficit involving both temporal fields
Tuber cinereum	Connects the hypothalamus to the pituitary stalk	Lesions cause hypopituitarism
Mammillary bodies	Ball-like inferior projections of the hypothalamus	Involved in memory and emotion as part of the limbic system
Cerebral peduncle	Contains the corticospinal tract	Cerebral peduncle and CN-III can be compressed by nearby uncus
Oculomotor nerve (CN-III)	Exits the midbrain ventrally	
Trochlear nerve (CN-IV)	Exits the midbrain dorsally, crosses midline, and loops around to the ventral surface	Only cranial nerve to exit dorsally; innervates superior oblique muscle
Basis pontis	Large "belly of the pons" is conspicuous on this view	Contains motor fibers from the corticospinal tract
Trigeminal nerve (CN-V)	Pierces and exits the basis pontis	Controls sensations of the face, mouth, tongue, and teeth as well as muscles of mastication
Abducens nerve (CN-VI)	Exits pons inferomedially	Innervates lateral rectus muscle
Facial and vestibulo-cochlear nerves (CN-VII and CN-VIII)	Exit together at the cerebellopontine angle	Facial nerve innervates most facial muscles Vestibulocochlear nerve mediates hearing and balance
Pyramid	Medial bulge of medulla *Note:* The two pyramids decussate in inferior medulla	Contains fibers of corticospinal tract
Olive (inferior)	Conspicuous lateral bulge of medulla	Involved in important cerebellar pathway, called *triangle of Guillain and Mollaret*
Glossopharyngeal, vagus and spinal accessory nerves (CN-IX, -X, and -XI)	Exit the medulla, posterior and lateral to olive and anterior to fasciculus cuneatus, as individual rootlets, which join to form nerves	CN-IX and CN-X control swallowing; CN-X provides parasympathetic input to the heart, lungs, and gut; CN-XI innervates the sternocleidomastoid and trapezius
Hypoglossal nerve (CN-XII)	Exits between olive and pyramid as individual rootlets, which join to form the nerve	Innervates most muscles in the tongue

BRAINSTEM: ANTERIOR AND VENTRAL VIEWS *continued*

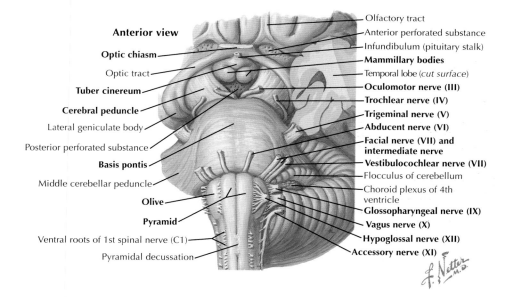

Olfactory tract
Anterior perforated substance
Infundibulum (pituitary stalk)
Mammillary bodies
Temporal lobe (*cut surface*)
Oculomotor nerve (III)
Trochlear nerve (IV)
Trigeminal nerve (V)
Abducent nerve (VI)
Facial nerve (VII) and intermediate nerve
Vestibulocochlear nerve (VII)
Flocculus of cerebellum
Choroid plexus of 4th ventricle
Glossopharyngeal nerve (IX)
Vagus nerve (X)
Hypoglossal nerve (XII)
Accessory nerve (XI)

Anterior view
Optic chiasm
Optic tract
Tuber cinereum
Cerebral peduncle
Lateral geniculate body
Posterior perforated substance
Basis pontis
Middle cerebellar peduncle
Olive
Pyramid
Ventral roots of 1st spinal nerve (C1)
Pyramidal decussation

BRAINSTEM: POSTEROLATERAL VIEW

STRUCTURE	ANATOMIC NOTES	FUNCTIONAL AND CLINICAL NOTES
Thalamus	Large structure composed of many nuclei; sets deep in the brain, above the brainstem	Most nuclei function as relay centers between the cortex and subcortical structures
Pulvinar	Posterior-most nucleus of the thalamus	Involved in central visual processing
Pineal gland	Midline structure, dorsal to the upper midbrain	Can compress the dorsal midbrain, causing Parinaud's syndrome: poor upgaze, nystagmus, and eyelid retraction
Superior colliculus	Upper bulge from the midbrain tectum	Functions in generation of saccades
Inferior colliculus	Lower bulge from the midbrain tectum	Part of auditory relay input from the inner ear to the temporal lobe
Trochlear nerve	Exits the midbrain in this view	Innervates superior oblique
Superior cerebellar peduncle (*cut*)	Upper of 3 large conduits of information between the cerebellum and other structures	Contains mainly cerebellar output to the thalamus and red nucleus
Middle cerebellar peduncle (*cut*)	Middle of 3 large conduits of information between the cerebellum and other structures	Contains mainly input fibers to the cerebellum from the pons
Inferior cerebellar peduncle	Lower of 3 large conduits of information between the cerebellum and other structures	Contains mainly input fibers to the cerebellum from vestibular systems and spinal cord
Rhomboid fossa of fourth ventricle	Forms floor of 4th ventricle; the 2 median eminences bulge into it	
Fasciculus gracilis	Medial-most tract in the medulla	Contains fibers from medial portion of dorsal column of spinal cord; mediates discriminative touch, joint position, and vibration from legs
Fasciculus cuneatus	Lies lateral to the fasciculus gracilis in medulla	Contains fibers from the lateral portion of dorsal column of spinal cord; mediates discriminative touch, joint position, and vibration from arms
Cuneate and gracile tubercles	Visible bulge of respective nuclei	

BRAINSTEM: POSTEROLATERAL VIEW *continued*

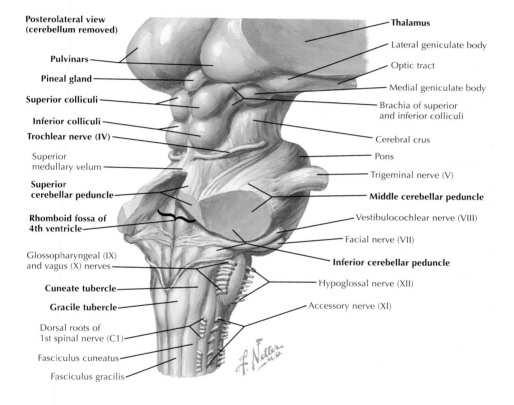

Posterolateral view (cerebellum removed)

Pulvinars

Pineal gland

Superior colliculi

Inferior colliculi

Trochlear nerve (IV)

Superior medullary velum

Superior cerebellar peduncle

Rhomboid fossa of 4th ventricle

Glossopharyngeal (IX) and vagus (X) nerves

Cuneate tubercle

Gracile tubercle

Dorsal roots of 1st spinal nerve (C1)

Fasciculus cuneatus

Fasciculus gracilis

Thalamus

Lateral geniculate body

Optic tract

Medial geniculate body

Brachia of superior and inferior colliculi

Cerebral crus

Pons

Trigeminal nerve (V)

Middle cerebellar peduncle

Vestibulocochlear nerve (VIII)

Facial nerve (VII)

Inferior cerebellar peduncle

Hypoglossal nerve (XII)

Accessory nerve (XI)

CEREBELLUM: SUPERIOR AND INFERIOR SURFACES

The cerebellum is formed by two hemispheres and a single median vermis.

CEREBELLAR LOBE	ANATOMIC NOTES	FUNCTIONAL SIGNIFICANCE
Anterior	Separated from the middle lobe by primary fissure	Becomes atrophic in alcoholics
Middle	Lies posterior and inferior to anterior lobe; separated from it by primary fissure Tonsil is its inferior and medial-most projection	Cerebellar tonsil lies just lateral to the medulla; if displaced by pressure, can compress medulla, causing death; called *tonsillar herniation*
Flocculonodular	Flocculus is separated from the middle lobe by postero-lateral fissure Nodule is part of the vermis	Involved in balance by communicating with the vestibular system

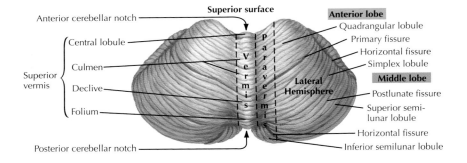

Superior surface

Anterior cerebellar notch
Central lobule
Superior vermis {
Culmen
Declive
Folium
Posterior cerebellar notch

Anterior lobe
Quadrangular lobule
Primary fissure
Horizontal fissure
Simplex lobule
Middle lobe
Postlunate fissure
Superior semi-lunar lobule
Horizontal fissure
Inferior semilunar lobule

Paravermis
Vermis
Lateral Hemisphere

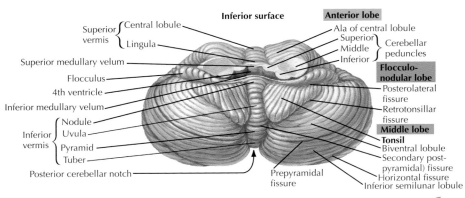

Inferior surface

Superior vermis { Central lobule / Lingula
Superior medullary velum
Flocculus
4th ventricle
Inferior medullary velum
Inferior vermis { Nodule / Uvula / Pyramid / Tuber
Posterior cerebellar notch

Anterior lobe
Ala of central lobule
Superior / Middle / Inferior } Cerebellar peduncles
Flocculo-nodular lobe
Posterolateral fissure
Retrotonsillar fissure
Middle lobe
Tonsil
Biventral lobule
Secondary post-pyramidal) fissure
Horizontal fissure
Inferior semilunar lobule

Prepyramidal fissure

PRINCIPAL TRACTS OF THE SPINAL CORD *continued*

**Principal fiber tracts
of spinal cord**

■ Ascending pathways
■ Descending pathways
■ Fibers passing in both directions

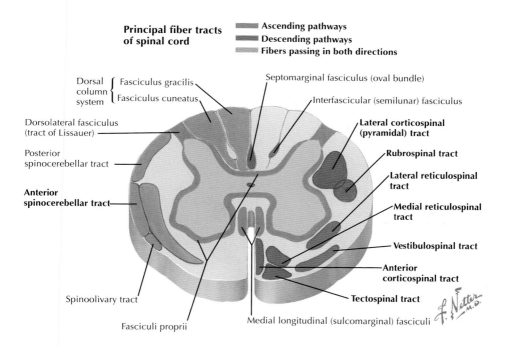

Dorsal
column { Fasciculus gracilis
system { Fasciculus cuneatus

Dorsolateral fasciculus
(tract of Lissauer)

Posterior
spinocerebellar tract

**Anterior
spinocerebellar tract**

Spinoolivary tract

Fasciculi proprii

Septomarginal fasciculus (oval bundle)

Interfascicular (semilunar) fasciculus

**Lateral corticospinal
(pyramidal) tract**

Rubrospinal tract

**Lateral reticulospinal
tract**

**Medial reticulospinal
tract**

Vestibulospinal tract

**Anterior
corticospinal tract**

Tectospinal tract

Medial longitudinal (sulcomarginal) fasciculi

Blood Vessels of the Brain and Spinal Cord

3 Blood Vessels of the Brain and Spinal Cord

BRANCHES OF THE AORTA

ORDER	ARTERY	ANATOMIC NOTES	FUNCTIONAL SIGNIFICANCE
1st	Left subclavian	1st branch is left vertebral artery	Atherosclerosis can lead to shunting of blood away from the vertebral artery and to the arm, leading to symptoms of vertebral insufficiency and possible stroke. This is known as *subclavian steal.*
2nd	Left common carotid	Ascends the neck in carotid sheath before dividing into external and internal carotid arteries (bifurcation)	Atherosclerosis can occur at bifurcation, a common cause of stroke.
3rd	Brachiocephalic trunk	Divides to form right common carotid and right subclavian arteries Right vertebral artery is a branch of right subclavian artery	

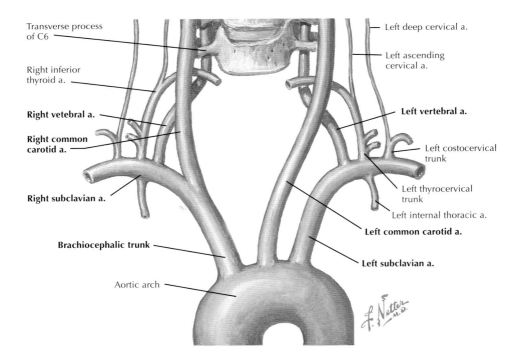

Blood Vessels of the Brain and Spinal Cord 3

ARTERIAL SUPPLY TO BRAIN AND MENINGES

The brain and meninges derive all arterial supply via two arterial systems: carotid and vertebrobasilar.

ARTERY	ANATOMIC NOTES	FUNCTIONAL SIGNIFICANCE
External carotid (ECA)	Has multiple extracranial branches	Supplies the face, tongue, and anterior meninges
Internal carotid (ICA)	Has no extracranial branches Segments: • Cervical: ascends the neck posterior and medial to ECA • Petrous: bends to assume horizontal position, traversing the petrous portion of temporal bone • Cavernous: runs in cavernous sinus near CN-III, -IV, -V, and -VI • Supraclinoid: ascends posteriorly and laterally and terminates as middle and anterior cerebral arteries	Via its branches, supplies anterior circulation of the brain, including frontal, parietal, most of temporal lobes, and basal ganglia
Vertebral artery	Arises from subclavian artery Segments: • Prevertebral: ascends neck muscles to enter the bony canal within the spine at C6 through the foramen transversarium • Cervical: ascends the cervical spine through foramina in transverse processes • Atlantic: exits cervical spine at level of atlas (C1) and bends posteriorly to reach the dura • Intracranial: ascends anterior to the medulla and joins the contralateral vertebral artery to form basilar artery	Via its branches, supplies posterior circulation of the brain, including brainstem, cerebellum, thalamus, and occipital and inferior temporal lobes

3 Blood Vessels of the Brain and Spinal Cord

ARTERIAL SUPPLY TO BRAIN AND MENINGES *continued*

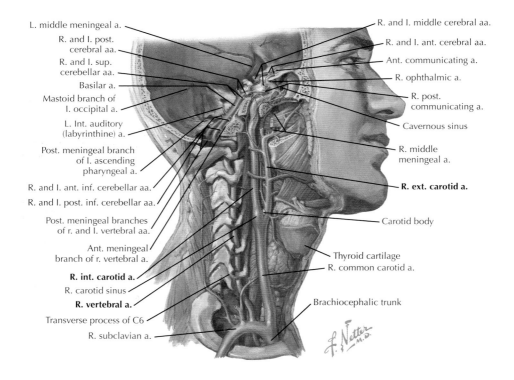

L. middle meningeal a.

R. and I. post. cerebral aa.

R. and I. sup. cerebellar aa.

Basilar a.

Mastoid branch of I. occipital a.

L. Int. auditory (labyrinthine) a.

Post. meningeal branch of I. ascending pharyngeal a.

R. and I. ant. inf. cerebellar aa.

R. and I. post. inf. cerebellar aa.

Post. meningeal branches of r. and I. vertebral aa.

Ant. meningeal branch of r. vertebral a.

R. int. carotid a.

R. carotid sinus

R. vertebral a.

Transverse process of C6

R. subclavian a.

R. and I. middle cerebral aa.

R. and I. ant. cerebral aa.

Ant. communicating a.

R. ophthalmic a.

R. post. communicating a.

Cavernous sinus

R. middle meningeal a.

R. ext. carotid a.

Carotid body

Thyroid cartilage

R. common carotid a.

Brachiocephalic trunk

MENINGEAL ARTERIES

Meningeal arteries supply the dura mater and are located in the outer portion of the dura mater.

ARTERY	ANATOMIC NOTES	FUNCTIONAL SIGNIFICANCE
Middle meningeal	Branch of the ECA system via maxillary artery Enters skull via foramen spinosum Has frontal and parietal branches	Injury to this vessel from head trauma can cause an epidural hematoma, which can lead to death by downward displacement of brain structures; known as **herniation**
Accessory meningeal and anterior meningeal	Arise from ECA system	Supply portions of dura
Tentorial and meningeal branches of the meningohypophyseal trunk	Arise from ICA system	Supply a small segment of dura
Anterior and posterior meningeal branches of vertebral artery		Supply dura in posterior fossa, below the tentorium cerebelli

MENINGEAL ARTERIES *continued*

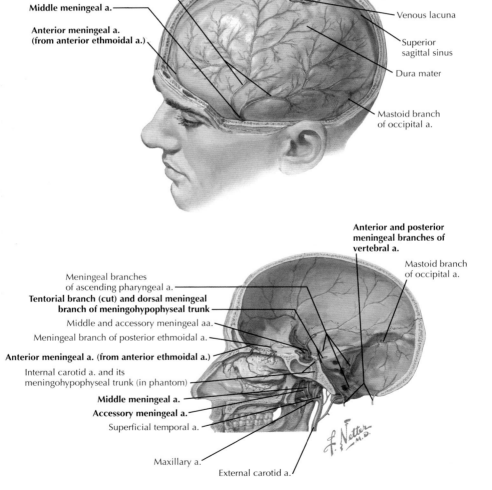

Parietal (post.) and frontal (ant.)
branches of middle meningeal a.

Middle meningeal a.

Anterior meningeal a.
(from anterior ethmoidal a.)

Arachnoid granulations

Opening of
superior cerebral v.

Venous lacuna

Superior
sagittal sinus

Dura mater

Mastoid branch
of occipital a.

Anterior and posterior
meningeal branches of
vertebral a.

Mastoid branch
of occipital a.

Meningeal branches
of ascending pharyngeal a.

Tentorial branch (cut) and dorsal meningeal
branch of meningohypophyseal trunk

Middle and accessory meningeal aa.

Meningeal branch of posterior ethmoidal a.

Anterior meningeal a. (from anterior ethmoidal a.)

Internal carotid a. and its
meningohypophyseal trunk (in phantom)

Middle meningeal a.

Accessory meningeal a.

Superficial temporal a.

Maxillary a.

External carotid a.

THE CIRCLE OF WILLIS

The circle of Willis is an anastomotic arterial network located at the base of the brain, surrounding the optic tracts, pituitary stalk, and basal hypothalamus. Major arterial feeders are the ICA and basilar artery.

ARTERY	ANATOMIC NOTES	FUNCTIONAL SIGNIFICANCE
Superior and inferior hypophyseal	Early branches of ICA	Supplies pituitary gland
Ophthalmic	Branch of ICA; runs with optic nerve into orbit	Supplies optic nerve and retina Embolus from ICA can lodge in this artery, causing monocular blindness
Posterior communicating	Connects ICA to posterior cerebral artery (PCA)	Connects anterior circulation to posterior circulation Runs parallel and near CN-III; so aneurysms can lead to pupillary and oculomotor problems
Anterior choroidal	Branch of ICA	Supplies optic tract, posterior limb of internal capsule, and lateral geniculate body
Anterior cerebral	Terminal branch of ICA	Supplies medial cortical structures and caudate
Middle cerebral	Terminal branch of ICA	Supplies lateral cortical structures and most of basal ganglia and posterior limb of internal capsule
Anterior communicating	Connects the two anterior cerebral arteries (ACAs)	Forms anterior-most portion of circle of Willis
Posterior cerebral	Terminal branch of the basilar system	Supplies occipital and inferior temporal lobe and the thalamus

THE CIRCLE OF WILLIS *continued*

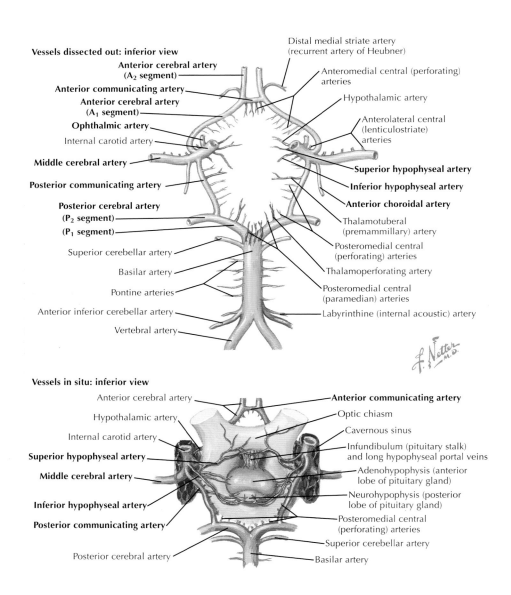

Vessels dissected out: inferior view

- **Anterior cerebral artery (A_2 segment)**
- **Anterior communicating artery**
- **Anterior cerebral artery (A_1 segment)**
- **Ophthalmic artery**
- Internal carotid artery
- **Middle cerebral artery**
- **Posterior communicating artery**
- **Posterior cerebral artery (P_2 segment)** **(P_1 segment)**
- Superior cerebellar artery
- Basilar artery
- Pontine arteries
- Anterior inferior cerebellar artery
- Vertebral artery

- Distal medial striate artery (recurrent artery of Heubner)
- Anteromedial central (perforating) arteries
- Hypothalamic artery
- Anterolateral central (lenticulostriate) arteries
- **Superior hypophyseal artery**
- **Inferior hypophyseal artery**
- **Anterior choroidal artery**
- Thalamotuberal (premammillary) artery
- Posteromedial central (perforating) arteries
- Thalamoperforating artery
- Posteromedial central (paramedian) arteries
- Labyrinthine (internal acoustic) artery

Vessels in situ: inferior view

- Anterior cerebral artery
- Hypothalamic artery
- Internal carotid artery
- **Superior hypophyseal artery**
- **Middle cerebral artery**
- **Inferior hypophyseal artery**
- **Posterior communicating artery**
- Posterior cerebral artery

- **Anterior communicating artery**
- Optic chiasm
- Cavernous sinus
- Infundibulum (pituitary stalk) and long hypophyseal portal veins
- Adenohypophysis (anterior lobe of pituitary gland)
- Neurohypophysis (posterior lobe of pituitary gland)
- Posteromedial central (perforating) arteries
- Superior cerebellar artery
- Basilar artery

ARTERIES OF THE BRAIN: BASAL VIEW

ARTERY	ANATOMIC NOTES	FUNCTIONAL SIGNIFICANCE
Vertebral	The paired vertebral arteries ascend the medulla ventrally and join at the pontomedullary junction to form the basilar artery	Dissection and thrombosis of the vertebral artery in the neck can cause strokes by occlusion or dislodgement of embolic material
Posterior inferior cerebellar (PICA)	Long, circumferential artery, branch of the vertebral artery	Supplies a portion of the cerebellum and dorsolateral medulla Strokes in this distribution cause crossed sensory loss, vertigo, dysarthria, dysphagia, and Horner's syndrome
Basilar	Ascends basis pontis ventrally Gives off small penetrating branches to basis pontis Terminates by dividing into the 2 PCAs	Basilar occlusion can lead to infarction of basis pontis, causing a "locked-in" syndrome
Anterior inferior cerebellar (AICA)	Long circumferential artery, branch of the basilar artery	Supplies a portion of the cerebellum and dorsolateral pons
Superior cerebellar (SCA)	Long circumferential artery, branch of the basilar artery	Supplies superior surface of cerebellum and part of midbrain

ARTERIES OF THE BRAIN: BASAL VIEW *continued*

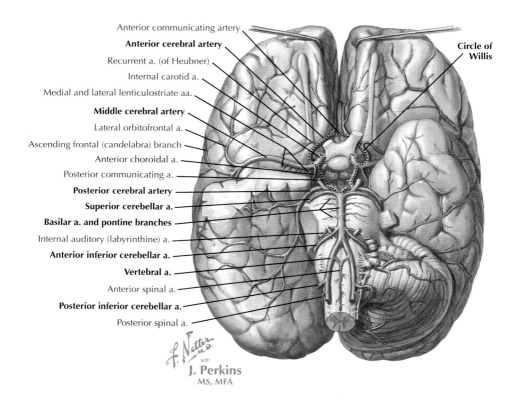

Anterior communicating artery

Anterior cerebral artery

Recurrent a. (of Heubner)

Internal carotid a.

Medial and lateral lenticulostriate aa.

Middle cerebral artery

Lateral orbitofrontal a.

Ascending frontal (candelabra) branch

Anterior choroidal a.

Posterior communicating a.

Posterior cerebral artery

Superior cerebellar a.

Basilar a. and pontine branches

Internal auditory (labyrinthine) a.

Anterior inferior cerebellar a.

Vertebral a.

Anterior spinal a.

Posterior inferior cerebellar a.

Posterior spinal a.

Circle of Willis

with
J. Perkins
MS, MFA

ARTERIES OF THE BRAIN: FRONTAL VIEW

STRUCTURE	ANATOMIC NOTES	FUNCTIONAL SIGNIFICANCE
Oculomotor nerve (CN-III)	Exits upper midbrain ventrally, between the PCA and SCA; then runs parallel to the posterior communicating artery	Aneurysms of the posterior communicating artery can compress CN-III, causing a dilated pupil on that side.
Middle cerebral artery (MCA)	Courses through the sylvian fissure, exiting laterally over the frontal, parietal, and temporal cortex	MCA has a large area of distribution along lateral cortex. Deep branches supply the basal ganglia and internal capsule.
Anterior cerebral arteries	Paired ACAs run in parallel and loop around the midline just above the corpus callosum	ACA has a large area of distribution along the medial frontal and parietal cortex.

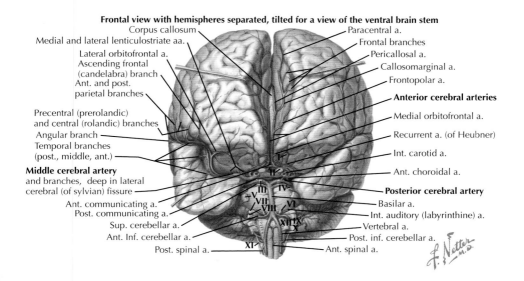

Frontal view with hemispheres separated, tilted for a view of the ventral brain stem

Corpus callosum
Medial and lateral lenticulostriate aa.
Lateral orbitofrontal a.
Ascending frontal (candelabra) branch
Ant. and post. parietal branches
Precentral (prerolandic) and central (rolandic) branches
Angular branch
Temporal branches (post., middle, ant.)
Middle cerebral artery and branches, deep in lateral cerebral (of sylvian) fissure
Ant. communicating a.
Post. communicating a.
Sup. cerebellar a.
Ant. Inf. cerebellar a.
Post. spinal a.

Paracentral a.
Frontal branches
Pericallosal a.
Callosomarginal a.
Frontopolar a.
Anterior cerebral arteries
Medial orbitofrontal a.
Recurrent a. (of Heubner)
Int. carotid a.
Ant. choroidal a.
Posterior cerebral artery
Basilar a.
Int. auditory (labyrinthine) a.
Vertebral a.
Post. inf. cerebellar a.
Ant. spinal a.

Blood Vessels of the Brain and Spinal Cord

ARTERIES OF THE BRAIN: CORONAL SECTION

ARTERY	ANATOMIC NOTES	FUNCTIONAL SIGNIFICANCE
Medial and lateral lenticulostriate	Thin, deep vessels that arise from the MCA in sylvian fissure	Supply basal ganglia and internal capsule
		Small vessels that can be occluded in diseases involving small vessels, such as diabetes and hypertension
Recurrent (of Heubner)	Small, deep branch of the ACA	Supplies a portion of the head of caudate and anterior limb of internal capsule
		May be damaged during surgery for ACA aneurysms

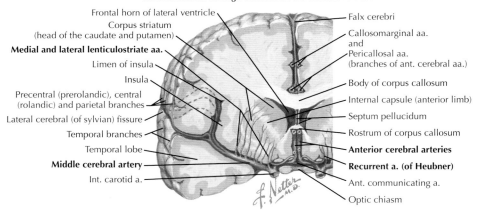

Coronal section through the head of the caudate nucleus

Frontal horn of lateral ventricle
Corpus striatum (head of the caudate and putamen)
Medial and lateral lenticulostriate aa.
Limen of insula
Insula
Precentral (prerolandic), central (rolandic) and parietal branches
Lateral cerebral (of sylvian) fissure
Temporal branches
Temporal lobe
Middle cerebral artery
Int. carotid a.

Falx cerebri
Callosomarginal aa. and Pericallosal aa. (branches of ant. cerebral aa.)
Body of corpus callosum
Internal capsule (anterior limb)
Septum pellucidum
Rostrum of corpus callosum
Anterior cerebral arteries
Recurrent a. (of Heubner)
Ant. communicating a.
Optic chiasm

VENOUS SINUSES

- Venous sinuses are located between the inner and outer layers of dura.
- Sinuses serve as conduits to drain venous blood from the brain to the jugular venous system.

VENOUS SINUS	ANATOMIC NOTES	FUNCTIONAL SIGNIFICANCE
Superior sagittal	Follows the interhemispheric fissure and joins the straight sinus at the confluence of sinuses	Drains venous blood from the scalp, skull, and the meningeal and cerebral veins Collects reabsorbed cerebrospinal fluid (CSF) from arachnoid granulations Thrombosis can cause increased intracranial pressure resulting from backup of venous drainage
Inferior sagittal	Follows the base of falx cerebri and joins the great cerebral vein of Galen to form the straight sinus	Drains deeper veins

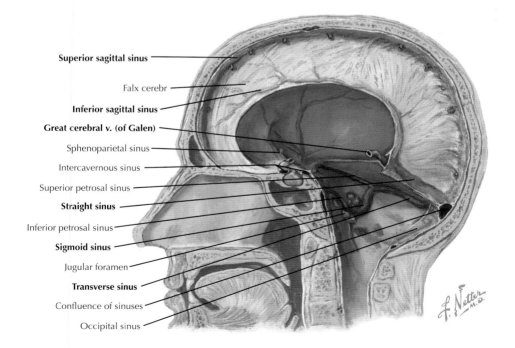

Superior sagittal sinus

Falx cerebr

Inferior sagittal sinus

Great cerebral v. (of Galen)

Sphenoparietal sinus

Intercavernous sinus

Superior petrosal sinus

Straight sinus

Inferior petrosal sinus

Sigmoid sinus

Jugular foramen

Transverse sinus

Confluence of sinuses

Occipital sinus

VENOUS SINUSES *continued*

VENOUS SINUS	ANATOMIC NOTES	FUNCTIONAL SIGNIFICANCE
Cavernous	Contains CN-III, -IV, -V and -VI Drains superior ophthalmic vein and drains into petrosal sinuses	Thrombosis can cause cranial nerve damage and venous backup in the retina.
Superior petrosal	Drains cavernous sinus and drains into transverse sinus	
Inferior petrosal	Drains venous blood from cavernous sinus and brainstem and drains into internal jugular vein	
Straight	Drains inferior sagittal sinus and great cerebral vein and then drains into the confluence of sinuses	
Transverse	Large structure that drains venous blood from the confluence of sinuses and drains into sigmoid sinus	Thrombosis can cause increased intracranial pressure due to backup of venous drainage.
Sigmoid	S-shaped sinus that drains blood from the transverse sinus. As it exits the jugular foramen, it becomes the internal jugular vein	

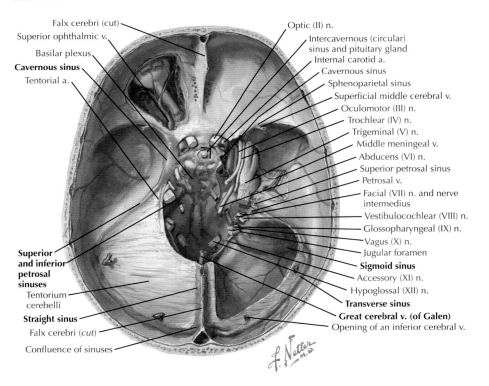

Falx cerebri (cut)
Superior ophthalmic v.
Basilar plexus
Cavernous sinus
Tentorial a.

Optic (II) n.
Intercavernous (circular) sinus and pituitary gland
Internal carotid a.
Cavernous sinus
Sphenoparietal sinus
Superficial middle cerebral v.
Oculomotor (III) n.
Trochlear (IV) n.
Trigeminal (V) n.
Middle meningeal v.
Abducens (VI) n.
Superior petrosal sinus
Petrosal v.
Facial (VII) n. and nerve intermedius
Vestibulocochlear (VIII) n.
Glossopharyngeal (IX) n.
Vagus (X) n.
Jugular foramen
Sigmoid sinus
Accessory (XI) n.
Hypoglossal (XII) n.
Transverse sinus
Great cerebral v. (of Galen)
Opening of an inferior cerebral v.

Superior and inferior petrosal sinuses
Tentorium cerebelli
Straight sinus
Falx cerebri (*cut*)
Confluence of sinuses

SUPERFICIAL VEINS

VEINS	ANATOMIC NOTES
Superficial cerebral	Located in the pia mater, they arise from the substance of brain and drain into venous sinuses
Meningeal	Follow meningeal arteries between the dura and skull and drain into venous sinuses
Diploic and emissary	Thin venous channels located between inner and outer layers of calvaria
	Include the frontal, anterior, and posterior temporal veins and the occipital diploic veins
	Drain into venous sinuses via small emissary veins

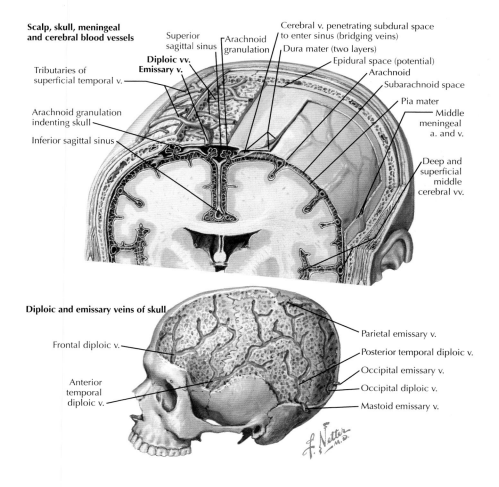

Scalp, skull, meningeal and cerebral blood vessels

Superior sagittal sinus

Arachnoid granulation

Cerebral v. penetrating subdural space to enter sinus (bridging veins)

Dura mater (two layers)

Epidural space (potential)

Diploic vv.
Emissary v.

Arachnoid

Tributaries of superficial temporal v.

Subarachnoid space

Pia mater

Arachnoid granulation indenting skull

Middle meningeal a. and v.

Inferior sagittal sinus

Deep and superficial middle cerebral vv.

Diploic and emissary veins of skull

Parietal emissary v.

Frontal diploic v.

Posterior temporal diploic v.

Occipital emissary v.

Anterior temporal diploic v.

Occipital diploic v.

Mastoid emissary v.

DEEP AND SUBEPENDYMAL VEINS

Deep veins collect venous blood from deep structures and eventually drain into venous sinuses.

VEINS	ANATOMIC NOTES
Anterior septal	Drains deep white matter of the frontal lobe
Thalamostriate	Drains caudate, internal capsule, and deep white matter of the parietal lobe
Internal cerebral	Formed by union of the anterior septal and thalamostriate veins
Basal vein of Rosenthal	Joins internal cerebral vein to form the great cerebral vein of Galen

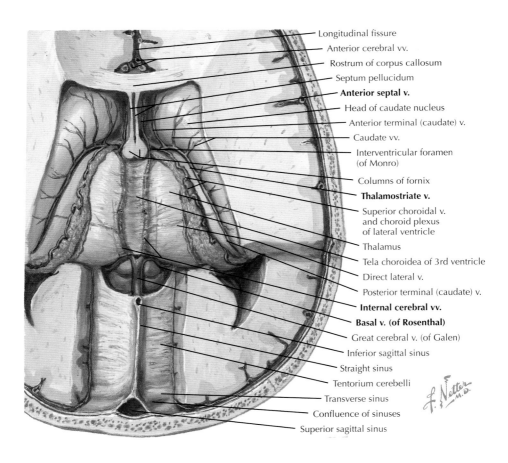

Longitudinal fissure
Anterior cerebral vv.
Rostrum of corpus callosum
Septum pellucidum
Anterior septal v.
Head of caudate nucleus
Anterior terminal (caudate) v.
Caudate vv.
Interventricular foramen (of Monro)
Columns of fornix
Thalamostriate v.
Superior choroidal v. and choroid plexus of lateral ventricle
Thalamus
Tela choroidea of 3rd ventricle
Direct lateral v.
Posterior terminal (caudate) v.
Internal cerebral vv.
Basal v. (of Rosenthal)
Great cerebral v. (of Galen)
Inferior sagittal sinus
Straight sinus
Tentorium cerebelli
Transverse sinus
Confluence of sinuses
Superior sagittal sinus

DEEP VEINS

VEINS	ANATOMIC NOTES
Subependymal	Drain venous blood from subependymal regions, which are adjacent to the ventricular wall. They all eventually drain into the great cerebral vein of Galen or the inferior sagittal sinus.
Anterior cerebral	Medial vein that drains the medial frontal lobe and anterior portion of corpus callosum and drains into the basal vein of Rosenthal

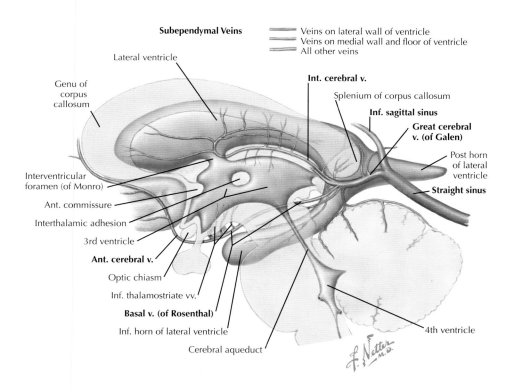

Subependymal Veins

Veins on lateral wall of ventricle
Veins on medial wall and floor of ventricle
All other veins

Lateral ventricle

Genu of
corpus
callosum

Int. cerebral v.

Splenium of corpus callosum

Inf. sagittal sinus

Great cerebral
v. (of Galen)

Post horn
of lateral
ventricle

Interventricular
foramen (of Monro)

Ant. commissure

Interthalamic adhesion

3rd ventricle

Ant. cerebral v.

Optic chiasm

Inf. thalamostriate vv.

Basal v. (of Rosenthal)

Inf. horn of lateral ventricle

Cerebral aqueduct

Straight sinus

4th ventricle

VEINS OF THE POSTERIOR CRANIAL FOSSA

GROUP	VEINS	STRUCTURES DRAINED
Superior	Precentral vein, which drains into the great cerebral vein Superior vermian vein, which drains into the great cerebral vein Posterior mesencephalic vein, which runs parallel to the basal vein Lateral mesencephalic vein, which drains into the basal or posterior mesencephalic vein	Drain superior cerebellum and upper brainstem
Anterior	Anterior spinal vein becomes anterior medullary vein, which becomes anterior pontomesencephalic vein, which drains into the anterior cerebral vein There are many other small named and unnamed veins that are not shown	Drain the anterior brainstem and cerebellar hemispheres
Posterior	Inferior vermian vein drains into straight sinus and forms anastomosis with the superior vermian vein Superior and inferior cerebellar hemispheric veins drain superomedial and inferomedial cerebellar surfaces, respectively	Drain the inferior vermis and cerebellar hemispheres

Veins of Posterior Cranial Fossa

L. sup and inf. colliculi
Left pulvinar
Basal v. (of Rosenthal)
Right thalamus
Int. cerebral vv.
Post. mesencephalic v.
Splenium of corpus callosum
Great cerebral v. (of Galen)
Medial geniculate body
Inf. sagittal sinus
Cut surface of left thalamus
Sup. cerebellar v. (inconstant)
Lateral mesencephalic v.
Sup. vermian v.
Inf. thalamostriate vv.
Straight sinus
Ant. cerebral v.
Falx cerebri
Optic (II) n.
Sup. sagittal sinus
Ant. ponto-mesencephalic v.
Tentorium cerebelli (cut)
Petrosal v.
Confluence of sinuses
Vein of lateral recess of 4th ventricle
L. transverse sinus
Ant. medullary v.
Inf. vermian v.
Sup., middle, and inf. cerebellar peduncles
Falx cerebelli (cut) and occipital sinus
Inf. cerebellar hemispheric vv.
4th ventricle
Precentral v.
Ant. spinal v.
Post. spinal v.

BLOOD SUPPLY TO THE SPINAL CORD

- Anterior and paired posterior spinal arteries branch off vertebral arteries.
- All spinal arteries receive additional supply from radicular arteries off the aorta.
- Major anterior radicular artery (of Adamkiewicz) supplies anterior spinal artery from T8 to the conus.
- Spinal cord segments from T3 to T7 are most vulnerable to ischemia because of the minimal arterial input from radicular vessels at these levels.

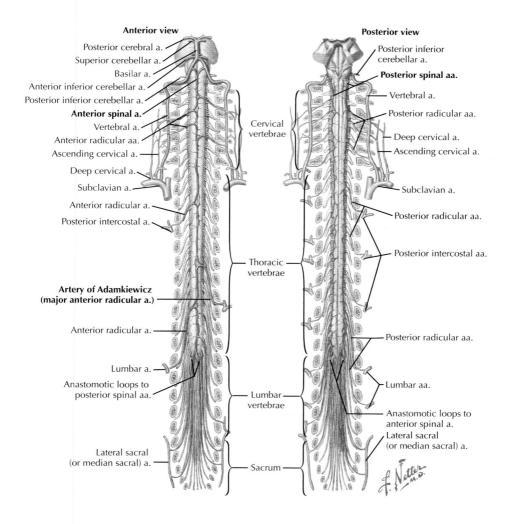

Anterior view

Posterior cerebral a.
Superior cerebellar a.
Basilar a.
Anterior inferior cerebellar a.
Posterior inferior cerebellar a.
Anterior spinal a.
Vertebral a.
Anterior radicular aa.
Ascending cervical a.
Deep cervical a.
Subclavian a.
Anterior radicular a.
Posterior intercostal a.
Artery of Adamkiewicz (major anterior radicular a.)
Anterior radicular a.
Lumbar a.
Anastomotic loops to posterior spinal aa.
Lateral sacral (or median sacral) a.

Cervical vertebrae

Thoracic vertebrae

Lumbar vertebrae

Sacrum

Posterior view

Posterior inferior cerebellar a.
Posterior spinal aa.
Vertebral a.
Posterior radicular aa.
Deep cervical a.
Ascending cervical a.
Subclavian a.
Posterior radicular aa.
Posterior intercostal aa.
Posterior radicular aa.
Lumbar aa.
Anastomotic loops to anterior spinal a.
Lateral sacral (or median sacral) a.

3 Blood Vessels of the Brain and Spinal Cord

DISTRIBUTION OF ANTERIOR AND POSTERIOR SPINAL ARTERIES

ARTERY	FUNCTIONAL SIGNIFICANCE
Anterior spinal	Supplies anterior $^2/_3$ of spinal cord Infarcts cause leg weakness and loss of pain sensation below the level of the lesion with spared vibration and proprioception (posterior column function)
Posterior spinal	Supplies posterior columns Occlusion would cause loss of vibration and proprioception below the level of the lesion

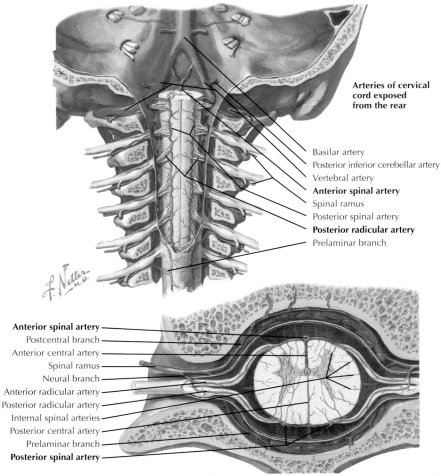

Arteries of cervical cord exposed from the rear

Basilar artery
Posterior inferior cerebellar artery
Vertebral artery
Anterior spinal artery
Spinal ramus
Posterior spinal artery
Posterior radicular artery
Prelaminar branch

Anterior spinal artery
Postcentral branch
Anterior central artery
Spinal ramus
Neural branch
Anterior radicular artery
Posterior radicular artery
Internal spinal arteries
Posterior central artery
Prelaminar branch
Posterior spinal artery

Arteries of spinal cord diagrammatically shown in horizontal section

RADICULAR ARTERIES

- Radicular arteries arise from the aorta in the thoracic region.
- They branch into anterior and posterior radicular arteries.
- Anterior radicular arteries supply the anterior spinal artery.
- Posterior radicular arteries supply the posterior spinal artery.

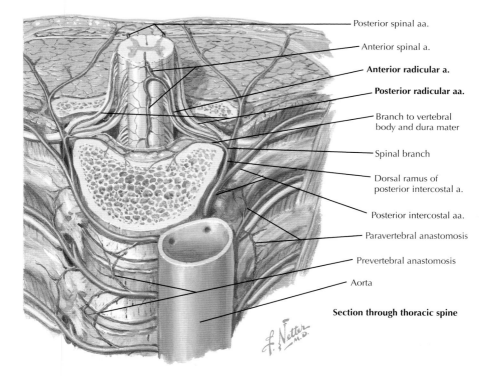

Posterior spinal aa.

Anterior spinal a.

Anterior radicular a.

Posterior radicular aa.

Branch to vertebral body and dura mater

Spinal branch

Dorsal ramus of posterior intercostal a.

Posterior intercostal aa.

Paravertebral anastomosis

Prevertebral anastomosis

Aorta

Section through thoracic spine

VEINS OF SPINAL CORD AND VERTEBRAE

VENOUS STRUCTURE	ANATOMIC NOTES	FUNCTIONAL SIGNIFICANCE
External venous plexus	Anterior external venous plexus lies anterior to the vertebral bodies Posterior external venous plexus lies over the vertebral laminae	Venous plexuses are valveless, allowing infection and malignant tissue access to the spine.
Internal venous plexus	A network of veins in the epidural space of the spinal cord Basivertebral veins drain the vertebral bodies and join the various plexus	
Anterior and posterior spinal veins	Adjacent to anterior and posterior spinal arteries	All spinal veins eventually drain into intervertebral veins, which exit the spinal canal via intervertebral foramina.
Anterior and posterior radicular veins	Adjacent to anterior and posterior radicular arteries.	

VEINS OF SPINAL CORD AND VERTEBRAE *continued*

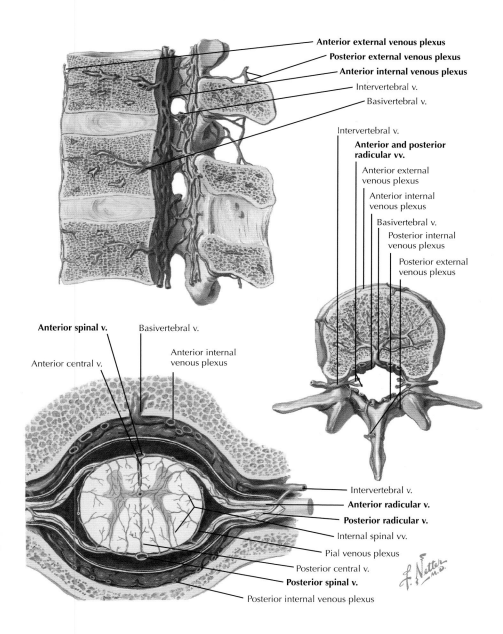

Anterior external venous plexus
Posterior external venous plexus
Anterior internal venous plexus
Intervertebral v.
Basivertebral v.

Intervertebral v.
Anterior and posterior radicular vv.
Anterior external venous plexus
Anterior internal venous plexus
Basivertebral v.
Posterior internal venous plexus
Posterior external venous plexus

Anterior spinal v.   Basivertebral v.
Anterior central v.   Anterior internal venous plexus

Intervertebral v.
Anterior radicular v.
Posterior radicular v.
Internal spinal vv.
Pial venous plexus
Posterior central v.
Posterior spinal v.
Posterior internal venous plexus

CHAPTER 4

Cerebrospinal Fluid and Coverings of the Brain

Cerebrospinal Fluid and Coverings of the Brain

MENINGES

In addition to the protection of the skull, the brain is protected and surrounded by a set of coverings known as the *meninges.*

LAYER	LOCATION	ANATOMIC NOTES	CLINICAL NOTES
Dura mater	Outermost layer	Leathery consistency Lies just under the inner surface of the skull Has 2 layers separated by potential space	Epidural hematomas form between the dura and the skull. They are typically caused by injury to the middle meningeal artery. Subdural hematomas form between the dura and the arachnoid. They are typically caused by rupture of bridging veins.
Arachnoid mater	Middle layer	Fine, lacy membrane, deep to the dura mater Contains cerebrospinal fluid (CSF) and cerebral arteries	Subarachnoid hemorrhages form between the arachnoid and the pia. They are most commonly caused by rupture of an aneurysm of a cerebral artery.
Pia mater	Inner layer	Thin membrane Adheres to contours of the cerebral cortex	

MENINGES *continued*

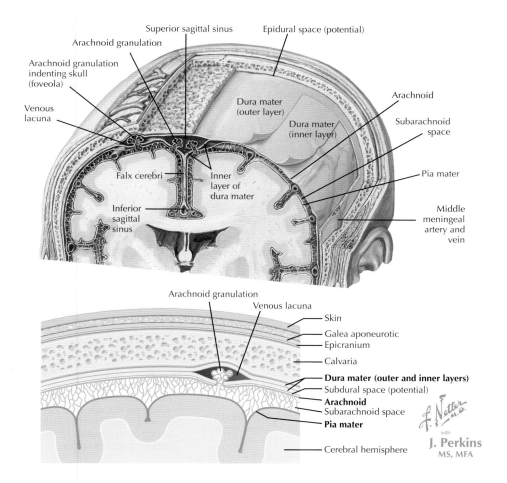

Superior sagittal sinus

Epidural space (potential)

Arachnoid granulation

Arachnoid granulation
indenting skull
(foveola)

Venous
lacuna

Dura mater
(outer layer)

Dura mater
(inner layer)

Arachnoid

Subarachnoid
space

Falx cerebri

Inner
layer of
dura mater

Pia mater

Inferior
sagittal
sinus

Middle
meningeal
artery and
vein

Arachnoid granulation

Venous lacuna

Skin

Galea aponeurotic
Epicranium

Calvaria

Dura mater (outer and inner layers)
Subdural space (potential)
Arachnoid
Subarachnoid space
Pia mater

Cerebral hemisphere

with
J. Perkins
MS, MFA

VENTRICULAR SYSTEM

VENTRICLE	ASSOCIATED STRUCTURE	ANATOMIC NOTES	CLINICAL NOTES
Lateral	Cortex	C-shaped structure Frontal horns are most anterior and are inferior to the corpus collosum Temporal horns are inferior and lie in close relationship to the hippocampus Occipital horns are small posterior extensions CSF exits into the third ventricle via paired foramina of Monro	Obstruction of flow at 1 or both foramina of Monro can cause enlargement of the ventricles called *noncommunicating hydrocephalus.*
Third	Thalamus and hypothalamus	Thin midline structure between the thalami Interrupted by the interthalamic adhesion, which connects the 2 thalami	
Cerebral aqueduct	Midbrain	Thin tubelike structure that connects 3rd to 4th ventricles	Because of its small size, it can be compressed, causing noncommunicating hydrocephalus.
Fourth	Pons and medulla	Rhombus-shaped structure Extends from the upper pons to lower medulla Roofed by the cerebellum	Hemorrhages or masses in the pons or cerebellum can compress the 4th ventricle, causing acute hydrocephalus, which causes headache and may progress to coma.

VENTRICULAR SYSTEM *continued*

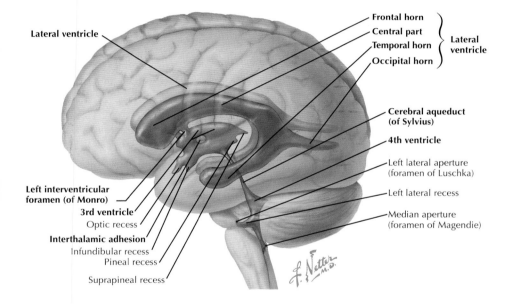

Lateral ventricle

Frontal horn
Central part
Temporal horn
Occipital horn
} Lateral ventricle

Cerebral aqueduct (of Sylvius)

4th ventricle

Left lateral aperture (foramen of Luschka)

Left lateral recess

Median aperture (foramen of Magendie)

Left interventricular foramen (of Monro)

3rd ventricle
Optic recess
Interthalamic adhesion
Infundibular recess
Pineal recess
Suprapineal recess

THE FOURTH VENTRICLE

FEATURE	DESCRIPTION
CSF entry	From the cerebral aqueduct
	CSF is also produced by the choroid plexus of the 4th ventricle
CSF exit	To the subarachnoid cisterns via laterally placed foramina of Luschka and medially placed foramen of Magendie
	Small amount of CSF continues into the central canal of the spinal cord
Roof	Formed by the superior and inferior medullar vela, which are thin white-matter structures that lie below the superior and inferior cerebellar peduncles
Floor	Shaped like a rhombus
	Most visible when the cerebellum and cerebellar peduncles are removed
	Important structures:
	• Striae medullares: separates the upper pontine portion from the lower medullary portion
	• Median sulcus: vertical sulcus that divides the floor symmetrically
	• Medial eminence: longitudinal elevation lateral to the medial sulcus. Its superior part is formed by the locus ceruleus, a bluish nucleus that produces norepinephrine
	• Facial colliculus: overlies the abducens nucleus and facial nerve in the pons
	• Sulcus limitans: a sulcus that lies lateral to the medial eminence
	• Vestibular area: overlies the vestibular nuclei in the pons and medulla
	• Hypoglossal trigone: overlies the hypoglossal nucleus in the medulla
	• Vagal trigone: overlies nuclei of the vagal and hypoglossal nerves

CHAPTER 5

Medulla Oblongata

GROSS BRAINSTEM: MIDSAGITTAL VIEW

STRUCTURE	ANATOMIC NOTES
Superior medullary velum	Roofs pontine part of ventricle
Inferior medullary velum	Roofs medullary part of ventricle
Fastigium	Apex in the cerebellum toward which superior and inferior medullary velum extend
Roof of 4th ventricle	Formed by the cerebellum and superior and inferior medullary velum

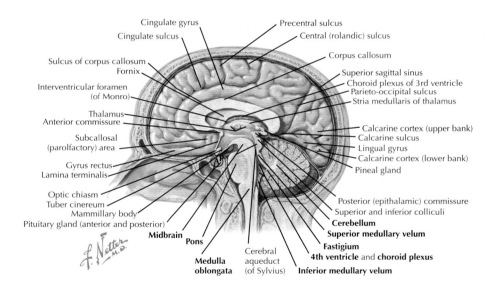

Cingulate gyrus
Cingulate sulcus
Precentral sulcus
Central (rolandic) sulcus
Sulcus of corpus callosum
Fornix
Corpus callosum
Superior sagittal sinus
Interventricular foramen (of Monro)
Choroid plexus of 3rd ventricle
Parieto-occipital sulcus
Stria medullaris of thalamus
Thalamus
Anterior commissure
Calcarine cortex (upper bank)
Subcallosal (parolfactory) area
Calcarine sulcus
Lingual gyrus
Gyrus rectus
Calcarine cortex (lower bank)
Lamina terminalis
Pineal gland
Optic chiasm
Tuber cinereum
Posterior (epithalamic) commissure
Mammillary body
Superior and inferior colliculi
Pituitary gland (anterior and posterior)
Cerebellum
Superior medullary velum
Midbrain Pons
Fastigium
Cerebral aqueduct (of Sylvius)
Medulla oblongata
4th ventricle and **choroid plexus**
Inferior medullary velum

GROSS BRAINSTEM: ANTERIOR VIEW

STRUCTURE	ANATOMIC NOTES
Pyramidal decussation	Marks the transition from spinal cord to lower medulla
Caudal medulla	Rostral to highest cervical rootlets
Inferior olivary nuclei	Oval eminences posterolateral to pyramids that give medulla characteristic appearance above the transition zone

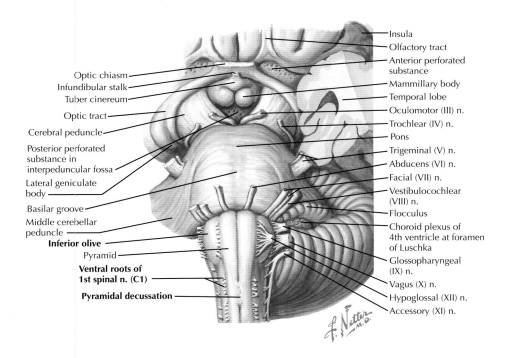

Insula
Olfactory tract
Anterior perforated substance
Optic chiasm
Infundibular stalk
Tuber cinereum
Mammillary body
Temporal lobe
Optic tract
Oculomotor (III) n.
Trochlear (IV) n.
Cerebral peduncle
Pons
Posterior perforated substance in interpeduncular fossa
Trigeminal (V) n.
Abducens (VI) n.
Lateral geniculate body
Facial (VII) n.
Vestibulocochlear (VIII) n.
Basilar groove
Flocculus
Middle cerebellar peduncle
Choroid plexus of 4th ventricle at foramen of Luschka
Inferior olive
Pyramid
Glossopharyngeal (IX) n.
Ventral roots of 1st spinal n. (C1)
Vagus (X) n.
Hypoglossal (XII) n.
Pyramidal decussation
Accessory (XI) n.

GROSS BRAINSTEM: POSTEROLATERAL VIEW

STRUCTURE	ANATOMIC NOTES
Rhomboid fossa	Forms floor of 4th ventricle, overlying the pons and medulla
Fourth ventricle	Extends from the central canal of the cervical cord to the cerebral aqueduct of the midbrain
Median sulcus	Divides the rhomboid fossa into symmetrical halves
Sulcus limitans	Divides each half of the rhomboid fossa into medial eminence and lateral vestibular area. Vestibular nuclei lie beneath the vestibular area
Obex	Caudal junction of walls of 4th ventricle
Cuneate and gracile tubercles	Lie caudal to 4th ventricle

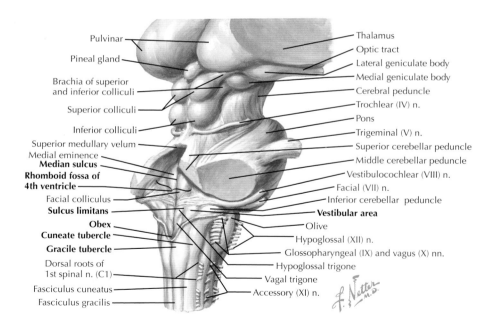

CRANIAL NERVES AND NUCLEI OF MEDULLA

STRUCTURE	ANATOMIC NOTES	FUNCTIONAL SIGNIFICANCE
Descending (spinal trigeminal) nucleus of CN-V	Continuation of substantia gelatinosa of cervical spinal cord	Conveys pain, thermal, and tactile sense from face, forehead, and mucous membranes of nose and mouth
Nucleus of the solitary tract	Solitary nuclei of both sides merge at obex to form commissural nucleus of vagus	Rostral part (*gustatory nucleus*) receives taste from CN-VII and CN-IX. Caudal part receives visceral afferents from CN-X (GI tract, pulmonary, and carotid sinus afferents)
Inferior (CN-IX) salivatory nucleus	Impossible to distinguish from reticular neurons	Innervates otic ganglion, via lesser petrosal nerve, to stimulate parotid gland
Dorsal vagal nucleus (CN-X)	Occupies medial portion of vagal trigone in floor of 4th ventricle	Gives rise to preganglionic parasympathetic fibers
Nucleus ambiguus	Column of cells in reticular formation, midway between spinal trigeminal nucleus and inferior olive	Caudal pole gives rise to cranial root of spinal accessory nerve (CN-XI)
Hypoglossal nerve (CN-XII)	18-mm column of motor cells in central grey of median eminence	Innervates somatic skeletal muscles of tongue

CRANIAL NERVES AND NUCLEI OF MEDULLA *continued*

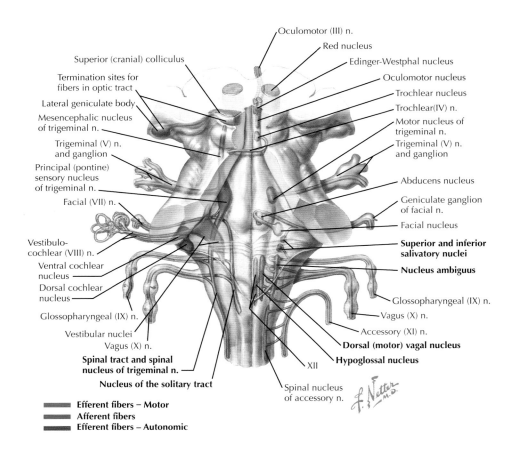

Oculomotor (III) n.

Red nucleus

Superior (cranial) colliculus

Edinger-Westphal nucleus

Termination sites for
fibers in optic tract

Oculomotor nucleus

Lateral geniculate body

Trochlear nucleus

Mesencephalic nucleus
of trigeminal n.

Trochlear(IV) n.

Motor nucleus of
trigeminal n.

Trigeminal (V) n.
and ganglion

Trigeminal (V) n.
and ganglion

Principal (pontine)
sensory nucleus
of trigeminal n.

Abducens nucleus

Facial (VII) n.

Geniculate ganglion
of facial n.

Facial nucleus

Vestibulo-
cochlear (VIII) n.

**Superior and inferior
salivatory nuclei**

Ventral cochlear
nucleus

Nucleus ambiguus

Dorsal cochlear
nucleus

Glossopharyngeal (IX) n.

Glossopharyngeal (IX) n.

Vagus (X) n.

Vestibular nuclei

Accessory (XI) n.

Vagus (X) n.

Dorsal (motor) vagal nucleus

**Spinal tract and spinal
nucleus of trigeminal n.**

XII

Hypoglossal nucleus

Nucleus of the solitary tract

Spinal nucleus
of accessory n.

━━━ Efferent fibers – Motor
━━━ Afferent fibers
━━━ Efferent fibers – Autonomic

MEDULLA: SPINAL CORD TRANSITION

STRUCTURE	ANATOMIC NOTES	FUNCTIONAL SIGNIFICANCE
Decussation of pyramids (corticospinal tracts)	Conspicuous external demarcation of medulla into the spinal cord	90% of each descending corticospinal tract crosses to the opposite side at this point
Spinal nucleus of CN-V	Rostral continuation of substantia gelatinosa of the cervical cord	Lesions here result in a loss of pain and thermal sense in the area innervated by the trigeminal nerve
Dorsal spinocerebellar tract	Uncrossed pathway from periphery to cerebellar vermis. Enters inferior cerebellar peduncle	Used in fine coordination of posture and movement of individual limb muscles
Ventral spinocerebellar tract	Predominantly crossed pathway (in cat) from periphery to anterior lobe of cerebellum. Ascends to pons and enters superior cerebellar peduncle	Conveys information regarding movement and posture of the whole limb
Spinothalamic tract	Crossed pathway of pain and temperature sense	Injury results in contralateral loss of pain and temperature sense
Nucleus CN-XI (spinal accessory nerve)	Spinal portion arises from the anterior horn cell column of C1-5, enters the skull through the foramen magnum, joins the cranial portion of nerve, and exits via the jugular foramen with CN-IX and CN-X	Innervates sternocleidomastoid and trapezius muscles

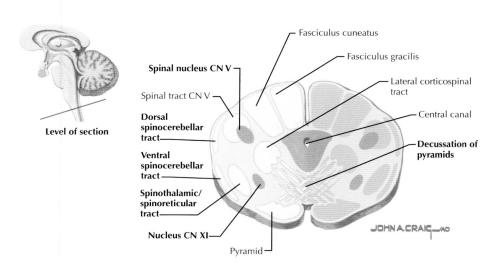

Level of section

Spinal nucleus CN V

Spinal tract CN V

Dorsal spinocerebellar tract

Ventral spinocerebellar tract

Spinothalamic/ spinoreticular tract

Nucleus CN XI

Pyramid

Fasciculus cuneatus

Fasciculus gracilis

Lateral corticospinal tract

Central canal

Decussation of pyramids

JOHN A.CRAIG—AD

MEDULLA: DORSAL COLUMN NUCLEI LEVEL

STRUCTURE	ANATOMIC NOTES	FUNCTIONAL SIGNIFICANCE
Nucleus gracilis	Fasciculus gracilis fibers synapse in this nucleus	Conveys position and vibration sensation from the leg
Nucleus cuneatus	Fasciculus cuneatus fibers synapse in this nucleus	Conveys position and vibration sensation from the arm
Tractus solitarius	Extends rostrally to lower pons	Vagal visceral afferents travel in the tractus solitarius and synapse in the nucleus solitarius
Nucleus solitarius (rostral)	Gustatory nucleus	Receives taste fibers from CN-VII and CN-IX
Nucleus solitarius (caudal)	Vagal visceral afferents synapse in the nucleus solitarius	Receives general visceral afferents from the vagus (carotid sinus, thoracic and abdominal viscera)
Dorsal motor nucleus of CN-X	Gives rise to efferent preganglionic parasympathetic fibers	Innervates thoracic and abdominal viscera
Spinothalamic tract	Posterolateral spinothalamic tract fibers are from the lower body; anteromedial fibers from the arm and neck	Injury results in contralateral loss of pain and temperature sense
Hypoglossal nucleus (CN-XII)	Forms column 18 mm long in central gray; fibers emerge from the medulla between pyramid and inferior olivary complex	Lesion results in weakness and atrophy of the ipsilateral half of the tongue

MEDULLA: DORSAL COLUMN NUCLEI LEVEL *continued*

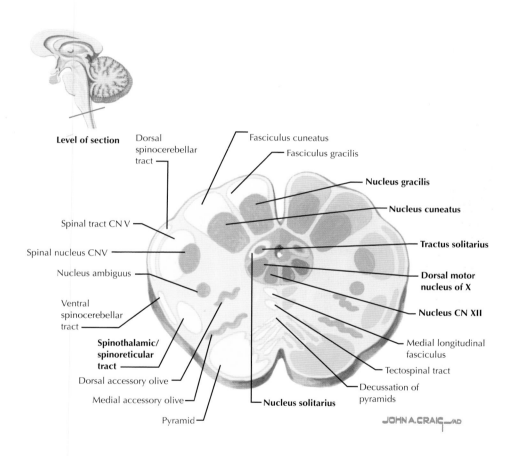

Level of section

Dorsal spinocerebellar tract

Fasciculus cuneatus

Fasciculus gracilis

Nucleus gracilis

Nucleus cuneatus

Spinal tract CN V

Spinal nucleus CN V

Nucleus ambiguus

Ventral spinocerebellar tract

Spinothalamic/ spinoreticular tract

Dorsal accessory olive

Medial accessory olive

Pyramid

Nucleus solitarius

Tractus solitarius

Dorsal motor nucleus of X

Nucleus CN XII

Medial longitudinal fasciculus

Tectospinal tract

Decussation of pyramids

JOHN A. CRAIG__AD

MEDULLA: OBEX LEVEL

STRUCTURE	ANATOMIC NOTES	FUNCTIONAL SIGNIFICANCE
Obex	Lies between the area postrema on each side of 4th ventricle	Area postrema is an emetic chemoreceptor trigger zone
Internal arcuate fibers	Myelinated fibers that sweep ventromedially from the nucleus gracilis and cuneatus to form contralateral ascending medial lemniscus	Crossing provides anatomic basis for sensory representation of half the body in the contralateral cerebral cortex
Medial longitudinal fasciculus (MLF)	Extends from the upper midbrain to spinal levels	Mediates conjugate horizontal eye movements
Tectospinal tract	Arises from the superior colliculus and terminates mostly in the upper 4 cervical segments	Mediates reflex postural movements in response to visual and perhaps auditory stimuli
Medial lemniscus	Contains 2nd-order neurons of the posterior column pathway	Mediates position and vibration sensation
Inferior olivary nucleus	Fibers enter the contralateral inferior cerebellar peduncle and end as climbing fibers in the cerebellar cortex	Largest medullary cerebellar relay nucleus, receiving input from cortex, red nucleus, pons, and spinal dorsal column
Nucleus ambiguus	Caudal pole of the nucleus ambiguus is nucleus of CN XI	Caudal parts give rise to cranial part of CN-XI fibers
		Rostral parts give rise to CN-IX fibers to stylopharyngeus
External (lateral) cuneate nucleus	Medullary equivalent of the dorsal nucleus of Clarke of spinal cord (which gave rise to uncrossed fibers of the dorsal spinocerebellar tract)	Gives rise to cuneocerebellar tract, the upper-limb equivalent of the dorsal spinocerebellar tract

MEDULLA: OBEX LEVEL *continued*

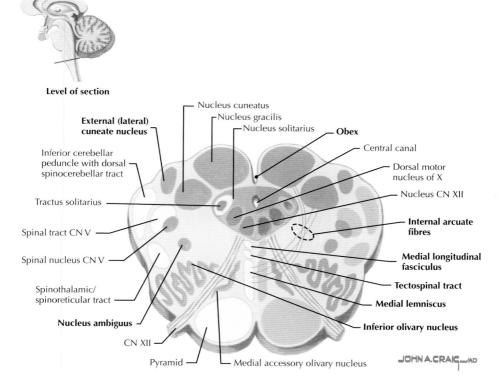

Level of section

Nucleus cuneatus
Nucleus gracilis
Nucleus solitarius
Obex

External (lateral) cuneate nucleus

Inferior cerebellar peduncle with dorsal spinocerebellar tract

Tractus solitarius

Spinal tract CN V

Spinal nucleus CN V

Spinothalamic/ spinoreticular tract

Nucleus ambiguus

CN XII

Pyramid

Medial accessory olivary nucleus

Central canal

Dorsal motor nucleus of X

Nucleus CN XII

Internal arcuate fibres

Medial longitudinal fasciculus

Tectospinal tract

Medial lemniscus

Inferior olivary nucleus

JOHN A.CRAIG—AD

MEDULLA: INFERIOR OLIVE LEVEL

STRUCTURE	ANATOMIC NOTES	FUNCTIONAL SIGNIFICANCE
External cuneate nucleus	Medullary equivalent of the dorsal nucleus of Clarke; gives rise to uncrossed cuneocerebellar fibers	Upper-limb equivalent of the posterior spinocerebellar tract
Spinal tract of CN-V	Afferent trigeminal fibers enter the upper pons and descend the dorsolateral brainstem as spinal trigeminal tract	Tractotomy may relieve severe pain of trigeminal neuralgia
Dorsal accessory olivary nucleus	Project largely to the cerebellar vermis	Modulates cerebellar processing
Medial accessory olivary nucleus	Project largely to the cerebellar vermis	Modulates cerebellar processing
Pyramid	Conveys descending corticospinal fibers	Lesion results in contralateral hemiparesis
Choroid plexus	Projects into the caudal part of the 4th ventricle	Main site of cerebrospinal fluid (CSF) formation Renews entire CSF 4-5 times per day

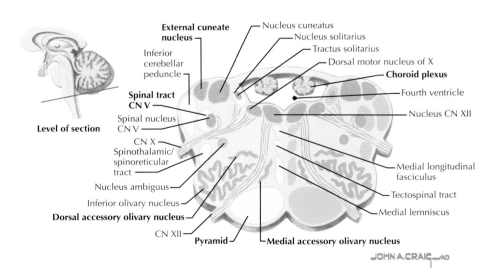

TRIGEMINAL SYSTEM: LONGITUDINAL BRAINSTEM VIEW

STRUCTURE	ANATOMIC NOTES	FUNCTIONAL SIGNIFICANCE
Spinal (descending) trigeminal nucleus	Merges with the substantia gelatinosa in dorsal spinal gray matter	Mediates pain, temperature, and tactile sense from the face, forehead, muscosa of the nose and mouth
Spinal (descending) trigeminal tract	Close to the spinothalamic tract	Due to the proximity of these 2 tracts, injury to this area (stroke) results in crossed hemianalgesia of the face and body (one side of the face and the opposite side of the body have impaired pain sensation)

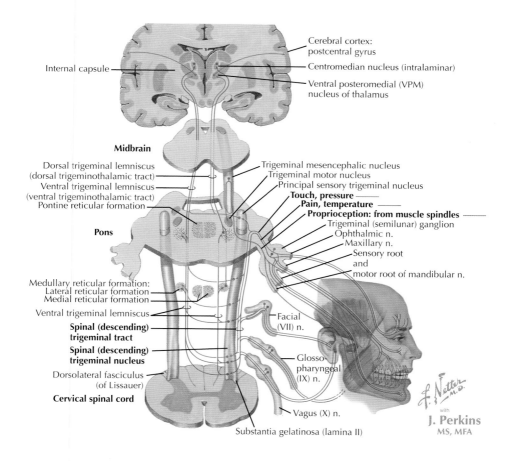

MEDULLA: VESTIBULAR NUCLEI LEVEL

STRUCTURE	ANATOMIC NOTES	FUNCTIONAL SIGNIFICANCE
Reticular formation	Constitutes a matrix throughout the lower brainstem, within which nuclei and tracts are embedded	Involved in consciousness and alertness Brainstem stroke results in coma due to injury of this region
Tractus solitarius	Constitutes a descending bundle of visceral afferents comparable to the spinal trigeminal tract, which contains general somatic afferents	Surrounded by, and synapses in, the nucleus solitarius, which rostrally subserves taste (i.e., the gustatory nucleus), and caudally subserves cardiorespiratory function and general visceral sensation
Inferior and medial vestibular nuclei	Two of the 4 vestibular nuclei. Due to the rostrocaudal extent of nuclei, only 2 can be seen in any single section	Innervate semicircular canals, utricle, and saccule Involved in balance and orientation in space
Inferior cerebellar peduncle	Formed by tracts and fibers from the medulla and spinal cord: the spinocerebellar and olivocerebellar tracts, lateral reticular, arcuate, and cuneate nuclei fibers	Most cerebellar afferents enter via inferior and middle cerebellar peduncles, conveying stretch, vestibular, visual, and other impulses
Medial lemniscus	Carries dorsal column sensation to the ventroposterlateral nucleus of the thalamus	Lesion results in contralateral loss of position and vibration sensation
Tectospinal tract	Originates in the superior colliculus, crosses in the midbrain, descends through anterior funiculus of the cervical spinal cord	Believed to play a role in head turning in response to light stimulation
Medial longitudinal fasciculus (MLF)	Contains fibers from all vestibular nuclei: descending vestibular MLF fibers project mainly to cervical spinal levels, ascending vestibular MLF fibers project to nuclei of extraocular muscles	Ascending MLF fibers in the pons also contain CN-VI internuclear neurons that cross to the contralateral CN-III nucleus to mediate conjugate horizontal eye movements

MEDULLA: VESTIBULAR NUCLEI LEVEL *continued*

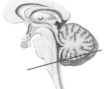

Level of section

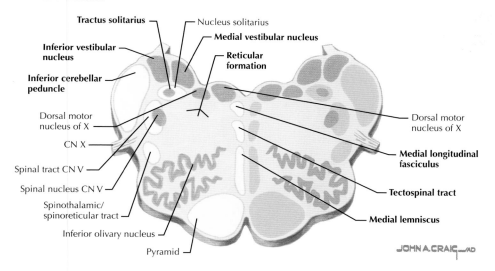

Tractus solitarius

Nucleus solitarius

Medial vestibular nucleus

Inferior vestibular nucleus

Reticular formation

Inferior cerebellar peduncle

Dorsal motor nucleus of X

Dorsal motor nucleus of X

CN X

Medial longitudinal fasciculus

Spinal tract CN V

Spinal nucleus CN V

Tectospinal tract

Spinothalamic/ spinoreticular tract

Medial lemniscus

Inferior olivary nucleus

Pyramid

JOHN A.CRAIG—AD

INTRACRANIAL OCCLUSION OF VERTEBRAL ARTERY

Lateral medullary infarction is due to vertebral artery (80%) or posterior inferior cerebellar artery (20%) occlusion and involves a wedge of medulla posterior to inferior olives. Characteristic of medullary lesions is crossed sensory disturbance: loss of pain and temperature on one side of the face and on the opposite side of the body. This is accounted for by involvement of descending trigeminal tract or nucleus and crossed lateral spinothalamic tract on one side of the brainstem. This crossed phenomenon would not occur with involvement in the upper medulla, pons, and midbrain because at these levels the crossed trigeminothalamic tract and lateral spinothalamic tract run together. A lesion at these levels will cause pain and temperature loss of both the face and body on the side opposite the lesion.

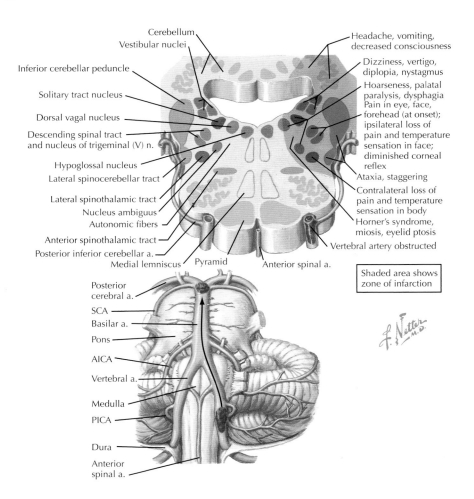

MEDULLA: BRAINSTEM RETICULAR FORMATION

STRUCTURE	ANATOMIC NOTES	FUNCTIONAL SIGNIFICANCE
Reticular formation	Morphologic region from the low medulla through the hypothalamus into the septal region	Constitutes a matrix embedded with nuclei and tracts
Medullary reticular formation	Consists of paramedian, central, and lateral nuclear groups	Reticular formation is involved in wakefulness
	Afferent fibers from spinothalamic, auditory, trigeminal, and vestibular pathways spinoreticular, cerebelloreticular, and corticoreticular projections	Brainstem infarction involving reticular formation results in coma
	Efferent fibers from medullary reticular formation project to the thalamus, cerebellum, and spinal cord	

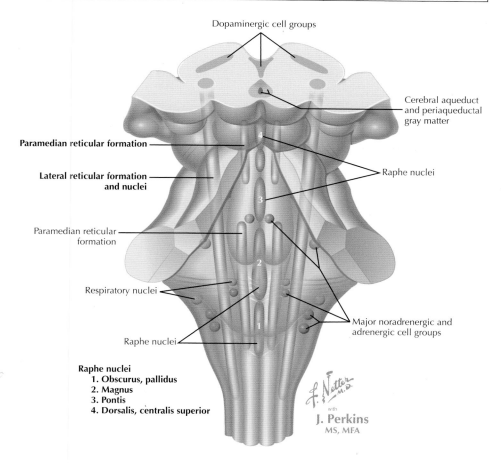

Dopaminergic cell groups

Cerebral aqueduct and periaqueductal gray matter

Paramedian reticular formation

Lateral reticular formation and nuclei

Raphe nuclei

Paramedian reticular formation

Respiratory nuclei

Major noradrenergic and adrenergic cell groups

Raphe nuclei

Raphe nuclei
1. Obscurus, pallidus
2. Magnus
3. Pontis
4. Dorsalis, centralis superior

J. Perkins
MS, MFA

MEDULLA-PONTINE JUNCTION: COCHLEAR NUCLEI LEVEL

- Raphe nuclei are situated along midline of medulla, pons, and midbrain.
- Midbrain and pontine serotonergic cells project to the diencephalon and cerebral cortex.

STRUCTURE	ANATOMIC NOTES	FUNCTIONAL SIGNIFICANCE
Medullary raphe nuclei	Include nucleus raphe magnus, obscurus, pallidus	Synthesize serotonin, project to the spinal cord
Inferior cerebellar peduncle	Contains mostly crossed olivocerebellar fibers, also posterior spinocerebellar tract	Olivocerebellar fibers may convey information regarding interneuron activity at spinal and brainstem levels
		Posterior spinocerebellar tract conveys impulses from muscle stretch receptors and touch and pressure receptors in the skin

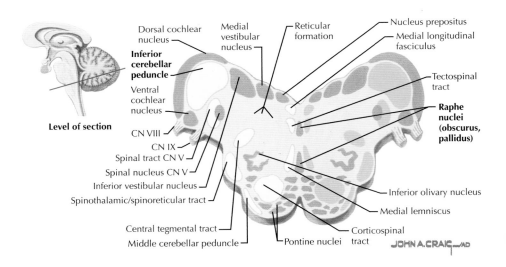

LOWER MOTOR NEURON ORGANIZATION IN MEDULLA

- Lower motor neurons (LMNs) are found in the spinal cord, medulla, pons, and midbrain.
- LMNs send axons into the cranial nerves, terminating on skeletal muscle fibers, and allow for voluntary movement.

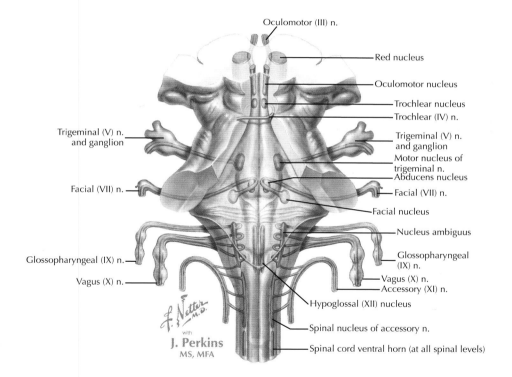

Oculomotor (III) n.

Red nucleus

Oculomotor nucleus

Trochlear nucleus

Trochlear (IV) n.

Trigeminal (V) n. and ganglion

Trigeminal (V) n. and ganglion

Motor nucleus of trigeminal n.

Abducens nucleus

Facial (VII) n.

Facial (VII) n.

Facial nucleus

Nucleus ambiguus

Glossopharyngeal (IX) n.

Glossopharyngeal (IX) n.

Vagus (X) n.

Vagus (X) n.

Accessory (XI) n.

Hypoglossal (XII) nucleus

Spinal nucleus of accessory n.

Spinal cord ventral horn (at all spinal levels)

with
J. Perkins
MS, MFA

GROSS BRAINSTEM: MIDSAGITTAL VIEW

STRUCTURE	ANATOMIC NOTES	FUNCTIONAL SIGNIFICANCE
Pons (metencephalon)	Separated from the midbrain by superior pontine sulcus and from the medulla by inferior pontine sulcus	Largest portion of the brainstem
Basis pontis	Massive ventral portion; composed of descending tracts, pontine nuclei, and transversely oriented fibers projecting to the cerebellum	Among most common sites for hypertensive bleed; results in locked-in state
Tegmentum (anterior to ventricle)	Smaller dorsal part; contains reticular formation as central core, continuous with reticular formation of medulla and midbrain	Reticular formation is crucial for maintenance of awake state

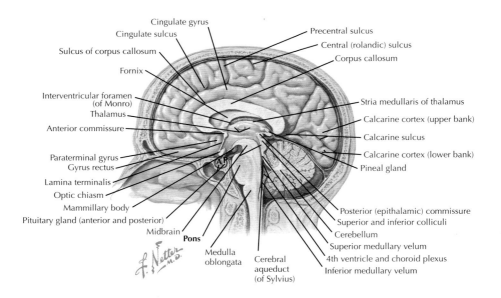

GROSS BRAINSTEM: ANTERIOR VIEW

STRUCTURE	ANATOMIC NOTES	FUNCTIONAL SIGNIFICANCE
Basilar groove (sulcus)	Anterior midline depression	Indicates position of basilar artery
Middle cerebellar peduncle	Formed by predominantly transverse fibers in the ventral pons	Most important pathway from cerebral cortex to contralateral cerebellum, via pontine relay nuclei
Trigeminal nerve (CN-V)	Largest cranial nerve Passes through rostral parts of the middle cerebellar peduncle to reach its nuclei	Supplies muscles of mastication, tensor tympani, tensor veli palatini, mylohyoid, anterior belly of digastric, and facial sensation
Abducens nerve (CN-VI)	Nucleus lies in floor of 4th ventricle	Nerve often is stretched with increased intracranial pressure, resulting in horizontal diplopia
Facial nerve (CN-VII) and vestibulocochlear nerve (CN-VIII)	Exit and enter at cerebellopontine angle (junction of pons, medulla, and cerebellum)	May be compressed with cerebellopontine angle tumors

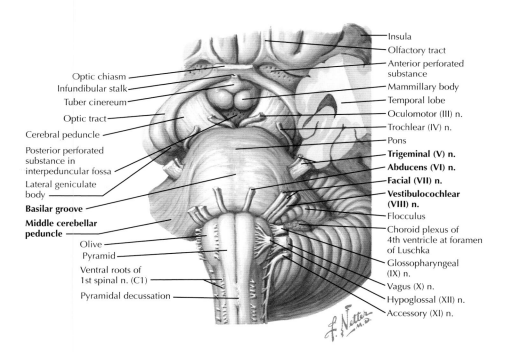

Optic chiasm
Infundibular stalk
Tuber cinereum
Optic tract
Cerebral peduncle
Posterior perforated substance in interpeduncular fossa
Lateral geniculate body
Basilar groove
Middle cerebellar peduncle
Olive
Pyramid
Ventral roots of 1st spinal n. (C1)
Pyramidal decussation

Insula
Olfactory tract
Anterior perforated substance
Mammillary body
Temporal lobe
Oculomotor (III) n.
Trochlear (IV) n.
Pons
Trigeminal (V) n.
Abducens (VI) n.
Facial (VII) n.
Vestibulocochlear (VIII) n.
Flocculus
Choroid plexus of 4th ventricle at foramen of Luschka
Glossopharyngeal (IX) n.
Vagus (X) n.
Hypoglossal (XII) n.
Accessory (XI) n.

GROSS BRAINSTEM: POSTEROLATERAL VIEW

STRUCTURE	ANATOMIC NOTES
Rhomboid fossa	Forms floor of 4th ventricle, overlying pons and medulla
Fourth ventricle	Extends from the central canal of the cervical cord to the cerebral aqueduct of the midbrain
Vestibular nuclei	Lie beneath the vestibular area
Facial colliculus, hypoglossal trigone	Lie within the medial eminence
Lateral portion of medial eminence	Formed by the abducens nucleus

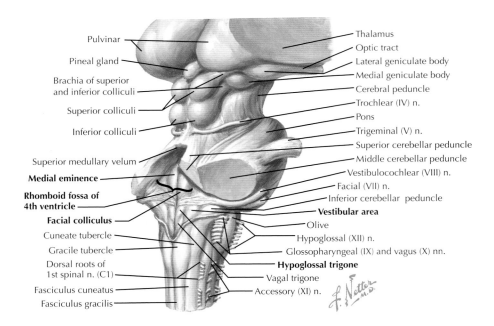

Pulvinar

Pineal gland

Brachia of superior and inferior colliculi

Superior colliculi

Inferior colliculi

Superior medullary velum

Medial eminence

Rhomboid fossa of 4th ventricle

Facial colliculus

Cuneate tubercle

Gracile tubercle

Dorsal roots of 1st spinal n. (C1)

Fasciculus cuneatus

Fasciculus gracilis

Thalamus

Optic tract

Lateral geniculate body

Medial geniculate body

Cerebral peduncle

Trochlear (IV) n.

Pons

Trigeminal (V) n.

Superior cerebellar peduncle

Middle cerebellar peduncle

Vestibulocochlear (VIII) n.

Facial (VII) n.

Inferior cerebellar peduncle

Vestibular area

Olive

Hypoglossal (XII) n.

Glossopharyngeal (IX) and vagus (X) nn.

Hypoglossal trigone

Vagal trigone

Accessory (XI) n.

CRANIAL NERVES OF PONS

- Lower motor neurons of pons are localized in the following:
  - Medial column (CN-VI)
  - Lateral column (CN-V, -VII)
- Preganglionic parasympathetic nuclei are located laterally in the superior (CN-VII) salivatory nucleus.
- Secondary sensory nuclei include the following:
  - Main sensory nucleus of CN-V
  - Descending nucleus of CN-V
  - Vestibular and cochlear nuclei (CN-VIII)
  - Nucleus solitarius (CN-VII, -IX, -X)

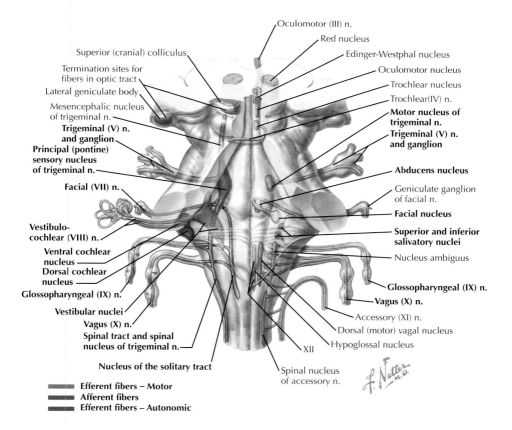

Oculomotor (III) n.
Red nucleus
Superior (cranial) colliculus
Edinger-Westphal nucleus
Termination sites for fibers in optic tract
Oculomotor nucleus
Lateral geniculate body
Trochlear nucleus
Mesencephalic nucleus of trigeminal n.
Trochlear(IV) n.
Trigeminal (V) n. and ganglion
Motor nucleus of trigeminal n.
Principal (pontine) sensory nucleus of trigeminal n.
Trigeminal (V) n. and ganglion
Facial (VII) n.
Abducens nucleus
Vestibulo-cochlear (VIII) n.
Geniculate ganglion of facial n.
Facial nucleus
Ventral cochlear nucleus
Superior and inferior salivatory nuclei
Dorsal cochlear nucleus
Nucleus ambiguus
Glossopharyngeal (IX) n.
Glossopharyngeal (IX) n.
Vestibular nuclei
Vagus (X) n.
Vagus (X) n.
Accessory (XI) n.
Spinal tract and spinal nucleus of trigeminal n.
Dorsal (motor) vagal nucleus
XII
Hypoglossal nucleus
Nucleus of the solitary tract
Spinal nucleus of accessory n.

▬▬▬ **Efferent fibers – Motor**
▬▬▬ **Afferent fibers**
▬▬▬ **Efferent fibers – Autonomic**

LEVEL OF THE COCHLEAR NUCLEUS

STRUCTURE	ANATOMIC NOTES	FUNCTIONAL SIGNIFICANCE
CN-VIII	Runs from the internal auditory meatus to the cerebellopontine angle Cochlear division enters the brainstem lateral and caudal to vestibular division	Vestibular nerve mediates equilibrium and spatial orientation; cochlear nerve mediates audition.
Cochlear nerve (division)	Fibers terminate in the dorsal and ventral cochlear nuclei, on the lateral surface of the inferior cerebellar peduncle	Basal cochlear fibers (high tones) end in the dorsal part of the dorsal cochlear nucleus. Apical cochlear fibers (low tones) end in the ventral part of the dorsal cochlear nucleus and in the ventral nucleus.
Dorsal and ventral cochlear nuclei	Fibers project bilaterally to the superior olive, trapezoid body, and lateral lemniscus	Once fibers project bilaterally, unilateral lesion will not result in deafness.
Vestibular nerve (division)	Enters the cerebellopontine angle medial to the cochlear nerve Passes dorsally between the inferior cerebellar peduncle and spinal trigeminal tract Distributes to vestibular nuclei: inferior (largest number), superior, medial, lateral	Acoustic neuromas almost always originate on this division of the 8th nerve.

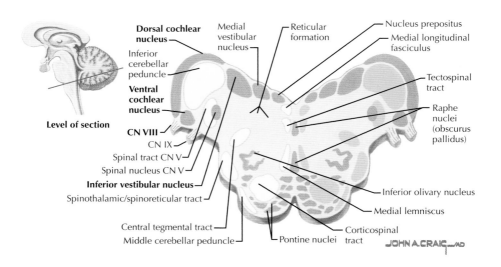

LEVEL OF THE FACIAL NUCLEUS

STRUCTURE	ANATOMIC NOTES	FUNCTIONAL SIGNIFICANCE
Dorsal pons (pontine tegmentum)	Rostral continuation of the medullary reticular formation	Contains cranial nuclei CN-V to CN-VIII, reticular nuclei, and ascending and descending tracts
Medial lemniscus	Lies anterior to the pontine tegmentum	Second-order neurons for position and vibration sensation
Vestibular nuclei	Present in floor of 4th ventricle throughout caudal pons	Posterior circulation ischemia affecting these nuclei result in vertigo, nausea, and vomiting
CN-VII motor nucleus	Pear-shaped mass in the lateral part of the reticular formation	Bell's palsy results from inflammation of CN-VII axons after they leave brainstem
CN-VII root fibers	Form the intramedullary loop around the abducens nucleus, medial to lateral	Both CN-VI and CN-VII would be affected by a lesion in the intramedullary loop area, such as multiple sclerosis, stroke, or tumor
Medial longitudinal fasciculus (MLF)	*Contains:* Ascending fibers from vestibular nuclei projecting to extraocular muscle nuclei, CN-VI internuclear neurons that cross and terminate in CN-III nuclear complex	Lesions of MLF most commonly seen in multiple sclerosis
Intermediate nerve	Enters pons between CN-VII and vestibular nerve (hence "intermediate")	Conveys taste from anterior $2/3$ of the tongue via chorda tympani nerve, terminating on rostral part of solitary (gustatory) nucleus (nucleus solitarius)
Ventral pons	Consists of transverse and longitudinal fiber bundles between pontine nuclei	Longitudinal: corticospinal, corticobulbar, corticopontine Transverse: axons of pontine nuclei crossing to the other side to form middle cerebellar peduncle
Pontine nuclei	Grouped into lateral, medial, dorsal, and ventral nuclear masses	Functions vary from balance to wakefulness

LEVEL OF THE FACIAL NUCLEUS *continued*

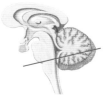

Level of section

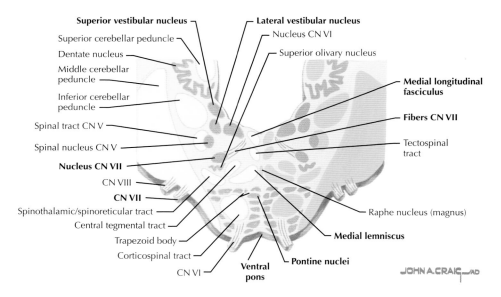

Superior vestibular nucleus

Superior cerebellar peduncle

Dentate nucleus

Middle cerebellar peduncle

Inferior cerebellar peduncle

Spinal tract CN V

Spinal nucleus CN V

Nucleus CN VII

CN VIII

CN VII

Spinothalamic/spinoreticular tract

Central tegmental tract

Trapezoid body

Corticospinal tract

CN VI

Ventral pons

Lateral vestibular nucleus

Nucleus CN VI

Superior olivary nucleus

Medial longitudinal fasciculus

Fibers CN VII

Tectospinal tract

Raphe nucleus (magnus)

Medial lemniscus

Pontine nuclei

JOHN A.CRAIG—AD

CENTRAL CONTROL OF EYE MOVEMENTS

STRUCTURE	ANATOMIC NOTES	FUNCTIONAL SIGNIFICANCE
Paramedian pontine reticular formation (PPRF)	Projects directly to the abducens nucleus Input: • Vestibular nuclei • Superior colliculus • Frontal eye fields • Interstitial nucleus of Cajal Supplies: • Ipsilateral CN VI • Contralateral CN III via MLF • VI nuclear interneurons for medial rectus	Horizontal gaze center Unilateral lesion causes paralysis of ipsilateral gaze Bilateral PPRF lesions may impair both horizontal and vertical gaze
Interstitial nucleus of Cajal	Lies lateral to the MLF in rostral midbrain	Coordinates vertical and oblique eye movements

CENTRAL CONTROL OF EYE MOVEMENTS *continued*

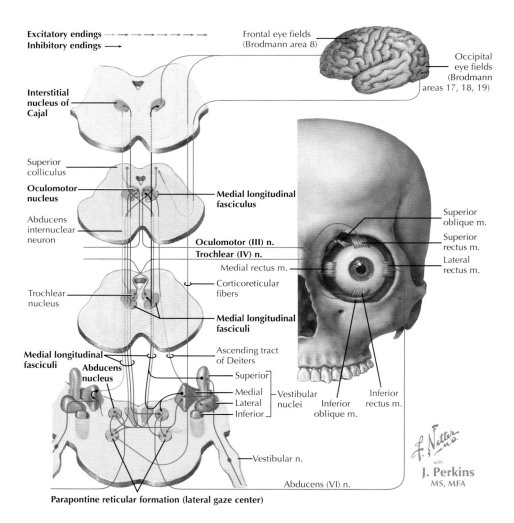

Excitatory endings
Inhibitory endings

Frontal eye fields
(Brodmann area 8)

Occipital
eye fields
(Brodmann
areas 17, 18, 19)

Interstitial
nucleus of
Cajal

Superior
colliculus

Oculomotor
nucleus

Medial longitudinal
fasciculus

Abducens
internuclear
neuron

Oculomotor (III) n.

Trochlear (IV) n.

Superior
oblique m.

Superior
rectus m.

Lateral
rectus m.

Medial rectus m.

Corticoreticular
fibers

Trochlear
nucleus

Medial longitudinal
fasciculi

Medial longitudinal
fasciculi

Ascending tract
of Deiters

Abducens
nucleus

Superior

Medial
Lateral
Inferior

Vestibular
nuclei

Inferior
oblique m.

Inferior
rectus m.

Vestibular n.

Abducens (VI) n.

Parapontine reticular formation (lateral gaze center)

J. Perkins
MS, MFA

NYSTAGMUS

- Alternating back and forth eye movement
- Optokinetic nystagmus: activated by tracking mechanisms
- Vestibular nystagmus: involves vestibular projections via MLF
- Slow phase (drift): caused by asymmetrical input from the following:
  - Semicircular canals
  - Vestibular nuclei
  - Vestibular cerebellum
  - Fast phase (saccade): provoked return to forward position

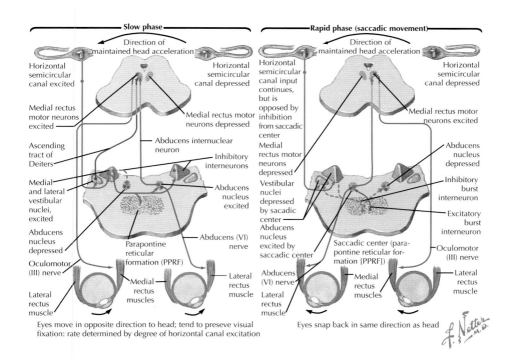

Slow phase

Direction of maintained head acceleration

Horizontal semicircular canal excited

Horizontal semicircular canal depressed

Medial rectus motor neurons excited

Medial rectus motor neurons depressed

Ascending tract of Deiters

Abducens internuclear neuron

Inhibitory interneurons

Medial and lateral vestibular nuclei, excited

Abducens nucleus excited

Abducens nucleus depressed

Parapontine reticular formation (PPRF)

Abducens (VI) nerve

Oculomotor (III) nerve

Lateral rectus muscle

Medial rectus muscles

Lateral rectus muscle

Eyes move in opposite direction to head; tend to preseve visual fixation: rate determined by degree of horizontal canal excitation

Rapid phase (saccadic movement)

Direction of maintained head acceleration

Horizontal semicircular canal input continues, but is opposed by inhibition from saccadic center

Horizontal semicircular canal depressed

Medial rectus motor neurons excited

Medial rectus motor neurons depressed

Vestibular nuclei depressed by sacadic center

Abducens nucleus excited by saccadic center

Abducens (VI) nerve

Lateral rectus muscle

Abducens nucleus depressed

Inhibitory burst interneuron

Excitatory burst interneuron

Oculomotor (III) nerve

Saccadic center (parapontine reticular formation [PPRF])

Medial rectus muscles

Lateral rectus muscle

Eyes snap back in same direction as head

LEVEL OF FACIAL GENU

STRUCTURE	ANATOMIC NOTES	FUNCTIONAL SIGNIFICANCE
Trapezoid body	Transverse fibers in ventral pontine tegmentum Fibers arise from ventral cochlear nucleus Most fibers cross to the other side, through the medial lemniscus Reach the ventrolateral tegmentum, turn sharply longitudinally Form lateral lemniscus Lateral lemniscus terminates in the inferior colliculus	Second-order neurons from the cochlear nuclei
Motor nucleus of CN-VII	Forms column in ventrolateral tegmentum, dorsal to superior olive, ventromedial to spinotrigeminal nucleus	Supplies axons to the muscles of facial expression
CN-VII root fibers	Make sharp lateral bend around rostral abducens nucleus Pass ventrolaterally, medial to the spinotrigeminal complex, lateral to the superior olive	Emerge from brainstem near caudal pons, at CP angle, where may be compressed by CP angle tumors
Spinal trigeminal nucleus (CN-V)	Forms long column medial to spinal trigeminal tract Rostrally merges with main sensory nucleus of CN-V Caudally blends into *substantia gelatinosa* Axons cross to contralateral medial lemniscus Terminate in the ventroposteromedial (VPM) nucleus of thalamus	Mediates pain sensation to face. Throughout, face is upside down: jaw dorsal, forehead ventral

LEVEL OF FACIAL GENU *continued*

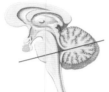

Level of section

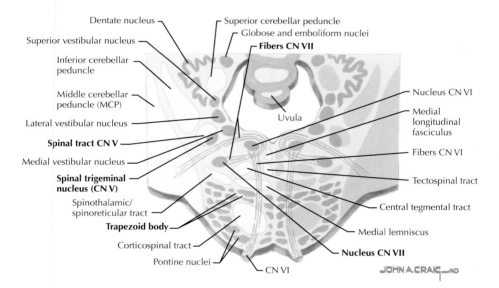

Dentate nucleus

Superior vestibular nucleus

Inferior cerebellar peduncle

Middle cerebellar peduncle (MCP)

Lateral vestibular nucleus

Spinal tract CN V

Medial vestibular nucleus

Spinal trigeminal nucleus (CN V)

Spinothalamic/ spinoreticular tract

Trapezoid body

Corticospinal tract

Pontine nuclei

Superior cerebellar peduncle

Globose and emboliform nuclei

Fibers CN VII

Uvula

Nucleus CN VI

Medial longitudinal fasciculus

Fibers CN VI

Tectospinal tract

Central tegmental tract

Medial lemniscus

Nucleus CN VII

CN VI

JOHN A. CRAIG—MD

LEVEL OF THE TRIGEMINAL NUCLEI

STRUCTURE	ANATOMIC NOTES	FUNCTIONAL SIGNIFICANCE
Main sensory nucleus of CN-V	Axons travel crossed and uncrossed to VPM nucleus of thalamus	Mediates touch and pressure, distributed as in spinal trigeminal nucleus
Mesencephalic nucleus of CN-V	Slender cell column near lateral margin of the central gray of the upper 4th ventricle and cerebral aqueduct Unique because primary sensory neurons are in this brainstem nucleus, not in the trigeminal ganglion Central pathway remains obscure	Mediates proprioception from teeth, periodontium, muscles of mastication, and joint capsules; controls force of bite
Motor nucleus of CN-V	Ovoid column medial to main sensory nucleus and motor root	Supplies muscles of mastication (masseter, temporalis, medial and lateral pterygoids), tensor tympani and veli palatini, mylohyoid, and anterior belly of digastric
Parabrachial nuclei	Juxtaposed to brachium conjunctivum (superior cerebellar peduncle)	Synaptic station for gustatory pathways

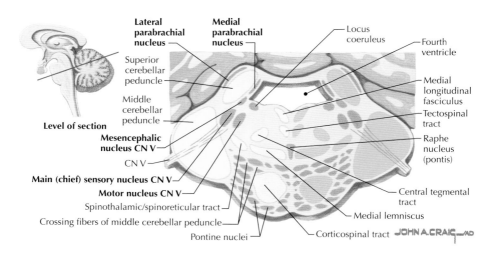

PARABRACHIAL NUCLEI: CONTROL OF RESPIRATION

STRUCTURE	ANATOMIC NOTES	FUNCTIONAL SIGNIFICANCE
Parabrachial nuclei (PBN)	Contains neuromelanin-containing catecholamine neurons Fibers connect with hypothalamus, amygdala, stria medullaris, brainstem nuclei	Believed to play a role in autonomic regulation
Medial PBN	Together with a lateral segment, makes up PBN	Acts as respiratory pacemaker to regulate dorsal respiratory nucleus (DRN) (lateral nucleus solitarius) and ventral respiratory nucleus (VRN) (nucleus retroambiguus)
Dorsal respiratory nucleus axons	Cross and terminate on phrenic nerve cervical cord motor neurons and thoracic cord motor neurons	Supplying inspiratory respiratory muscles
Ventral respiratory nucleus axons	Cross and terminate on thoracic cord motor neurons	Supplying expiratory respiratory muscles

PARABRACHIAL NUCLEI: CONTROL OF RESPIRATION *continued*

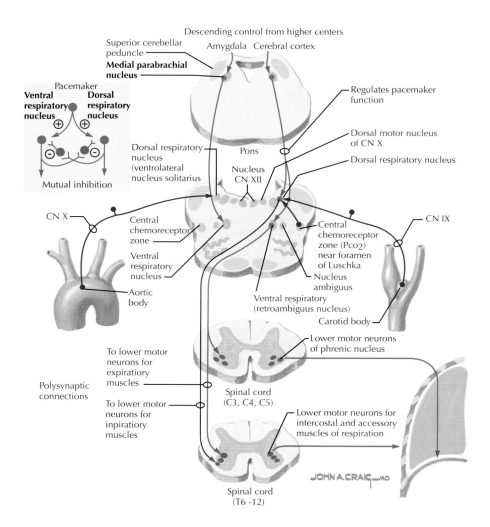

Descending control from higher centers

Superior cerebellar peduncle

Amygdala   Cerebral cortex

Medial parabrachial nucleus

Pacemaker

Ventral respiratory nucleus   **Dorsal respiratory nucleus**

Mutual inhibition

Regulates pacemaker function

Dorsal motor nucleus of CN X

Dorsal respiratory nucleus (ventrolateral nucleus solitarius)

Pons

Nucleus CN XII

Dorsal respiratory nucleus

CN X

Central chemoreceptor zone

Ventral respiratory nucleus

Aortic body

Central chemoreceptor zone (Pco2) near foramen of Luschka

Nucleus ambiguus

Ventral respiratory (retroambiguus nucleus)

CN IX

Carotid body

To lower motor neurons for expiratiory muscles

Polysynaptic connections

To lower motor neurons for inpiratiory muscles

Lower motor neurons of phrenic nucleus

Spinal cord (C3, C4, C5)

Lower motor neurons for intercostal and accessory muscles of respiration

JOHN A.CRAIG—AD

Spinal cord (T6 -12)

PONS-MIDBRAIN JUNCTION: CN-IV

STRUCTURE	ANATOMIC NOTES	FUNCTIONAL SIGNIFICANCE
Pons-midbrain junction (isthmus rhombencephali)	Fourth ventricle narrows, resembles cerebral aqueduct Roof consists of superior medullary velum	Coma and central neurogenic hyperventilation result with pathology at this level
CN-IV	Decussates in the superior medullary velum	Supplies superior oblique muscle
Superior cerebellar peduncle	Lies medial to the lateral lemniscus Arises from dentate, emboliform, and globose nuclei of cerebellum Decussates in midbrain, ends in red nucleus and VL nucleus of thalamus	Forms the most important efferent system from the cerebellum
Locus ceruleus	Pigmented cells near periventricular gray of upper 4th ventricle	Lost in Parkinson's disease
Nuclei of raphe region	Part of brainstem nuclei of reticular formation, which also include parmedian, medial, and lateral reticular nuclear groups	Contain serotonin (5-hydroxytryptamine, 5-HT).

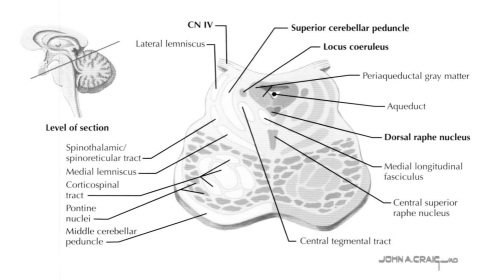

Level of section

CN IV

Lateral lemniscus

Superior cerebellar peduncle

Locus coeruleus

Periaqueductal gray matter

Aqueduct

Dorsal raphe nucleus

Medial longitudinal fasciculus

Central superior raphe nucleus

Central tegmental tract

Spinothalamic/spinoreticular tract

Medial lemniscus

Corticospinal tract

Pontine nuclei

Middle cerebellar peduncle

JOHN A.CRAIG—AD

RAPHE NUCLEI

STRUCTURE	ANATOMIC NOTES	FUNCTIONAL SIGNIFICANCE
Raphe nuclei	Situated along the midline of medulla, pons, midbrain	Caudal group involved in pain mechanisms; rostral group involved with wakefulness, alertness, and sleep
Inferior central nucleus	Appears at the pontomedullary junction and caudal pons; represents the rostral part of the nucleus raphe magnus	Electrical stimulation of this nucleus inhibits spontaneous activity of thalamic neurons in cats
Nucleus raphe pontis	Rostral to the inferior central nucleus	Receives vestibular input and is involved in the generation of saccadic eye movements
Superior central nucleus (i.e., median raphe nucleus)	Rostral extension of the pontine raphe nuclei	Together with dorsal nucleus, give rise to principal serotonin ascending fibers
Dorsal nucleus of raphe	On each side of midline, dorsal to MLF, merges with dorsal tegmental nucleus	Together with superior central nucleus, give rise to principal serotonin ascending fibers

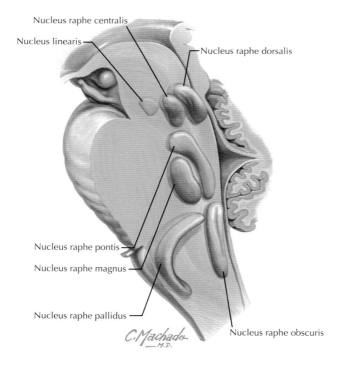

Nucleus raphe centralis
Nucleus linearis
Nucleus raphe dorsalis
Nucleus raphe pontis
Nucleus raphe magnus
Nucleus raphe pallidus
Nucleus raphe obscuris

C. Machado
—M.D.

ROSTRAL PONS

MAGNETIC RESONANCE IMAGING: CROSS–SECTIONAL CORRELATION

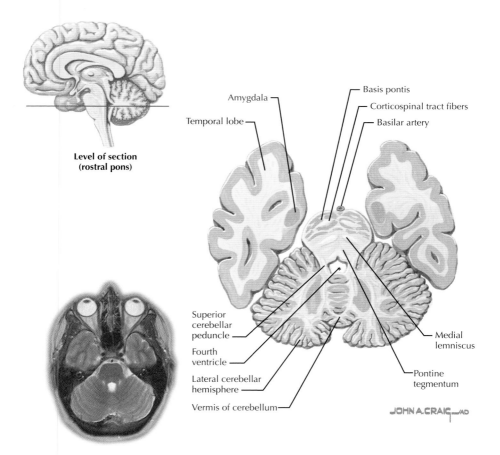

**Level of section
(rostral pons)**

Amygdala

Temporal lobe

Basis pontis

Corticospinal tract fibers

Basilar artery

Superior cerebellar peduncle

Fourth ventricle

Lateral cerebellar hemisphere

Vermis of cerebellum

Medial lemniscus

Pontine tegmentum

JOHN A.CRAIG—MD

CHAPTER 7
Midbrain (Mesencephalon)

7 Midbrain (Mesencephalon)

MIDBRAIN IN SITU

STRUCTURE	ANATOMIC NOTES	FUNCTIONAL SIGNIFICANCE
Tectum	Dorsal to cerebral aqueduct	Lesions here cause pupils to be in midposition and light-fixed, but to spontaneously fluctuate in size.
Crura cerebri	Separated from tegmentum by pigmented nuclear mass, the substantia nigra	Loss of pigmented cells characteristic of Parkinson's disease
Tegmentum	Located centrally Cerebral aqueduct is surrounded by central gray matter that separates tectum from tegmentum	Rostral continuation of the pontine tegmentum
Cerebral peduncle	Dorsal part is tegmentum Ventral part is crus cerebri	Denotes $\frac{1}{2}$ of the midbrain, excluding tectum

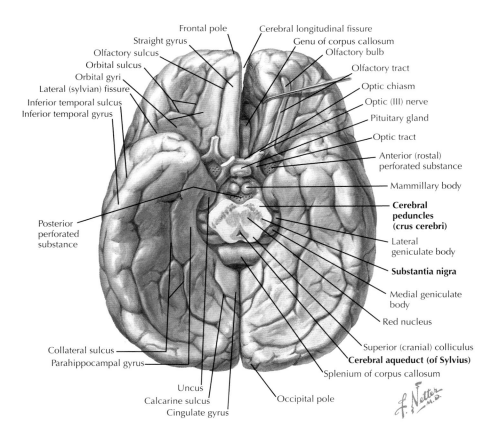

Frontal pole
Straight gyrus
Olfactory sulcus
Orbital sulcus
Orbital gyri
Lateral (sylvian) fissure
Inferior temporal sulcus
Inferior temporal gyrus

Cerebral longitudinal fissure
Genu of corpus callosum
Olfactory bulb
Olfactory tract
Optic chiasm
Optic (III) nerve
Pituitary gland
Optic tract
Anterior (rostal) perforated substance
Mammillary body

Posterior perforated substance

Cerebral peduncles (crus cerebri)
Lateral geniculate body
Substantia nigra
Medial geniculate body
Red nucleus

Collateral sulcus
Parahippocampal gyrus

Superior (cranial) colliculus
Cerebral aqueduct (of Sylvius)
Splenium of corpus callosum

Uncus
Calcarine sulcus
Cingulate gyrus
Occipital pole

GROSS BRAINSTEM: MIDSAGITTAL VIEW

STRUCTURE	ANATOMIC NOTES	FUNCTIONAL SIGNIFICANCE
Superior colliculus region	Known as *pretectum*	Superior colliculi influence the position of the head and eyes in response to visual, auditory, and somatic stimuli
Inferior colliculi	3 main nuclei: • Central • Pericentral • External	Relay nuclei transmitting auditory information to medial geniculate body, thence to primary auditory cortex
Pretectal region	Immediately rostral to superior colliculus at the posterior commisure level	Principal midbrain center involved in pupillary light reflex
Posterior commisure	Region of transition from midbrain to diencephalon	Lesions here produce bilateral eyelid retraction and impaired vertical eye movement
Subcommisural organ	Modified ependymal plate in the roof of the cerebral aqueduct, immediately beneath posterior commisure	Function in humans is unknown

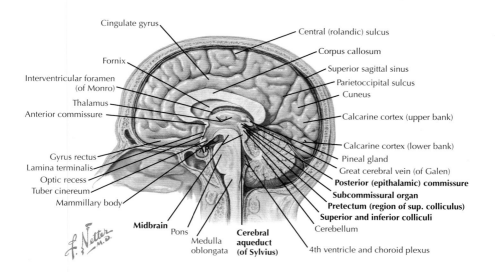

Cingulate gyrus

Central (rolandic) sulcus

Corpus callosum

Fornix

Superior sagittal sinus

Interventricular foramen (of Monro)

Parietoccipital sulcus

Cuneus

Thalamus

Anterior commissure

Calcarine cortex (upper bank)

Calcarine cortex (lower bank)

Gyrus rectus

Pineal gland

Lamina terminalis

Great cerebral vein (of Galen)

Optic recess

Posterior (epithalamic) commissure

Tuber cinereum

Subcommissural organ

Mammillary body

Pretectum (region of sup. colliculus)

Superior and inferior colliculi

Cerebellum

Midbrain Pons

Medulla oblongata

Cerebral aqueduct (of Sylvius)

4th ventricle and choroid plexus

GROSS BRAINSTEM: ANTERIOR VIEW

STRUCTURE	ANATOMIC NOTES	FUNCTIONAL SIGNIFICANCE
Basilar groove (sulcus)	Anterior midline depression	Indicates position of basilar artery
Oculomotor nerve (cranial nerve [CN]-III)	Emerges from interpeduncular fossa between the crura cerebri	Weber syndrome: CN-III palsy with contralateral hemiparesis resulting from involvement of CN-III and crus cerebri (descending corticospinal tract)
Trochlear nerve (CN-IV)	Exits dorsal midbrain, crosses in superior medullary velum, and courses anteriorly around brainstem	Longest, most delicate cranial nerve Often injured in head trauma, causing diplopia and head tilt

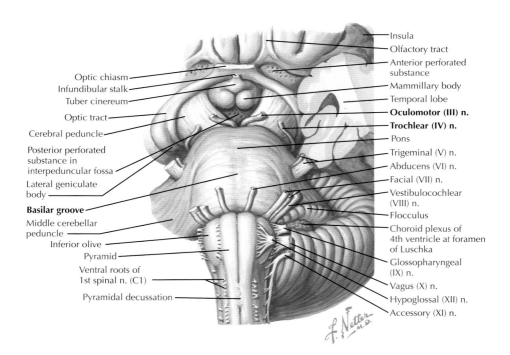

CRANIAL NERVES OF MIDBRAIN

STRUCTURE	ANATOMIC NOTES	FUNCTIONAL SIGNIFICANCE
Nucleus of Edinger-Westphal (CN-III)	Preganglionic parasympathetic nucleus Gives rise to uncrossed parasympathetic fibers	Involved in accommodation and pupillary light reflex
Superior colliculus	Receive input from optic tract	Visual way station, together with lateral geniculate body
Inferior colliculus	Receives input from cochlear nuclei and other accessory auditory nuclei	Auditory way station, together with medial geniculate body

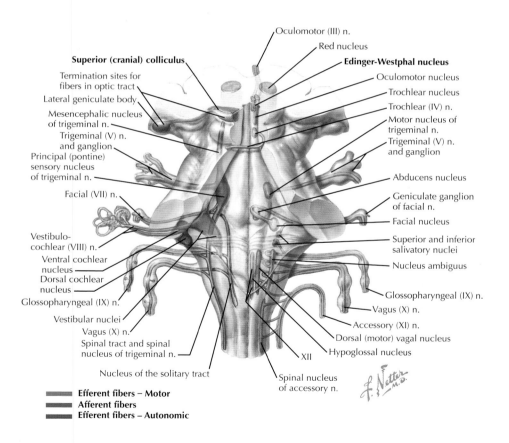

Efferent fibers – Motor
Afferent fibers
Efferent fibers – Autonomic

LOWER MIDBRAIN

MAGNETIC RESONANCE IMAGING (MRI): CROSS-SECTIONAL CORRELATION

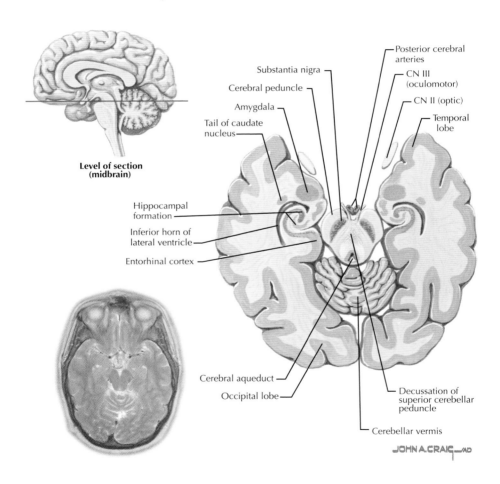

Level of section (midbrain)

Substantia nigra

Cerebral peduncle

Amygdala

Tail of caudate nucleus

Posterior cerebral arteries

CN III (oculomotor)

CN II (optic)

Temporal lobe

Hippocampal formation

Inferior horn of lateral ventricle

Entorhinal cortex

Cerebral aqueduct

Occipital lobe

Decussation of superior cerebellar peduncle

Cerebellar vermis

JOHN A. CRAIG—MD

UPPER MIDBRAIN

MRI: CROSS-SECTIONAL CORRELATION

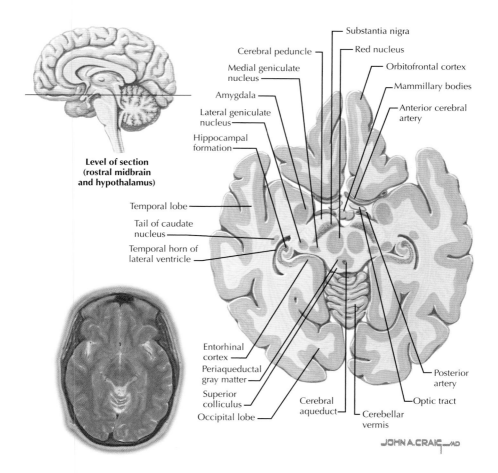

Substantia nigra

Cerebral peduncle

Red nucleus

Medial geniculate nucleus

Orbitofrontal cortex

Amygdala

Mammillary bodies

Lateral geniculate nucleus

Anterior cerebral artery

Hippocampal formation

Level of section (rostral midbrain and hypothalamus)

Temporal lobe

Tail of caudate nucleus

Temporal horn of lateral ventricle

Entorhinal cortex

Periaqueductal gray matter

Superior colliculus

Occipital lobe

Cerebral aqueduct

Posterior artery

Optic tract

Cerebellar vermis

JOHN A.CRAIG—AD

CORONAL SECTION THROUGH SUBSTANTIA NIGRA

MRI: CROSS-SECTIONAL CORRELATION

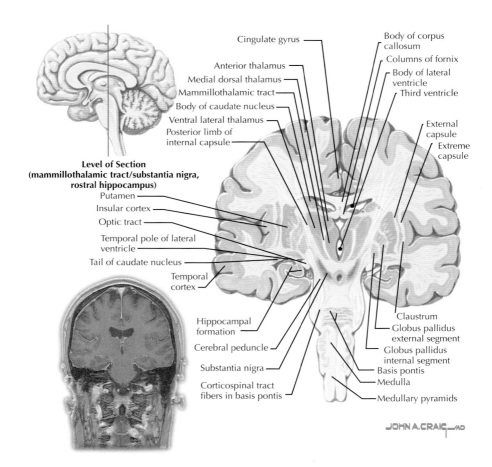

Cingulate gyrus

Anterior thalamus

Medial dorsal thalamus

Mammillothalamic tract

Body of caudate nucleus

Ventral lateral thalamus

Posterior limb of internal capsule

Level of Section (mammillothalamic tract/substantia nigra, rostral hippocampus)

Putamen

Insular cortex

Optic tract

Temporal pole of lateral ventricle

Tail of caudate nucleus

Temporal cortex

Hippocampal formation

Cerebral peduncle

Substantia nigra

Corticospinal tract fibers in basis pontis

Body of corpus callosum

Columns of fornix

Body of lateral ventricle

Third ventricle

External capsule

Extreme capsule

Claustrum

Globus pallidus external segment

Globus pallidus internal segment

Basis pontis

Medulla

Medullary pyramids

JOHN A. CRAIG—AD

THALAMUS IN HORIZONTAL SECTION

- Thalami form the lateral walls of the third ventricle.
- Posterior limb of the internal capsule separates thalamus from the lentiform nucleus.
- Pulvinar is demonstrated in the artwork below.

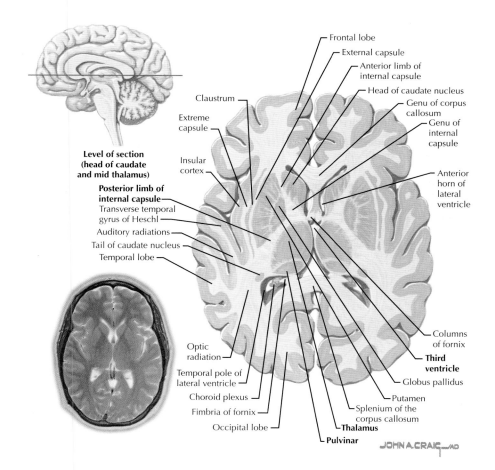

Frontal lobe
External capsule
Anterior limb of internal capsule
Head of caudate nucleus
Genu of corpus callosum
Genu of internal capsule
Anterior horn of lateral ventricle

Claustrum
Extreme capsule
Insular cortex

Level of section (head of caudate and mid thalamus)

Posterior limb of internal capsule
Transverse temporal gyrus of Heschl
Auditory radiations
Tail of caudate nucleus
Temporal lobe

Columns of fornix
Third ventricle
Globus pallidus
Putamen
Splenium of the corpus callosum
Thalamus

Optic radiation
Temporal pole of lateral ventricle
Choroid plexus
Fimbria of fornix
Occipital lobe
Pulvinar

JOHN A. CRAIG—AD

THALAMUS IN CORONAL SECTION

STRUCTURE	ANATOMIC NOTES	FUNCTIONAL SIGNIFICANCE
Thalamus	Individual nuclei are anatomically separated. The thalamus defines the borders of the 3rd ventricle	
LGN of the thalamus	Comma-shaped, lateral nucleus of the thalamus	Serves as the visual relay center from the optic tract to occipital cortex. Lesions can cause visual field defects
MGN of the thalamus	Medial to the lateral geniculate nucleus	Serves as the auditory relay center from the inferior colliculus to auditory cortex
MDN of the thalamus	Most dorsal and medial nucleus; forms part of the wall of the 3rd ventricle	Part of the limbic system
CM thalamus	Located ventral to the MDN	Involved in the central modulation and perception of pain
Lateral thalamus	Contains multiple nuclear structures, including the VL and VPL	Involved in motor and sensory relays

THALAMUS IN CORONAL SECTION *continued*

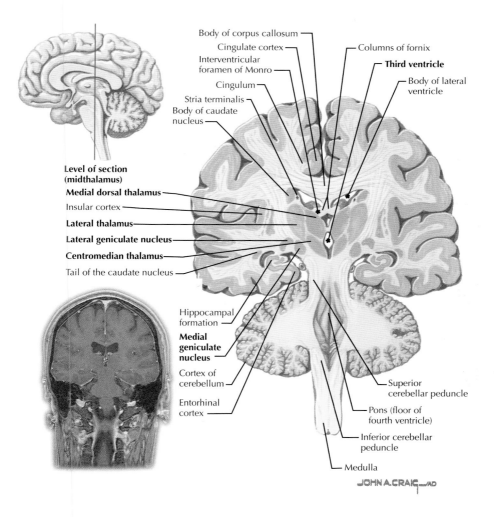

Body of corpus callosum

Cingulate cortex

Interventricular foramen of Monro

Cingulum

Stria terminalis

Body of caudate nucleus

Columns of fornix

Third ventricle

Body of lateral ventricle

Level of section (midthalamus)

Medial dorsal thalamus

Insular cortex

Lateral thalamus

Lateral geniculate nucleus

Centromedian thalamus

Tail of the caudate nucleus

Hippocampal formation

Medial geniculate nucleus

Cortex of cerebellum

Entorhinal cortex

Superior cerebellar peduncle

Pons (floor of fourth ventricle)

Inferior cerebellar peduncle

Medulla

JOHN A. CRAIG—AD

Basal Ganglia

BASAL GANGLIA: OVERVIEW

Function	Involved in the initiation and modulation of movement
Organization	Deep set of nuclear structures
	Receive input from the cerebral cortex, process it, and relay back to the cerebral cortex via the thalamus
Structures	Caudate nucleus, putamen, globus pallidus (internal and external segments), subthalamic nucleus, substantia nigra
Disease Status	Diseases can lead to a paucity of movement (hypokinetic states) or abnormal movements (hyperkinetic states)

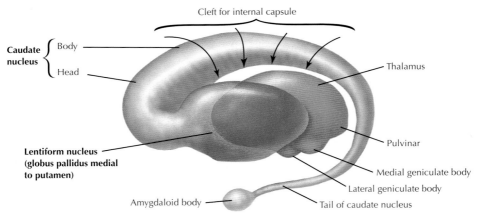

Schematic illustration showing interrelationship of thalamus, lentiform nucleus, caudate nucleus and amygdaloid body (viewed from side)

AXIAL VIEW OF THE BRAIN AT THE LEVEL OF THE BASAL GANGLIA

STRUCTURE	ANATOMIC NOTES	FUNCTIONAL SIGNIFICANCE
Caudate nucleus*	C-shaped structure that is lateral to the lateral ventricle The *head of the caudate* bulges into the frontal horn of the lateral ventricle The *body of the caudate* sweeps into a C shape with the lateral ventricle The *tail of the caudate* is located in the temporal lobe superior and lateral to the temporal horn of the lateral ventricle	Serves as the major input nucleus of the basal ganglia Degeneration of the caudate is typical of Huntington's disease and can be easily appreciated on computed tomography scans, with loss of the normal indentation into the lateral ventricle
Internal capsule	U-shaped in axial sections The anterior limb separates the head of the caudate nucleus from the lentiform nucleus (putamen and globus pallidus) The posterior limb separates the thalamus from the globus pallidus The genu is the bend that connects the anterior and posterior limbs	Important white matter structure that conduits information from the basal ganglia, thalamus, and cerebellum to cortex The posterior limb contains the descending upper motor neurons from the cortex
Putamen*	Lens-shaped structure lateral to the globus pallidus Anteriorly and inferiorly, it is connected to the caudate Together the putamen and caudate are called the *corpus striatum*	Although separated by the internal capsule, the putamen is histologically and functionally equivalent to the caudate
Globus pallidus (GPe and GPi)*	Composed of an internal (GPi) and an external (GPe) segment Conspicuously pale, hence the name, which means "pale globe" Together, putamen and globus pallidus are called the *lentiform nucleus*	The GPi serves as the major output nucleus of the basal ganglia system The GPe is part of the internal circuitry of the basal ganglia
External capsule	Thin white matter band lateral to putamen	
Claustrum	Thin gray matter band lateral to the external capsule	Function not well elucidated
Extreme capsule	Thin white matter band lateral to claustrum	

*Structures of the basal ganglia

AXIAL VIEW OF BRAIN AT THE LEVEL OF THE BASAL GANGLIA *continued*

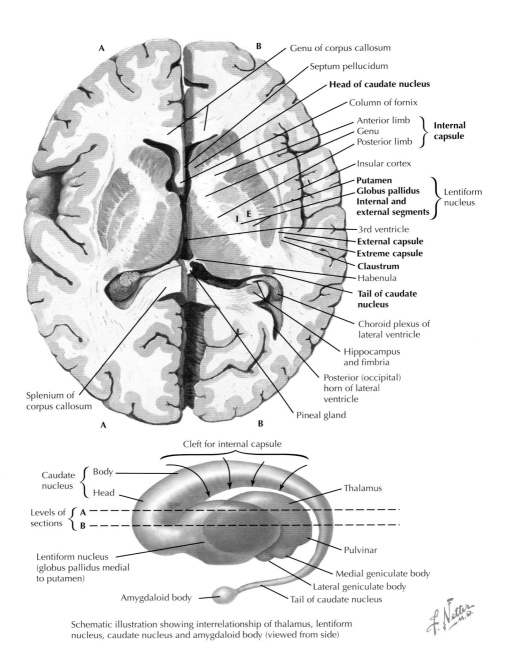

A B Genu of corpus callosum

Septum pellucidum

Head of caudate nucleus

Column of fornix

Anterior limb
Genu — **Internal capsule**
Posterior limb

Insular cortex

Putamen
Globus pallidus — Lentiform nucleus
Internal and external segments

3rd ventricle
External capsule
Extreme capsule
Claustrum
Habenula

Tail of caudate nucleus

Choroid plexus of lateral ventricle

Hippocampus and fimbria

Posterior (occipital) horn of lateral ventricle

Splenium of corpus callosum

A B Pineal gland

Cleft for internal capsule

Caudate nucleus — Body, Head

Thalamus

Levels of sections — A, B

Lentiform nucleus (globus pallidus medial to putamen)

Pulvinar

Medial geniculate body
Lateral geniculate body
Amygdaloid body — Tail of caudate nucleus

Schematic illustration showing interrelationship of thalamus, lentiform nucleus, caudate nucleus and amygdaloid body (viewed from side)

CORONAL VIEW OF THE BRAIN AT THE LEVEL OF THE HEAD OF THE CAUDATE

STRUCTURE	ANATOMIC NOTES	FUNCTIONAL SIGNIFICANCE
Nucleus accumbens	Ventral nuclear structure located at the junction of the caudate and putamen	Involved in modulation of emotions by communicating with the limbic system Implicated in addiction behaviors
Head of the caudate nucleus	Note again that it bulges into the frontal horn of the lateral ventricle	
Anterior limb of the internal capsule	In this coronal view, it can be seen separating the caudate and putamen Note the bands of gray matter connecting the caudate and putamen	Contains fibers traveling from cerebellum and basal ganglia to the cortex
Putamen	At this anterior level, the globus pallidus is not yet visible	
External capsule, claustrum, extreme capsule	Again, note the relationship of these 3 structures to each other	

CORONAL VIEW OF THE BRAIN AT THE LEVEL OF THE HEAD OF THE CAUDATE
continued

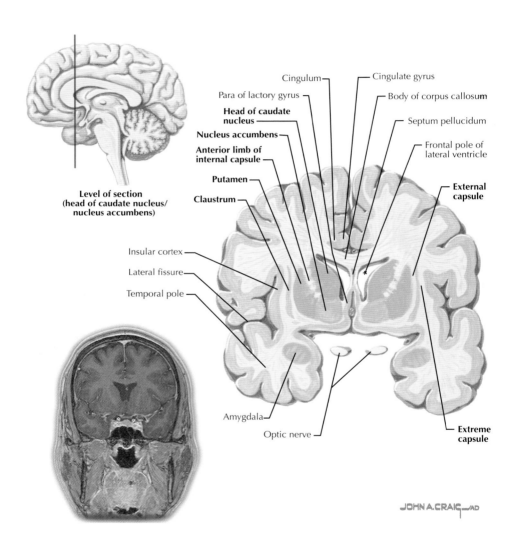

Level of section
(head of caudate nucleus/
nucleus accumbens)

Cingulum

Para of lactory gyrus

Head of caudate nucleus

Nucleus accumbens

Anterior limb of internal capsule

Putamen

Claustrum

Insular cortex

Lateral fissure

Temporal pole

Amygdala

Optic nerve

Cingulate gyrus

Body of corpus callosum

Septum pellucidum

Frontal pole of lateral ventricle

External capsule

Extreme capsule

JOHN A.CRAIG AD

CORONAL VIEW OF THE BRAIN AT THE LEVEL OF THE ANTERIOR LIMB OF THE INTERNAL CAPSULE

STRUCTURE	ANATOMIC NOTES	FUNCTIONAL SIGNIFICANCE
Body of caudate	Note that the caudate tapers in size from the head to the body	The body and head have similar functions as the input zone of the basal ganglia
GPi segment	The innermost segment of the globus pallidus	Functions as an output nucleus of the basal ganglia to thalamus, en route to the cortex
GPe segment	The outermost segment of the globus pallidus	Functions as an intrinsic nucleus, relaying information from striatum to other structures in basal ganglia
Putamen	Lateral to the globus pallidus Note that the putamen and globus pallidus are closely positioned and lens-shaped, known together as the *lentiform nucleus*	Although close to globus pallidus, the putamen is histologically and functionally equivalent to the caudate

CORONAL VIEW OF THE BRAIN AT THE LEVEL OF THE ANTERIOR LIMB OF THE INTERNAL CAPSULE *continued*

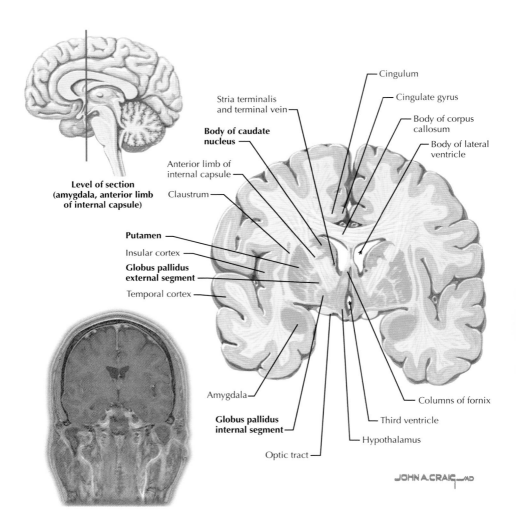

Cingulum

Stria terminalis and terminal vein

Cingulate gyrus

Body of caudate nucleus

Body of corpus callosum

Body of lateral ventricle

Anterior limb of internal capsule

Level of section (amygdala, anterior limb of internal capsule)

Claustrum

Putamen

Insular cortex

Globus pallidus external segment

Temporal cortex

Amygdala

Globus pallidus internal segment

Columns of fornix

Third ventricle

Hypothalamus

Optic tract

JOHN A.CRAIG—MD

AXIAL VIEW OF THE BRAIN THROUGH THE MIDBRAIN

STRUCTURE	ANATOMIC NOTES	FUNCTIONAL SIGNIFICANCE
Substantia nigra	Located in the ventral midbrain Appears brown owing to neuromelanin pigmentation Has two internal subdivisions called the *pars compacta* and *pars reticularis*	Pars compacta has dopamine-producing neurons, which project to the striatum and facilitate movement. Pars reticularis, like the GPi, is an output nucleus of the basal ganglia. Degeneration of the substantia nigra causes Parkinson's disease.
Tail of the caudate nucleus	Can be seen here in its expected location, superior and lateral to the temporal horn of the lateral ventricle	

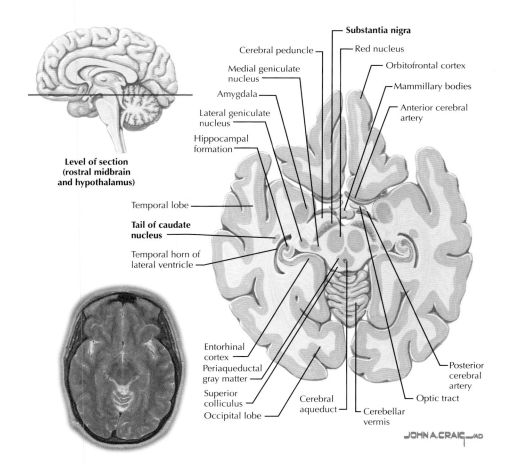

Substantia nigra

Cerebral peduncle — Red nucleus

Medial geniculate nucleus — Orbitofrontal cortex

Amygdala — Mammillary bodies

Lateral geniculate nucleus — Anterior cerebral artery

Hippocampal formation

Level of section (rostral midbrain and hypothalamus)

Temporal lobe

Tail of caudate nucleus

Temporal horn of lateral ventricle

Entorhinal cortex

Periaqueductal gray matter — Posterior cerebral artery

Superior colliculus

Cerebral aqueduct — Optic tract

Occipital lobe — Cerebellar vermis

JOHN A. CRAIG—AD

9 Basal Ganglia

CONNECTIONS OF THE BASAL GANGLIA

ANATOMIC NOTES	PATHWAYS	FUNCTIONAL SIGNIFICANCE
Basal ganglia are involved in a complex set of loop pathways Basic principle is that all loops follow the following general path: cortex→basal ganglia→thalamus→cortex *Input* All input to basal ganglia goes to striatum (caudate, putamen, nucleus accumbens) *Output* All output from basal ganglia comes from GPi and substantia nigra pars reticulata (SNr)	Two distinct pathways through basal ganglia: *Direct pathway* Facilitates movement cortex→striatum→GPi + SNr→thalamus→cortex *Indirect pathway* Inhibits movement cortex→striatum→GPe→subthalamic nucleus→GPi + SNr→cortex	Dopamine from pars compacta of the substantia nigra facilitates movement by exciting direct pathway and suppressing indirect pathway. In Parkinson's disease, dopaminergic neurons in the pars compacta of substantia nigra degenerate, causing decreased speed of movements, known as *bradykinesia.*

Connections of Basal Ganglia

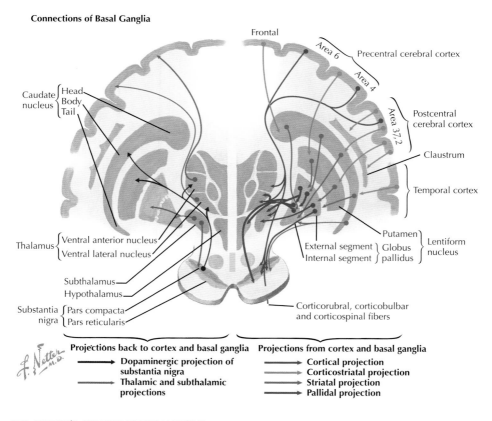

Frontal

Area 6   Precentral cerebral cortex

Area 4

Area 37,2

Caudate nucleus { Head, Body, Tail

Postcentral cerebral cortex

Claustrum

Temporal cortex

Thalamus { Ventral anterior nucleus / Ventral lateral nucleus

Putamen } Lentiform nucleus
External segment } Globus
Internal segment } pallidus

Subthalamus
Hypothalamus

Substantia nigra { Pars compacta / Pars reticularis

Corticorubral, corticobulbar and corticospinal fibers

Projections back to cortex and basal ganglia
→ **Dopaminergic projection of substantia nigra**
→ **Thalamic and subthalamic projections**

Projections from cortex and basal ganglia
→ **Cortical projection**
→ **Corticostriatal projection**
→ **Striatal projection**
→ **Pallidal projection**

CHAPTER 10
Cerebellum

OVERVIEW OF THE CEREBELLUM

Location	Posterior fossa, below the tentorium cerebelli
Architecture	Similar to cerebrum, contains folded cortex, white matter, and deep nuclear structures
Function	Major function is to coordinate and stabilize movement
	Important in maintenance of balance
Clinical Significance	Cerebellar diseases can cause poor coordination, slurred speech, and gait imbalance
	Midline lesions tend to cause more gait problems

Midsagittal View of Brain

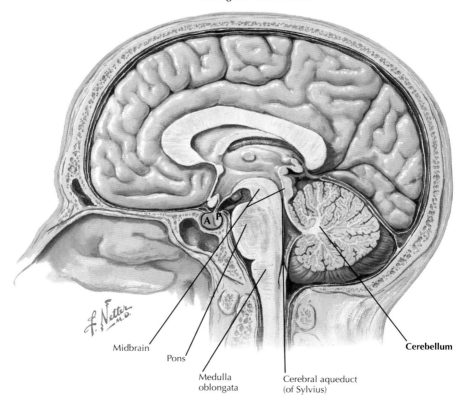

Midbrain

Pons

Medulla oblongata

Cerebral aqueduct (of Sylvius)

Cerebellum

CEREBELLAR PEDUNCLES

- In this dorsal view of the brainstem, the cerebellum has been removed to expose its three peduncles.
- Cerebellum communicates with rest of the nervous system through its peduncles.

PEDUNCLE	ALTERNATE NAME	FUNCTIONAL SIGNIFICANCE
Superior cerebellar peduncle	Brachium conjuctivum	Primarily carries output from cerebellum
Middle cerebellar peduncle	Brachium pontis	Exclusively carries input to cerebellum
Inferior cerebellar peduncle	Restiform body	Primarily carries input to cerebellum

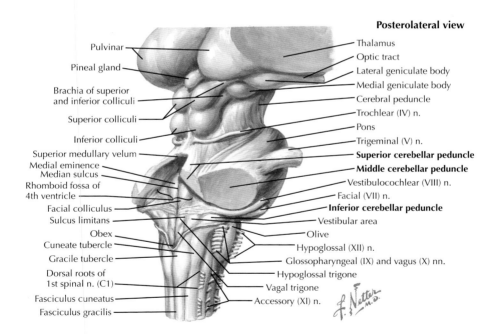

Posterolateral view

Pulvinar
Pineal gland
Brachia of superior and inferior colliculi
Superior colliculi
Inferior colliculi
Superior medullary velum
Medial eminence
Median sulcus
Rhomboid fossa of 4th ventricle
Facial colliculus
Sulcus limitans
Obex
Cuneate tubercle
Gracile tubercle
Dorsal roots of 1st spinal n. (C1)
Fasciculus cuneatus
Fasciculus gracilis

Thalamus
Optic tract
Lateral geniculate body
Medial geniculate body
Cerebral peduncle
Trochlear (IV) n.
Pons
Trigeminal (V) n.
Superior cerebellar peduncle
Middle cerebellar peduncle
Vestibulocochlear (VIII) n.
Facial (VII) n.
Inferior cerebellar peduncle
Vestibular area
Olive
Hypoglossal (XII) n.
Glossopharyngeal (IX) and vagus (X) nn.
Hypoglossal trigone
Vagal trigone
Accessory (XI) n.

10 Cerebellum

CEREBELLAR ANATOMY

CEREBELLAR SURFACE ANATOMY			
Cerebellar Lobe	Associated Lobules	Anatomic Notes	Functional Significance
Anterior lobe	Quadrangular Ala of central lobule	Separated from the middle lobe by primary fissure	Becomes atrophic in alcoholics
Middle lobe	Simplex Superior semilunar Inferior semilunar Biventral Tonsil	Lies posterior and inferior to anterior lobe, separated from it by primary fissure Tonsil is its inferior and medial-most projection	Cerebellar tonsils lie just lateral to the medulla and, if displaced by pressure, can compress the medulla, causing death, called tonsillar herniation
Flocculonodular lobe	Flocculus Nodule of the vermis	Flocculus is separated from the middle lobe by posterolateral fissure	Involved in balance by communicating with vestibular system

FISSURES OF THE MIDDLE LOBE	
Fissure	Anatomic Notes
Postlunate	Separates simplex from superior semilunar lobule
Horizontal	Separates superior and inferior semilunar lobules
Prepyramidal	Separates inferior semilunar from biventral lobule
Retrotonsillar	Separates biventral lobule from tonsil

CEREBELLAR ANATOMY *continued*

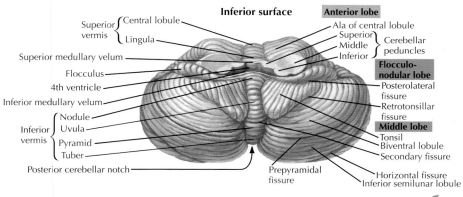

Superior surface

Anterior cerebellar notch

Central lobule

Superior vermis {
Culmen

Declive

Folium
}

Posterior cerebellar notch

Vermis

Paravermis

Lateral Hemisphere

Anterior lobe
Quadrangular lobule
Primary fissure
Horizontal fissure
Simplex lobule
Middle lobe
Postlunate fissure
Superior semi-lunar lobule
Horizontal fissure
Inferior semilunar lobule

Inferior surface

Superior vermis {
Central lobule
Lingula
}

Superior medullary velum

Flocculus

4th ventricle

Inferior medullary velum

Inferior vermis {
Nodule
Uvula
Pyramid
Tuber
}

Posterior cerebellar notch

Prepyramidal fissure

Anterior lobe
Ala of central lobule
Superior
Middle
Inferior
} Cerebellar peduncles
Flocculo-nodular lobe
Posterolateral fissure
Retrotonsillar fissure
Middle lobe
Tonsil
Biventral lobule
Secondary fissure
Horizontal fissure
Inferior semilunar lobule

INTERIOR OF CEREBELLUM

- The cerebellum has cortex, white matter, and deep nuclei.
- The cerebellar cortex is folded into folia, collectively forming the arbor vitae cerebelli.
- Input to the cerebellum goes mainly to the cerebellar cortex.
- Output from the cerebellum comes from deep nuclei.

DEEP NUCLEUS	ANATOMIC NOTES	FUNCTIONAL SIGNIFICANCE
Dentate nucleus	Largest, lateral-most, deep nucleus	Receives input from the lateral hemispheres and outputs via the superior cerebellar peduncle
Globose nuclei Emboliform nucleus	Collectively known as the *interposed nuclei*	Receive input from paravermian regions and send output via the superior cerebellar peduncle
Fastigial nucleus	Medial-most deep nucleus	Receives input from the vermis and flocculonodular lobe and outputs via the juxtarestiform body of the inferior cerebellar peduncle

Section in plane of superior cerebellar peduncle

Decussation of superior cerebellar peduncles
Cerebral peduncle
Medial longitudinal fasciculus
4th ventricle
Superior medullary velum
Superior cerebellar peduncle
Fastigial nucleus
Globose nuclei
Dentate nucleus
Emboliform nucleus
Lingula
Cerebellar cortex
Vermis

CEREBELLAR CORTEX TYPES

STRUCTURE	ANATOMIC NOTES	FUNCTIONAL SIGNIFICANCE
Purkinje cell	Large, flask-shaped cells uniformly arranged along the upper margin of granular layer	All impulses entering the cerebellar cortex must converge on these cells to reach efferent cerebellar pathways
	Purkinje cell axons are the only ones to emerge from the cerebellar cortex and enter the white matter	γ-aminobutric acid (GABA) is neurotransmitter released at synapse
Basket cell	Situated in the molecular layer, in the vicinity of Purkinje cell bodies	Gives rise to branching dendrites, which ascend in the molecular layer to produce a fan-shaped field in sagittal plane, and to axons which arborize around somata of 10 Purkinje cells
Granule cell	Fills granular layer which has appearance of packed chromatic nuclei with irregular light spaces called cerebellar islands or glomeruli which are complex synaptic structures	Prodigious in number (3-7 million granule cells/mm³ of granular layer)
Outer stellate cell	Situated in molecular layer	Establish synaptic contacts with Purkinje cell dendrites

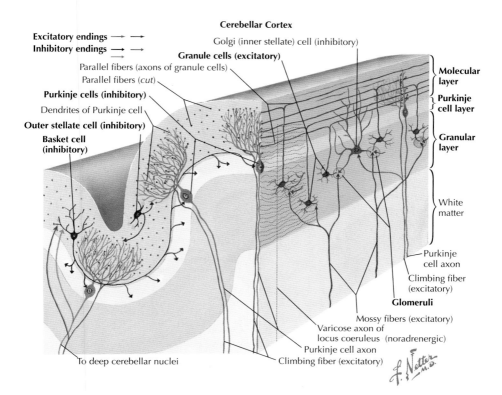

Cerebellar Cortex

Excitatory endings → →
Inhibitory endings → →

Golgi (inner stellate) cell (inhibitory)

Granule cells (excitatory)

Parallel fibers (axons of granule cells)
Parallel fibers (cut)

Purkinje cells (inhibitory)
Dendrites of Purkinje cell

Outer stellate cell (inhibitory)
Basket cell (inhibitory)

Molecular layer
Purkinje cell layer
Granular layer

White matter

Purkinje cell axon
Climbing fiber (excitatory)

Glomeruli

Mossy fibers (excitatory)
Varicose axon of locus coeruleus (noradrenergic)
Purkinje cell axon
To deep cerebellar nuclei
Climbing fiber (excitatory)

FUNCTIONAL SUBDIVISIONS OF THE CEREBELLUM

The cerebellum can be divided into functional lobes:
- Lateral hemispheres
- Paravermis
- Vermis and flocculonodular lobe

The cerebellum has somatotopic organization:
- Body is represented three times
- Each hemisphere and the vermis have a somatotopic map

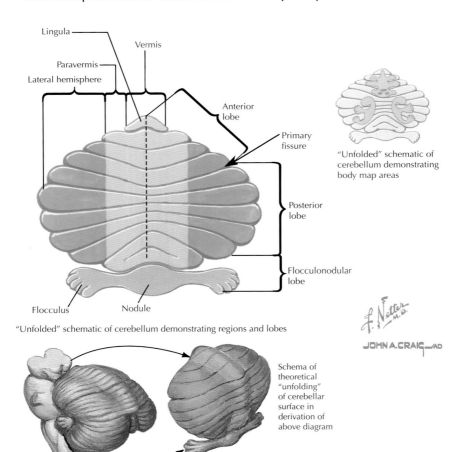

"Unfolded" schematic of cerebellum demonstrating body map areas

"Unfolded" schematic of cerebellum demonstrating regions and lobes

Schema of theoretical "unfolding" of cerebellar surface in derivation of above diagram

CEREBELLAR INPUT

- Input to the cerebellum arises from multiple locations in the nervous system.
- Input from the spinocerebellar tracts provides unconscious proprioception.
- Inputs from the vestibular system provides information about acceleration and head position.
- Inputs from the motor cortex provides information about motor function.
- Cerebellum uses all input to assist in coordinating smooth motor function and balance.
- All input to the cerebellum from spinal cord is from the ipsilateral body.
- The ventral spinocerebellar tract double crosses.

PEDUNCLE	INPUT(S) TO CEREBELLUM
Superior	Ventral spinocerebellar tract
	Midbrain tectum (colliculi)
	Trigeminal system
Middle	Cerebral cortex (motor and sensory) via pontine nuclei
Inferior	Dorsal spinocerebellar tract
	Rostral spinocerebellar tract
	Cuneocerebellar tract
	Reticulocerebellar tract
	Inferior olive
	Trigeminal system
	Vestibular system

CEREBELLAR INPUT *continued*

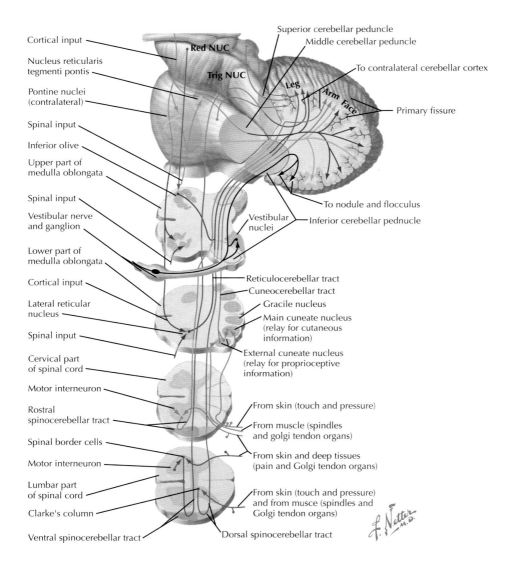

Cortical input

Nucleus reticularis tegmenti pontis

Pontine nuclei (contralateral)

Spinal input

Inferior olive

Upper part of medulla oblongata

Spinal input

Vestibular nerve and ganglion

Lower part of medulla oblongata

Cortical input

Lateral reticular nucleus

Spinal input

Cervical part of spinal cord

Motor interneuron

Rostral spinocerebellar tract

Spinal border cells

Motor interneuron

Lumbar part of spinal cord

Clarke's column

Ventral spinocerebellar tract

Red NUC

Trig NUC

Leg

Arm

Face

Superior cerebellar peduncle

Middle cerebellar peduncle

To contralateral cerebellar cortex

Primary fissure

To nodule and flocculus

Vestibular nuclei

Inferior cerebellar pednucle

Reticulocerebellar tract

Cuneocerebellar tract

Gracile nucleus

Main cuneate nucleus (relay for cutaneous information)

External cuneate nucleus (relay for proprioceptive information)

From skin (touch and pressure)

From muscle (spindles and golgi tendon organs)

From skin and deep tissues (pain and Golgi tendon organs)

From skin (touch and pressure) and from musce (spindles and Golgi tendon organs)

Dorsal spinocerebellar tract

CEREBELLAR OUTPUT

- Output from the cerebellum comes from deep nuclei.
- The flocculonodular cortex also outputs directly to vestibular nuclei.

PEDUNCLE	CEREBELLAR OUTPUT(S)
Superior	Thalamus (ventrolateral [VL] nucleus) Red nucleus Reticular formation
Middle	None
Inferior	Vestibular nuclei (via hook bundle of Russel) Reticular formation

CEREBELLAR CIRCUITRY BY FUNCTIONAL LOBE				
Functional Lobe	Input	Deep Nucleus	Output	Function
Lateral hemispheres	Motor and sensory cortex	Dentate	Thalamus VL to the premotor cortex	Coordinates movement by influencing the corticospinal tract
Paravermis	Muscle spindles and Golgi tendon organs via spinocerebellar tracts	Interposed (globose and emboliform)	Red nucleus	Modulates movement by influencing rubrospinal tract
Vermis and flocculonodular lobe	Vestibular system	Fastigial and vestibular nuclei	Vestibular system	Modulates balance and truncal stability

CEREBELLAR OUTPUT *continued*

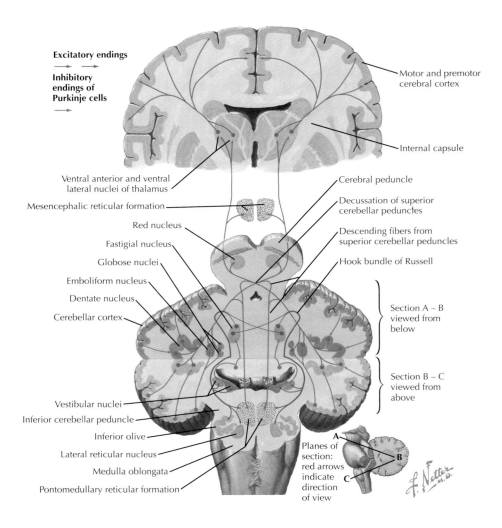

Excitatory endings

Inhibitory endings of Purkinje cells

Motor and premotor cerebral cortex

Internal capsule

Ventral anterior and ventral lateral nuclei of thalamus

Mesencephalic reticular formation

Red nucleus

Fastigial nucleus

Globose nuclei

Emboliform nucleus

Dentate nucleus

Cerebellar cortex

Cerebral peduncle

Decussation of superior cerebellar pedunctes

Descending fibers from superior cerebellar peduncles

Hook bundle of Russell

Section A – B viewed from below

Section B – C viewed from above

Vestibular nuclei

Inferior cerebellar peduncle

Inferior olive

Lateral reticular nucleus

Medulla oblongata

Pontomedullary reticular formation

Planes of section: red arrows indicate direction of view

A

B

C

Cerebral Cortex

LAYERS OF THE CEREBRAL CORTEX

STRUCTURE	ANATOMIC NOTES	FUNCTIONAL SIGNIFICANCE
Sensory cortex	Large granule cell layers (granular cortex) for receiving input	Receives afferent fibers and terminals from other parts of nervous system (e.g., thalamocortical)
Association cortex	Most association fibers arise from superficial layers of cortex	Axons interrelate cortical regions of same or opposite hemisphere
Motor cortex	Most projection neurons arise from deeper layers of cortex	Contains projection neurons to other parts of the neuraxis (e.g., corticospinal, corticobulbar)

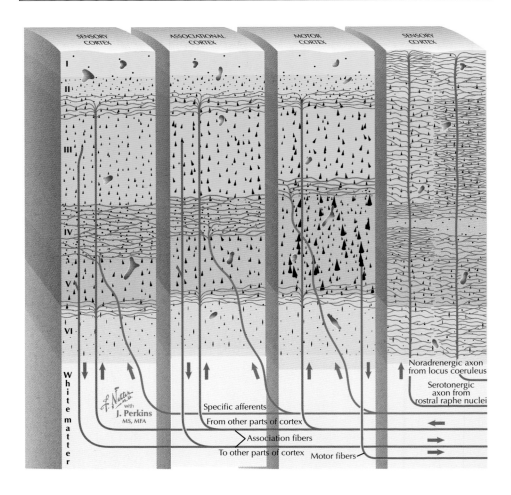

CORTICAL NEURONAL CELL TYPES

STRUCTURE	ANATOMIC NOTES	FUNCTIONAL SIGNIFICANCE
Stellate (granule) cells	Small bodies, localized dendritic trees All layers of cortex, most in layer IV	Receiving neurons for thalamic input Modulate excitability of other cortical neurons
Pyramidal cells	Varied cell bodies Large basal and apical dendritic branching patterns run perpendicular to the cortical surface and arborize in upper layers.	Projection neurons (e.g., corticobulbar, corticoreticular, corticothalamic tracts)
Cells of Martinotti	Small triangular cells present in all cortical layers	Intracortical neuron
Horizontal cell (of Cajal)	Small fusiform cells present mostly in superficial cortical layer	Intracortical neuron
Betz cell	Giant pyramidal cells	Concentrated in Brodmann area 4, primary motor cortex Give rise to corticospinal tract

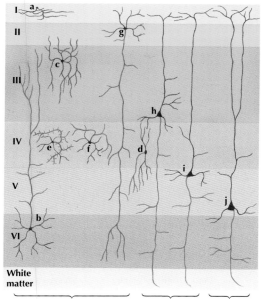

Key for Abbreviations
a Horizontal cell
b Cell of Martinotti
c Chandelier cell
d Aspiny granule cell
e Spiny granule cell
f Stellate (granule) cell
g Small pyramidal cell of layers II, III
h Small pyramidal association cell
i Small pyramidal association and projection cells of layer V
j Large pyramidal projection cell (Betz cell)

Cortical interneurons — Cortical association neurons — Efferent neuron

Black - cell bodies and dendrites
Brown - axons of interneurons and association neurons
Red - axons of efferent neurons

SENSORY CORTEX VERTICAL COLUMNS

STRUCTURE	ANATOMIC NOTES	FUNCTIONAL SIGNIFICANCE
Vertical cell columns in sensory and visual cortex	Neurons of particular column are all related to same peripheral receptive field	Constitute elementary functional cortical unit Neurons of same vertical column are activated by same peripheral stimulus

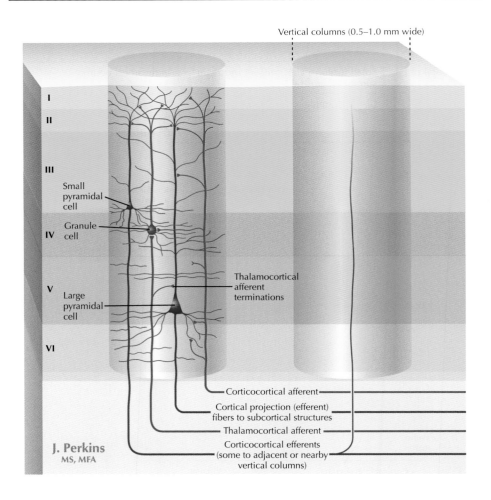

Vertical columns (0.5–1.0 mm wide)

I
II
III

Small pyramidal cell

Granule cell
IV

Thalamocortical afferent terminations

V
Large pyramidal cell

VI

Corticocortical afferent
Cortical projection (efferent) fibers to subcortical structures
Thalamocortical afferent
Corticocortical efferents (some to adjacent or nearby vertical columns)

J. Perkins
MS, MFA

NEURONAL ORIGINS OF EFFERENT CORTICAL CONNECTIONS

STRUCTURE	ANATOMIC NOTES	FUNCTIONAL SIGNIFICANCE
Corticocortical columns	Same size as functional columns of sensory cortex	Delineated by pattern of termination of association and commissural fibers Afferent fibers converge from multiple vertical columns to create vast mosaic of cortical connections

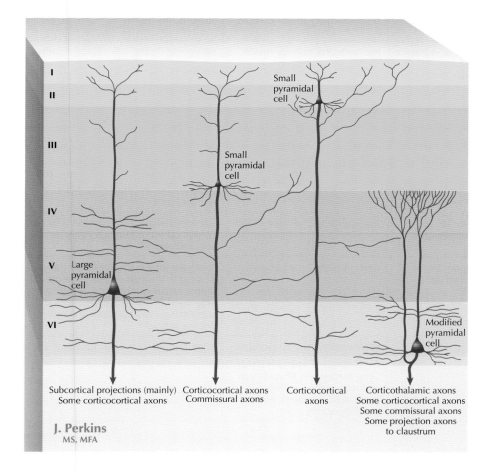

I

II

III

IV

V Large pyramidal cell

VI

Small pyramidal cell

Small pyramidal cell

Modified pyramidal cell

Subcortical projections (mainly)   Corticocortical axons   Corticocortical   Corticothalamic axons
Some corticocortical axons   Commissural axons   axons   Some corticocortical axons
Some commissural axons
Some projection axons
to claustrum

J. Perkins
MS, MFA

COMMISSURAL AND OTHER ASSOCIATION FIBER SYSTEMS

STRUCTURE	ANATOMIC NOTES	FUNCTIONAL SIGNIFICANCE
Corpus callosum: genu	Interconnects prefrontal cortex	Enables the reorganization of cerebral functions to compensate for disruption caused by lateralized brain insult
Corpus callosum: rostral part of body	Interconnects premotor and supplementary motor cortices	Callosotomy surgery for seizure control sections this region
Corpus callosum: middle part of body	Interconnects primary motor and primary and secondary somatic sensory areas	Sectioning during callosotomy results in left-sided neglect, aphasia, and disorders of visuospatial transfer
Corpus callosum: caudal part of body	Interconnects posterior parietal cortex	Interhemispheric transfer of tactile information
Corpus callosum: splenium	Interconnects temporal and occipital cortices	Lesion in splenium causes "pure" word blindness (alexia without agraphia): inability to read aloud, understand written script, and often to name colors Conversation, repetition, and writing remain intact
Anterior commissure	Interconnects 2 temporal lobes	Sectioned along with anterior $^2/_3$ of the corpus callosum during surgery for seizure control
Hippocampal commissure	Interconnects 2 hippocampi	Temporal lobe discharges may not propagate through corpus callosum or hippocampal commissure, resulting in little interhemispheric coherence, and supporting a multisynaptic route for seizure spread
Cingulum	White-matter core of cingulate gyrus Long-association fiber system connecting the anterior perforated substance and the parahippocampal gyrus	Important for emotional functions

HIPPOCAMPAL FORMATION *continued*

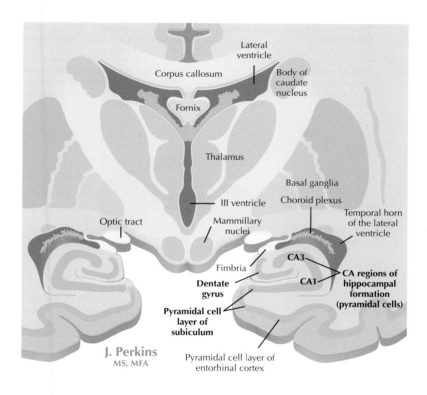

Lateral ventricle

Corpus callosum

Body of caudate nucleus

Fornix

Thalamus

Basal ganglia

III ventricle

Choroid plexus

Optic tract

Mammillary nuclei

Temporal horn of the lateral ventricle

CA3

Fimbria

CA1

CA regions of hippocampal formation (pyramidal cells)

Dentate gyrus

Pyramidal cell layer of subiculum

J. Perkins
MS, MFA

Pyramidal cell layer of entorhinal cortex

ENTORHINAL CORTEX

STRUCTURE	ANATOMIC NOTES	FUNCTIONAL SIGNIFICANCE
Alveus	Axons of pyramidal neurons gather at the ventricular surface of the hippocampus as alveus	Myelinated envelope surrounding the hippocampal formation
Fimbria	Alveus fibers converge to form flattened ribbon of white matter, the fimbria	Traced posteriorly, the fimbria, at posterior limit of hippocampus, arches under splenium of corpus callosum to form the crus of the fornix
Entorhinal cortex	Bulk of extrinsic input to hippocampal formation comes from the entorhinal cortex	Information from many cortical areas (visual, auditory, sensory) converge here and is conveyed to the hippocampus

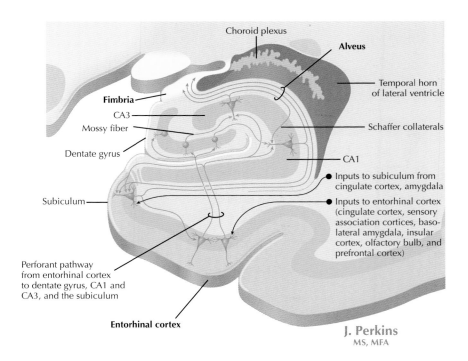

Choroid plexus

Alveus

Temporal horn of lateral ventricle

Fimbria

CA3

Mossy fiber

Schaffer collaterals

Dentate gyrus

CA1

Inputs to subiculum from cingulate cortex, amygdala

Subiculum

Inputs to entorhinal cortex (cingulate cortex, sensory association cortices, baso-lateral amygdala, insular cortex, olfactory bulb, and prefrontal cortex)

Perforant pathway from entorhinal cortex to dentate gyrus, CA1 and CA3, and the subiculum

Entorhinal cortex

J. Perkins
MS, MFA

OLFACTORY CORTEX

STRUCTURE	ANATOMIC NOTES	FUNCTIONAL SIGNIFICANCE
Olfactory cortex	Located in temporal lobe Composed of: • Pyriform cortex • Periamygdaloid area • Part of entorhinal area	Exceptionally small area in humans; concerned with conscious perception of olfactory stimuli
Pyriform cortex	Projects fibers to entorhinal cortex	Major link between the olfactory regions of the temporal and frontal lobes
Periamygdaloid area	Dorsal and rostral to the amygdala	Intimately related to the prepyriform area
Entorhinal area	Rostral part of parahippocampal gyrus, corresponding to Brodmann area 28	Constitutes a secondary olfactory cortex projecting to hippocampal formation, insula, and frontal cortex

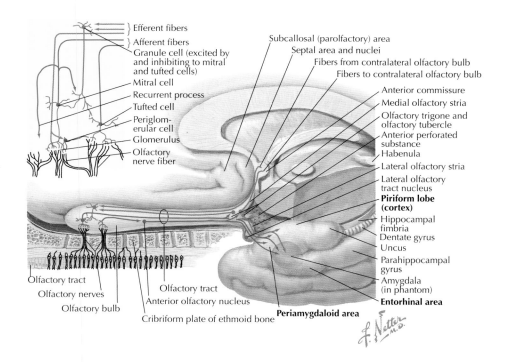

CHAPTER 12

Hypothalamus

ANATOMY OF THE HYPOTHALAMUS

Location	Located in ventral diencephalon along the walls of 3rd ventricle, below the hypothalamic sulcus and above the pituitary gland
	Anterior border is the lamina terminalis
	Lateral border is indistinct
Architecture	Composed of a collection of nuclei and fiber tracts
	In the sagittal plane can be divided into periventricular, medial, and lateral zones
	Connected to multiple parts of the nervous system
Function	Serves as a central regulator of homeostasis
	Controls the autonomic nervous system, visceral functions; participates in the limbic system
	Regulates appetite, temperature, thirst, stress response, lactation, and cardiorespiratory function
Clinical Significance	Lesions can lead to autonomic, emotional, or endocrine dysfunction, including precocious puberty

ANATOMY OF THE HYPOTHALAMUS *continued*

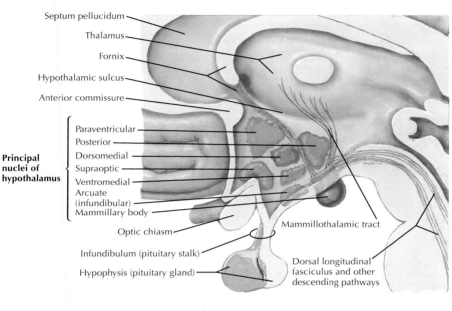

Septum pellucidum
Thalamus
Fornix
Hypothalamic sulcus
Anterior commissure

Principal nuclei of hypothalamus
Paraventricular
Posterior
Dorsomedial
Supraoptic
Ventromedial
Arcuate (infundibular)
Mammillary body

Optic chiasm
Infundibulum (pituitary stalk)
Hypophysis (pituitary gland)

Mammillothalamic tract
Dorsal longitudinal fasciculus and other descending pathways

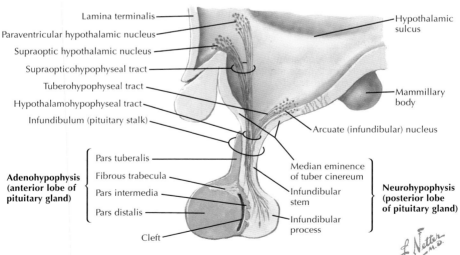

Lamina terminalis
Paraventricular hypothalamic nucleus
Supraoptic hypothalamic nucleus
Supraopticohypophyseal tract
Tuberohypophyseal tract
Hypothalamohypophyseal tract
Infundibulum (pituitary stalk)

Hypothalamic sulcus
Mammillary body
Arcuate (infundibular) nucleus

Adenohypophysis (anterior lobe of pituitary gland)
Pars tuberalis
Fibrous trabecula
Pars intermedia
Pars distalis
Cleft

Median eminence of tuber cinereum
Infundibular stem
Infundibular process

Neurohypophysis (posterior lobe of pituitary gland)

THE HYPOTHALAMUS IN RELATION TO OTHER MEDIAL STRUCTURES

STRUCTURE	ANATOMIC NOTES	FUNCTIONAL SIGNIFICANCE AND CLINICAL NOTES
Thalamus	Like the hypothalamus, the thalamus is a diencephalic structure Located above the hypothalamic sulcus lateral to the 3rd ventricle	As structures lining the 3rd ventricle, both the medial thalamus and hypothalamus can be damaged in thiamine deficiency
Hypothalamic sulcus	A groove in the wall of the 3rd ventricle, which separates the thalamus superiorly from the hypothalamus inferiorly	
Fornix	In sagittal section, it swings above and around the thalamus Separates medial from lateral hypothalamus. Carries hippocampal output to the hypothalamic mammillary body	Damage to this structure can cause problems with emotions and memory The pathway from the hippocampus to the mammillary bodies is part of the Papez circuit of the limbic system
Lamina terminalis	Represents the anterior end of the neural tube and the anterior border of the hypothalamus	Location of the rostral neural tube closure
Optic chiasm	Lies below the hypothalamus and above the pituitary	Pituitary lesions can compress the optic chiasm, causing visual-field deficits, specifically a bitemporal field cut
Tuber cinereum	Layer of hypothalamic gray matter that forms the floor of the 3rd ventricle and descends to form the infundibulum	
Anterior lobe of pituitary gland	The anterior portion of the pituitary gland Also known as adenohypophysis	Produces and secretes various hormones into the systemic circulation; regulates the endocrine system. Its function is regulated by releasing factors from the hypothalamus
Posterior lobe of pituitary gland	The posterior portion of the pituitary Also known as *neurohypophysis* Direct extension of the hypothalamus, connected via the infundibulum	Secretes 2 hormones, vasopressin and oxytocin, which are produced in the hypothalamus

THE HYPOTHALAMUS IN RELATION TO OTHER MEDIAL STRUCTURES *continued*

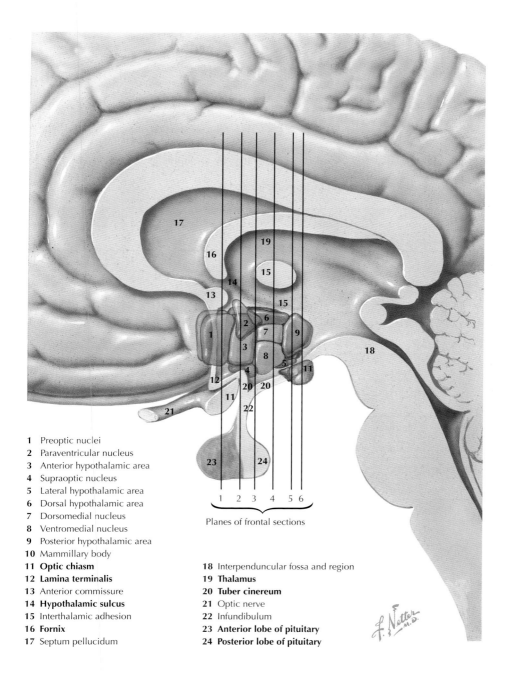

Planes of frontal sections

1 Preoptic nuclei
2 Paraventricular nucleus
3 Anterior hypothalamic area
4 Supraoptic nucleus
5 Lateral hypothalamic area
6 Dorsal hypothalamic area
7 Dorsomedial nucleus
8 Ventromedial nucleus
9 Posterior hypothalamic area
10 Mammillary body
11 **Optic chiasm**
12 **Lamina terminalis**
13 Anterior commissure
14 **Hypothalamic sulcus**
15 **Interthalamic adhesion**
16 **Fornix**
17 Septum pellucidum

18 Interpenduncular fossa and region
19 **Thalamus**
20 **Tuber cinereum**
21 Optic nerve
22 Infundibulum
23 **Anterior lobe of pituitary**
24 **Posterior lobe of pituitary**

HYPOTHALAMIC NUCLEI

- Composed of medial and lateral zones separated by the fornix as it traverses hypothalamus
- Can also be divided into anterior to posterior zones

NUCLEUS	ZONE
Medial preoptic	Preoptic
Lateral preoptic	Preoptic
Supraoptic	Anterior (supraoptic)
Suprachiasmatic	Anterior (supraoptic)
Anterior hypothalamic area	Anterior (supraoptic)
Paraventricular	Anterior (supraoptic)
Dorsomedial	Tuberal
Ventromedial	Tuberal
Arcuate	Tuberal
Dorsal hypothalamic area	Tuberal
Posterior hypothalamic area	Posterior (mammillary)
Mammillary bodies	Posterior (mammillary)
Lateral hypothalamic area	Spans anterior, tuberal, and posterior
Periventricular	Spans anterior and tuberal

HYPOTHALAMIC NUCLEI *continued*

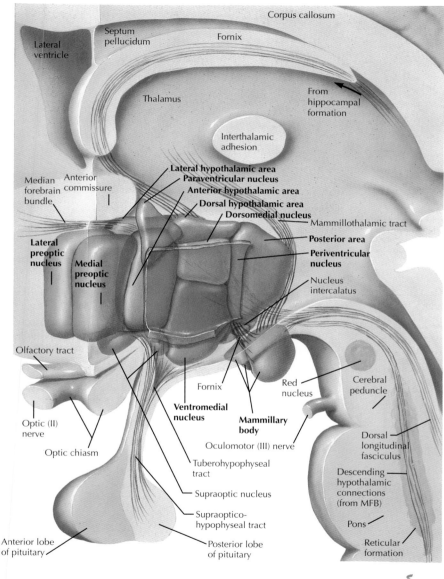

PREOPTIC AND ANTERIOR (SUPRAOPTIC) ZONE NUCLEI

NUCLEUS	FUNCTION
Medial preoptic	Regulates the parasympathetic nervous system
Lateral preoptic	Not clearly established; involved in sleep, sexual function, and reward behaviors
Supraoptic	Produces vasopressin (antidiuretic hormone), which is transported via axons to the posterior pituitary. Vasopressin causes vasoconstriction and water retention
Anterior hypothalamic area	Involved in temperature, appetite, and sexual regulation. Regulates the parasympathetic nervous system
Paraventricular	Produces oxytocin, which is transported via axons to the posterior pituitary; oxytocin causes uterine contractions and milk ejection
Suprachiasmatic (not shown)	Receives input from the retina; controls the circadian rhythm, partly by influencing the pineal gland
Lateral hypothalamic area	Involved in appetite, thirst, and temperature regulation

PREOPTIC AND ANTERIOR (SUPRAOPTIC) ZONE NUCLEI *continued*

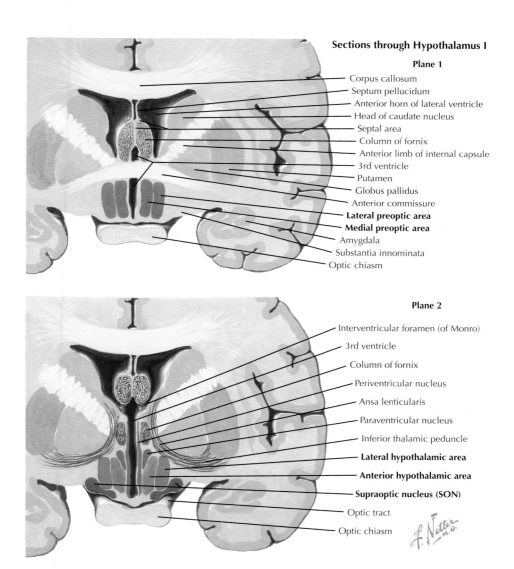

Sections through Hypothalamus I

Plane 1

Corpus callosum
Septum pellucidum
Anterior horn of lateral ventricle
Head of caudate nucleus
Septal area
Column of fornix
Anterior limb of internal capsule
3rd ventricle
Putamen
Globus pallidus
Anterior commissure
Lateral preoptic area
Medial preoptic area
Amygdala
Substantia innominata
Optic chiasm

Plane 2

Interventricular foramen (of Monro)
3rd ventricle
Column of fornix
Periventricular nucleus
Ansa lenticularis
Paraventricular nucleus
Inferior thalamic peduncle
Lateral hypothalamic area
Anterior hypothalamic area
Supraoptic nucleus (SON)
Optic tract
Optic chiasm

TUBERAL ZONE NUCLEI

NUCLEUS	FUNCTION
Dorsomedial	Represents the satiety center of the brain Lesions can lead to obesity
Ventromedial	Involved in emotions and rage responses
Arcuate	Produces dopamine which inhibits prolactin release from the anterior pituitary Involved in appetite regulation
Periarcuate area	Produces β-endorphins
Periventricular	Produces releasing and inhibiting factors, which are sent to the median eminence for release into hypothalamic-pituitary portal system and control hormone release from the anterior pituitary
Lateral hypothalamic area	Involved in appetite, thirst, and temperature regulation

TUBERAL ZONE NUCLEI *continued*

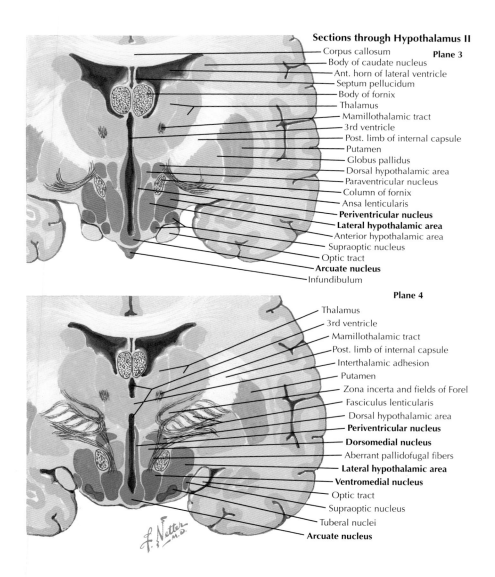

Sections through Hypothalamus II

Plane 3

- Corpus callosum
- Body of caudate nucleus
- Ant. horn of lateral ventricle
- Septum pellucidum
- Body of fornix
- Thalamus
- Mamillothalamic tract
- 3rd ventricle
- Post. limb of internal capsule
- Putamen
- Globus pallidus
- Dorsal hypothalamic area
- Paraventricular nucleus
- Column of fornix
- Ansa lenticularis
- **Periventricular nucleus**
- **Lateral hypothalamic area**
- Anterior hypothalamic area
- Supraoptic nucleus
- Optic tract
- **Arcuate nucleus**
- Infundibulum

Plane 4

- Thalamus
- 3rd ventricle
- Mamillothalamic tract
- Post. limb of internal capsule
- Interthalamic adhesion
- Putamen
- Zona incerta and fields of Forel
- Fasciculus lenticularis
- Dorsal hypothalamic area
- **Periventricular nucleus**
- **Dorsomedial nucleus**
- Aberrant pallidofugal fibers
- **Lateral hypothalamic area**
- **Ventromedial nucleus**
- Optic tract
- Supraoptic nucleus
- Tuberal nuclei
- **Arcuate nucleus**

POSTERIOR (MAMILLARY) ZONE NUCLEI

NUCLEUS	FUNCTION
Posterior hypothalamic area	Regulates the sympathetic nervous system; involved in the response to cold
Medial and lateral mammillary nuclei	Integral part of the limbic system
	Receive hippocampal input via the fornix and project to the anterior nucleus of the thalamus
	Damage causes inability to form new memories; can be damaged by thiamine deficiency, common in alcoholics, known as *Wernicke-Korsakoff syndrome*

POSTERIOR (MAMILLARY) ZONE NUCLEI *continued*

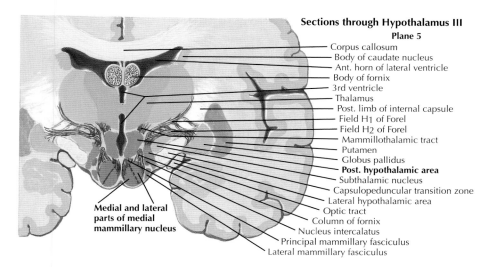

Sections through Hypothalamus III
Plane 5

- Corpus callosum
- Body of caudate nucleus
- Ant. horn of lateral ventricle
- Body of fornix
- 3rd ventricle
- Thalamus
- Post. limb of internal capsule
- Field H1 of Forel
- Field H2 of Forel
- Mammillothalamic tract
- Putamen
- Globus pallidus
- **Post. hypothalamic area**
- Subthalamic nucleus
- Capsulopeduncular transition zone
- Lateral hypothalamic area
- Optic tract
- Column of fornix
- Nucleus intercalatus
- Principal mammillary fasciculus
- Lateral mammillary fasciculus

Medial and lateral parts of medial mammillary nucleus

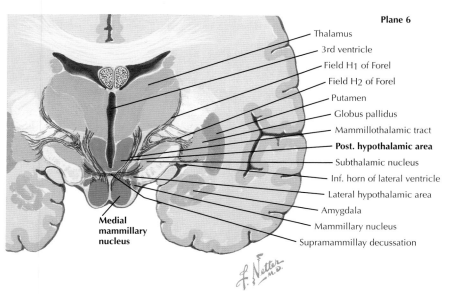

Plane 6

- Thalamus
- 3rd ventricle
- Field H1 of Forel
- Field H2 of Forel
- Putamen
- Globus pallidus
- Mammillothalamic tract
- **Post. hypothalamic area**
- Subthalamic nucleus
- Inf. horn of lateral ventricle
- Lateral hypothalamic area
- Amygdala
- Mammillary nucleus
- Supramammillay decussation

Medial mammillary nucleus

HYPOTHALAMIC PATHWAYS

The hypothalamus is integrally connected with multiple parts of the nervous system.

SELECTED AFFERENT PATHWAYS			
Input	Pathway	Destination	Function
Retina	Retinohypothalamic	Suprachiasmatic nucleus	Sets the circadian rhythm
Median dorsal thalamus		Multiple nuclei	Limbic-emotional modulation
Cerebral cortex	Median forebrain bundle	Lateral hypothalamus	Limbic-emotional modulation
Amygdala	Stria terminalis Ventral amygdalofugal	Multiple nuclei	Limbic-emotional modulation Olfactory input modulation
Hippocampus	Fornix	Medial mamillary	Memory formation Part of Papez circuit
Brainstem autonomic structures	Medial forebrain bundle Dorsal longitudinal fasciculus	Multiple nuclei	Autonomic modulation

SELECTED EFFERENT PATHWAYS			
Output Nucleus	Pathway	Destination	Function
Paraventricular and supraoptic	Supraopticohypophyseal tract	Posterior pituitary	Delivery of vasopressin and oxytocin
Multiple regions		Median eminence	Release of releasing and inhibiting factors for anterior pituitary
Lateral hypothalamus	Median forebrain bundle	Septal nuclei	Limbic-emotional modulation
Medial mammillary	Mammillothalamic tract	Thalamus (anterior nucleus)	Part of Papez circuit
Periarcuate area	β-endorphin pathway	Multiple subcortical and brainstem	Modulates stress responses
Multiple regions	Medial tegmental tract	Reticular formation, tegmental nuclei	Modulation of arousal and autonomic systems

HYPOTHALAMIC PATHWAYS *continued*

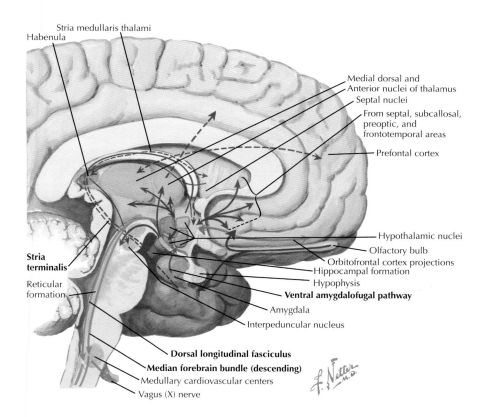

Stria medullaris thalami
Habenula
Medial dorsal and
Anterior nuclei of thalamus
Septal nuclei
From septal, subcallosal, preoptic, and frontotemporal areas
Prefontal cortex
Hypothalamic nuclei
Olfactory bulb
Orbitofrontal cortex projections
Hippocampal formation
Hypophysis
Ventral amygdalofugal pathway
Amygdala
Interpeduncular nucleus
Stria terminalis
Reticular formation
Dorsal longitudinal fasciculus
Median forebrain bundle (descending)
Medullary cardiovascular centers
Vagus (X) nerve

SUMMARY OF HYPOTHALAMIC INPUT AND OUTPUT

KEY HYPOTHALAMIC PATHWAYS

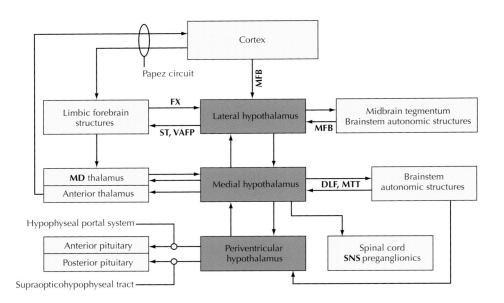

DLF = Dorsal longitudinal fasciculus

MFB = Median forebrain bundle

ST = Stria terminalis

VAFP = Ventral amygdalofugal pathway

MD = Medial dorsal nucleus of thalamus

FX = Fornix

MTT = Mammillothalamic tract

SNS = Sympathetic nervous system

POSTERIOR PITUITARY

Location	Is a direct extension of the hypothalamus, connected via the infundibulum
Architecture	Composed of descending axons from the supraoptic and paraventricular nuclei of hypothalamus
Function	Secretes oxytocin and vasopressin (antidiuretic hormone, or ADH) into the systemic circulation through fenestrated capillaries
Clinical Significance	Oxytocin causes uterine contractions during childbirth. Vasopressin causes water retention by the kidney and vasoconstriction. In severe brain injuries, damage can cause failure of ADH release, known as diabetes insipidus. Brain lesions can also cause the syndrome of inappropriate antidiuretic hormone (SIADH), leading to dilution of blood and low sodium

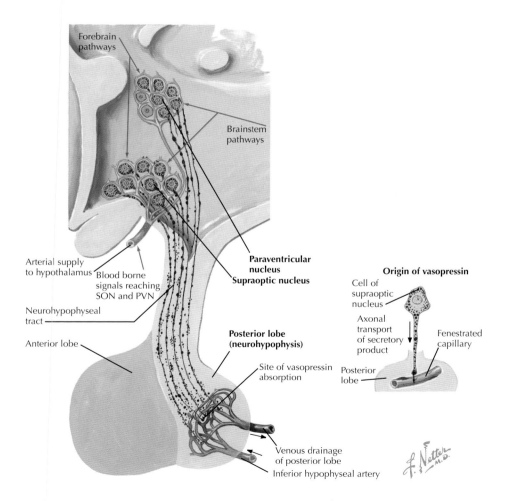

Forebrain pathways

Brainstem pathways

Arterial supply to hypothalamus

Blood borne signals reaching SON and PVN

Neurohypophyseal tract

Anterior lobe

Paraventricular nucleus

Supraoptic nucleus

Posterior lobe (neurohypophysis)

Site of vasopressin absorption

Origin of vasopressin

Cell of supraoptic nucleus

Axonal transport of secretory product

Fenestrated capillary

Posterior lobe

Venous drainage of posterior lobe

Inferior hypophyseal artery

ANTERIOR PITUITARY

- Diffuse hypothalamic neurons release factors that are transported to the median eminence.
- These factors are released into the hypophyseal portal veins and influence the anterior pituitary.
- Unlike the posterior pituitary, the anterior pituitary is not a direct extension of the hypothalamus.

HYPOTHALAMIC RELEASING FACTORS (SELECTED)		
Factor	Effect on Pituitary	Function
Thyrotropin-releasing hormone (TRH)	Stimulates release of thyroid-stimulating hormone (TSH)	Stimulates thyroid gland to secrete thyroxine and tri-iodothyronine
Growth hormone–releasing hormone (GHRH)	Stimulates release of growth hormone (GH)	Stimulates the liver to produce insulin-like growth factor I
Gonadotropin-releasing hormone (GnRH)	Stimulates release of luteinizing hormone (LH) and follicle-stimulating hormone (FSH)	Modulates puberty, menstrual cycle, menopause and sexual drive
Corticotropin-releasing hormone (CRH)	Stimulates release of adrenocorticotropic hormone (ACTH)	Stimulates the adrenal grand to secrete cortisol
Dopamine	Inhibits release of prolactin	Modulates lactation
Somatostatin	Inhibits release of GH and TSH	Regulates thyroid and growth hormones

ANTERIOR PITUITARY *continued*

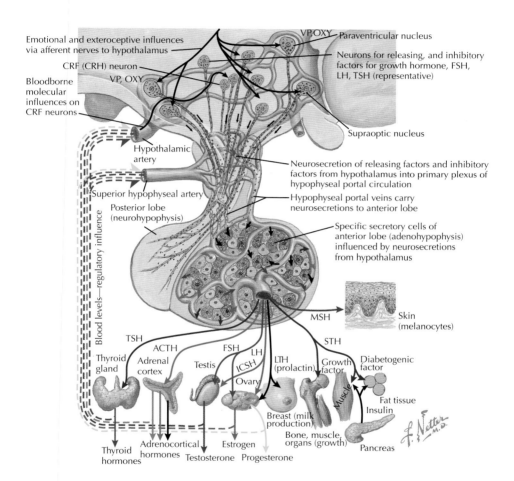

Emotional and exteroceptive influences via afferent nerves to hypothalamus

CRF (CRH) neuron

Bloodborne molecular influences on CRF neurons

VP, OXY

VP, OXY — Paraventricular nucleus

Neurons for releasing, and inhibitory factors for growth hormone, FSH, LH, TSH (representative)

Supraoptic nucleus

Hypothalamic artery

Neurosecretion of releasing factors and inhibitory factors from hypothalamus into primary plexus of hypophyseal portal circulation

Superior hypophyseal artery

Hypophyseal portal veins carry neurosecretions to anterior lobe

Posterior lobe (neurohypophysis)

Specific secretory cells of anterior lobe (adenohypophysis) influenced by neurosecretions from hypothalamus

Blood levels—regulatory influence

MSH

Skin (melanocytes)

TSH

ACTH

FSH LH

STH

Thyroid gland

Adrenal cortex

Testis

ICSH

Ovary

LTH (prolactin)

Growth factor

Diabetogenic factor

Fat tissue
Insulin

Breast (milk production)

Bone, muscle, organs (growth)

Pancreas

Thyroid hormones

Adrenocortical hormones

Testosterone

Estrogen

Progesterone

13 Limbic System

GENERAL FEATURES OF THE LIMBIC SYSTEM

Location	A system of nuclear structures and tracts found in a ring that encircles the thalamus
Architecture	Composed of multiple structures that interact with each other and have significant connections with other cortical and subcortical structures
Function	Serves a major central regulator of emotional control and memory encoding
Clinical Significance	Damage can lead to aggression, apathy, or anterograde amnesia (inability to form new memories).

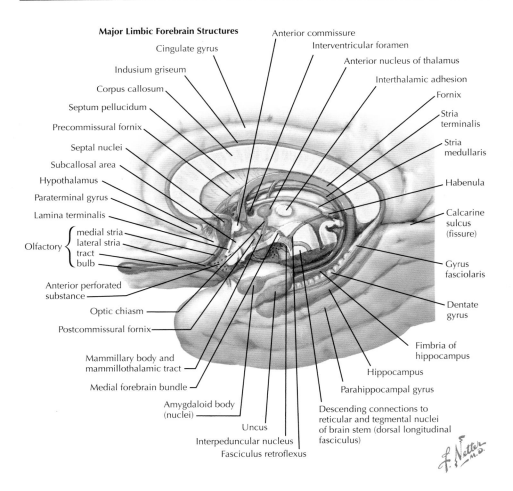

Major Limbic Forebrain Structures

Cingulate gyrus
Indusium griseum
Corpus callosum
Septum pellucidum
Precommissural fornix
Septal nuclei
Subcallosal area
Hypothalamus
Paraterminal gyrus
Lamina terminalis
Olfactory { medial stria / lateral stria / tract / bulb
Anterior perforated substance
Optic chiasm
Postcommissural fornix
Mammillary body and mammillothalamic tract
Medial forebrain bundle
Amygdaloid body (nuclei)
Uncus
Interpeduncular nucleus
Fasciculus retroflexus

Anterior commissure
Interventricular foramen
Anterior nucleus of thalamus
Interthalamic adhesion
Fornix
Stria terminalis
Stria medullaris
Habenula
Calcarine sulcus (fissure)
Gyrus fasciolaris
Dentate gyrus
Fimbria of hippocampus
Hippocampus
Parahippocampal gyrus
Descending connections to reticular and tegmental nuclei of brain stem (dorsal longitudinal fasciculus)

MAJOR LIMBIC FOREBRAIN STRUCTURES

STRUCTURE	ANATOMIC NOTES	FUNCTIONAL SIGNIFICANCE AND CLINICAL NOTES
Hippocampus	Lies deep in the medial temporal lobe, medial to the temporal horn of the lateral ventricle	Major regulator of the limbic system, especially memory encoding
Fornix	C-shaped structure that extends from the hippocampus, travels inferior to the corpus callosum, and dives down to mammillary bodies	Carries output from the hippocampus to mammillary bodies of the hypothalamus and to septal nuclei
Amygdala	Almond-shaped structure located anterior to the hippocampus deep in the temporal lobe	Involved in emotional responses, including rage Lesions can cause behavioral outbursts or docility
Stria terminalis	Thin C-shaped tract connecting amygdala to the hypothalamus and basal forebrain	Major output from amygdala Involved in autonomic response to fear, rage, and other emotions
Habenula	Small nuclear structure, rostral to the pineal gland	Part of the epithalamus; major input from the septal nucleus and thalamus via the stria medullaris Major output to the interpeduncular nucleus via the fasciculus retroflexus
Septal nuclei	Set of nuclear structures rostral to the anterior commissure	Functions as the pleasure center of the brain Communicates with the hippocampus, amygdala, and hypothalamus

MAJOR LIMBIC FOREBRAIN STRUCTURES *continued*

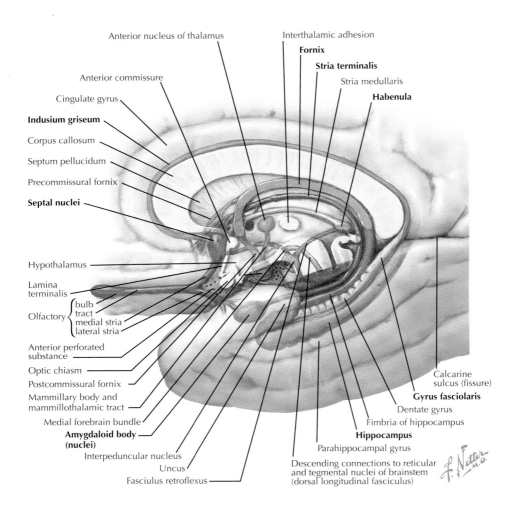

Anterior nucleus of thalamus

Interthalamic adhesion

Fornix

Stria terminalis

Stria medullaris

Anterior commissure

Habenula

Cingulate gyrus

Indusium griseum

Corpus callosum

Septum pellucidum

Precommissural fornix

Septal nuclei

Hypothalamus

Lamina terminalis

Olfactory { bulb / tract / medial stria / lateral stria }

Anterior perforated substance

Optic chiasm

Postcommissural fornix

Mammillary body and mammillothalamic tract

Medial forebrain bundle

Amygdaloid body (nuclei)

Interpeduncular nucleus

Uncus

Fasciulus retroflexus

Calcarine sulcus (fissure)

Gyrus fasciolaris

Dentate gyrus

Fimbria of hippocampus

Hippocampus

Parahippocampal gyrus

Descending connections to reticular and tegmental nuclei of brainstem (dorsal longitudinal fasciculus)

HIPPOCAMPUS

Location	Medial to the temporal horn of the lateral ventricle in the deep anterior temporal lobe
Architecture	Seahorse-shaped structure composed of the dentate gyrus, CA regions, and subiculum. Unlike most of the cortex, the hippocampus has 3 neuronal layers
Circuitry	Internal circuitry: entorhinal cortex→ dentate gyrus→ CA3→ CA1→subiculum→ entorhinal cortex
	Major external circuit (Papez circuit): hippocampus→ fornix→ mammillary bodies→ anterior nucleus of thalamus→ cingulate cortex→ temporal cortex→ hippocampus
	Other input and output involving the amygdala, olfactory system, septal nuclei, and sensory association areas
Function	Subserves memory encoding using Papez circuit
	Involved in emotional modulation, but this is not its major function
Clinical Significance	Bilateral hippocampal damage can occur with anoxia or paraneoplastic syndromes. Clinically, patients develop amnestic syndromes

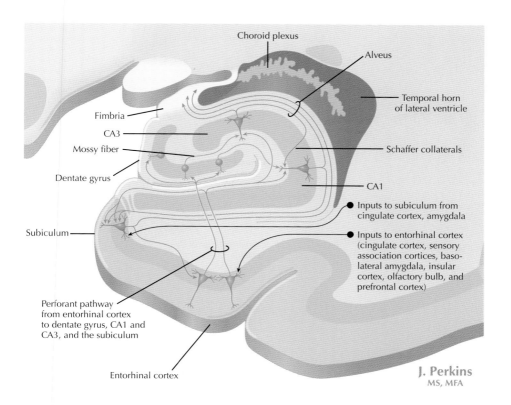

Choroid plexus

Alveus

Fimbria

CA3

Mossy fiber

Dentate gyrus

Temporal horn of lateral ventricle

Schaffer collaterals

CA1

Inputs to subiculum from cingulate cortex, amygdala

Inputs to entorhinal cortex (cingulate cortex, sensory association cortices, baso-lateral amygdala, insular cortex, olfactory bulb, and prefrontal cortex)

Subiculum

Perforant pathway from entorhinal cortex to dentate gyrus, CA1 and CA3, and the subiculum

Entorhinal cortex

J. Perkins
MS, MFA

HIPPOCAMPUS *continued*

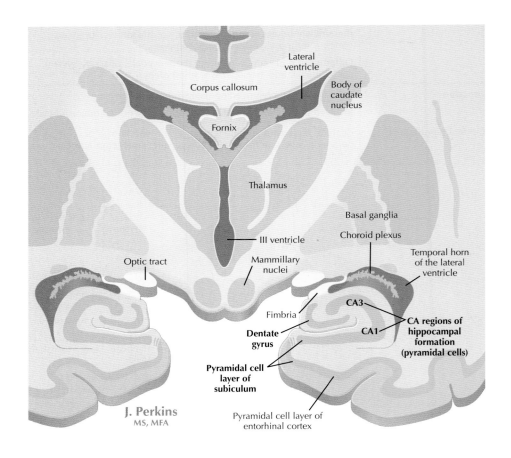

Lateral ventricle

Corpus callosum

Body of caudate nucleus

Fornix

Thalamus

Basal ganglia

Choroid plexus

III ventricle

Temporal horn of the lateral ventricle

Optic tract

Mammillary nuclei

CA3

Fimbria

CA regions of hippocampal formation (pyramidal cells)

Dentate gyrus

CA1

Pyramidal cell layer of subiculum

J. Perkins
MS, MFA

Pyramidal cell layer of entorhinal cortex

MAJOR HIPPOCAMPAL INPUTS AND OUTPUTS

HIPPOCAMPAL INPUTS	HIPPOCAMPAL OUTPUTS
Septal nuclei→fornix→dentate and CA regions (cholinergic input vital for memory and degenerates in Alzheimer's disease)	Subiculum→fornix→mammillary bodies
Multiple cortical areas→entorhinal cortex→ dentate gyrus	CA1/CA3→fornix→septal nuclei, nucleus accumbens, hypothalamus, cingulate cortex, frontal lobes

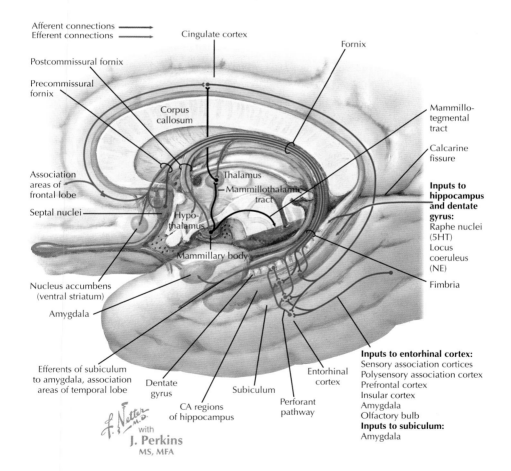

Afferent connections ⟶
Efferent connections ⟶

Cingulate cortex

Fornix

Postcommissural fornix

Precommissural fornix

Corpus callosum

Mammillo-tegmental tract

Calcarine fissure

Association areas of frontal lobe

Thalamus

Mammillothalamic tract

Inputs to hippocampus and dentate gyrus:
Raphe nuclei (5HT)
Locus coeruleus (NE)

Septal nuclei

Hypo-thalamus

Mammillary body

Nucleus accumbens (ventral striatum)

Fimbria

Amygdala

Efferents of subiculum to amygdala, association areas of temporal lobe

Dentate gyrus

CA regions of hippocampus

Subiculum

Perforant pathway

Entorhinal cortex

Inputs to entorhinal cortex:
Sensory association cortices
Polysensory association cortex
Prefrontal cortex
Insular cortex
Amygdala
Olfactory bulb
Inputs to subiculum:
Amygdala

AMYGDALA

Location	Almond-shaped structure located anterior to the hippocampus in the anterior portion of the medial temporal lobe
Architecture	Composed of 3 sets of nuclei: • Basolateral nuclei • Corticomedial nuclei • Central nucleus
Inputs	Major inputs include highly processed sensory stimuli from the temporal lobe, direct olfactory information, and limbic and autonomic information from the orbitofrontal lobe, cingulate gyrus, hypothalamus, and midbrain tegmentum
Outputs	Major outputs include the hypothalamus (via the ventral amygdalofugal pathway), thalamus, striatum, septal nuclei (via stria terminalis), hippocampus, and multiple cortical areas
Function	Regulates the emotional interpretation of environmental and internal stimuli, especially relating to fear and anger
Clinical Significance	Lesions of the amygdala can cause behavioral abnormalities. Bilateral amygdala damage causes emotional blunting, hyperphagia, and hypersexuality, known as Klüver-Bucy syndrome

AMYGDALA *continued*

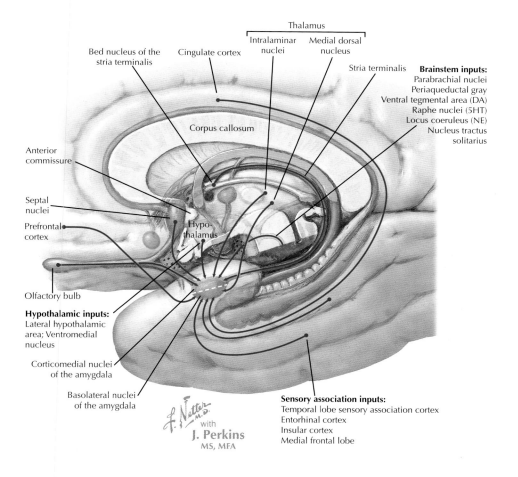

Thalamus
Intralaminar nuclei
Medial dorsal nucleus

Bed nucleus of the stria terminalis
Cingulate cortex
Stria terminalis

Brainstem inputs:
Parabrachial nuclei
Periaqueductal gray
Ventral tegmental area (DA)
Raphe nuclei (5HT)
Locus coeruleus (NE)
Nucleus tractus solitarius

Corpus callosum

Anterior commissure

Septal nuclei

Prefrontal cortex

Hypo-thalamus

Olfactory bulb

Hypothalamic inputs:
Lateral hypothalamic area; Ventromedial nucleus

Corticomedial nuclei of the amygdala

Basolateral nuclei of the amygdala

Sensory association inputs:
Temporal lobe sensory association cortex
Entorhinal cortex
Insular cortex
Medial frontal lobe

with
J. Perkins
MS, MFA

AMYGDALA *continued*

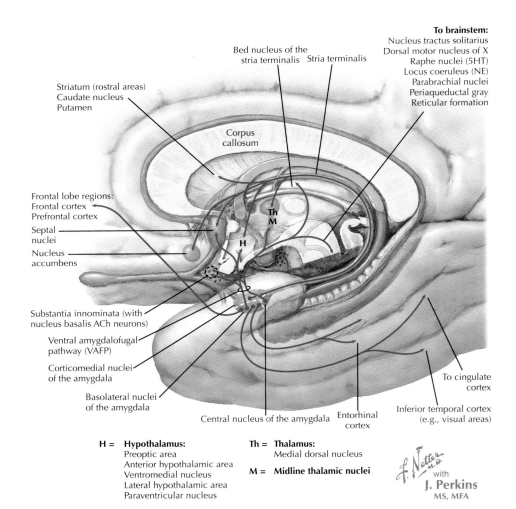

Striatum (rostral areas)
Caudate nucleus
Putamen

Bed nucleus of the
stria terminalis   Stria terminalis

To brainstem:
Nucleus tractus solitarius
Dorsal motor nucleus of X
Raphe nuclei (5HT)
Locus coeruleus (NE)
Parabrachial nuclei
Periaqueductal gray
Reticular formation

Corpus
callosum

Frontal lobe regions:
Frontal cortex
Prefrontal cortex

Septal
nuclei

Nucleus
accumbens

Th
M

H

Substantia innominata (with
nucleus basalis ACh neurons)

Ventral amygdalofugal
pathway (VAFP)

Corticomedial nuclei
of the amygdala

Basolateral nuclei
of the amygdala

Central nucleus of the amygdala   Entorhinal
cortex

To cingulate
cortex

Inferior temporal cortex
(e.g., visual areas)

H = **Hypothalamus:**
Preoptic area
Anterior hypothalamic area
Ventromedial nucleus
Lateral hypothalamic area
Paraventricular nucleus

Th = **Thalamus:**
Medial dorsal nucleus

M = **Midline thalamic nuclei**

with
J. Perkins
MS, MFA

CINGULATE CORTEX

Location	Located above the body of the corpus callosum
Architecture	C-shaped deep cortical structure
Inputs	Major input received from the anterior nucleus of the thalamus as a part of Papez circuit
	Receives input from association cortices, septal nuclei, and subiculum
Outputs	Output to the entorhinal cortex is part of the Papez circuit.
	Outputs to association cortices, septal nuclei, and thalamus
Function	Cortical regulation of basic autonomic functions, including respiration, circulation, and digestion. Also involved in behavior and emotional modulation of pain
Clinical Significance	Lesions can cause indifference to pain and social indifference. May be involved in depression

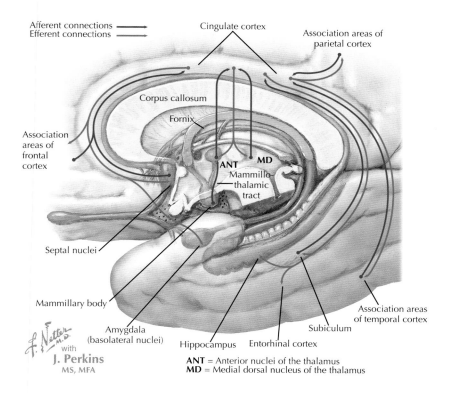

Afferent connections ⟶
Efferent connections ⟶

Cingulate cortex

Association areas of parietal cortex

Corpus callosum

Fornix

Association areas of frontal cortex

ANT   MD

Mammillo-thalamic tract

Septal nuclei

Mammillary body

Amygdala (basolateral nuclei)

Hippocampus   Entorhinal cortex

Subiculum

Association areas of temporal cortex

ANT = Anterior nuclei of the thalamus
MD = Medial dorsal nucleus of the thalamus

with
J. Perkins
MS, MFA

Cranial Nerves I-XII

CRANIAL NERVES: OVERVIEW

- So-called because they emerge from the cranium
- Carry 6 modalities, 3 motor and 3 sensory

ANATOMIC MODALITY	FUNCTIONAL SIGNIFICANCE
Somatic motor nerves	Innervate muscles that develop from somites
Branchial motor nerves	Innervate muscles that develop from branchial arches
Visceral motor nerves	Innervate viscera, including glands and smooth muscles
General sensory nerves	Mediate touch, pain, temperature, pressure, vibration, proprioception
Visceral sensory nerves	Sensory input from viscera
Special sensory nerves	Smell, vision, taste, hearing, balance

CRANIAL NERVES: OVERVIEW *continued*

Cranial Nerves (Motor and Sensory Distribution): Schema

- - - - Spinal nerve fibers
———— Efferent (motor) fibers
———— Afferent (sensory) fibers

I
Olfactory

II
Optic

III
Oculomotor
Ciliary muscle, sphincter of
pupil and all external eye
muscles except those below

Ophthalmic
Maxillary
Mandibular

IV
Trochlear
Superior oblique muscle

V
Trigeminal
Sensory—face
sinuses, teeth

Motor—muscles of
mastication

VI
Abducent
Lateral rectus
muscle

VII
Facial
Muscles of face

Intermediate nerve
Motor—submandibular,
sublingual, lacrimal glands
Taste—anterior 2/3 of
tongue, sensory soft palate

VIII
Vestibulocochlear
Cochlear   Vestibular

IX
Glossopharyngeal
Taste—posterior 1/3 of tongue
Sensory—tonsil, pharynx, middle ear
Motor—stylopharyngeus, upper
pharyngeal muscles, parotid gland

X
Vagus
Motor—heart, lungs, palate, pharynx,
larynx, trachea, bronchi, GI tract
Sensory—heart, lungs, trachea,
bronchi, larynx, pharynx,
GI tract, external ear

XII
Hypoglossal
Tongue
muscles

XI
Accessory
Sternocleidomastoid,
trapezius muscles

Strap
muscles
(C1, 2
fibers)

OLFACTORY NERVE (CN-I)

STRUCTURE	ANATOMIC NOTES	FUNCTIONAL SIGNIFICANCE
Olfactory nerves	Axons traverse the cribriform plate of ethmoid to synapse in the olfactory bulb	Special sensory—smell

Head trauma can shear the olfactory nerves as they traverse cribriform plate, resulting in a loss of sense of smell. More severe head trauma may fracture cribriform plate, again resulting in transection of the olfactory nerves with loss of sense of smell.

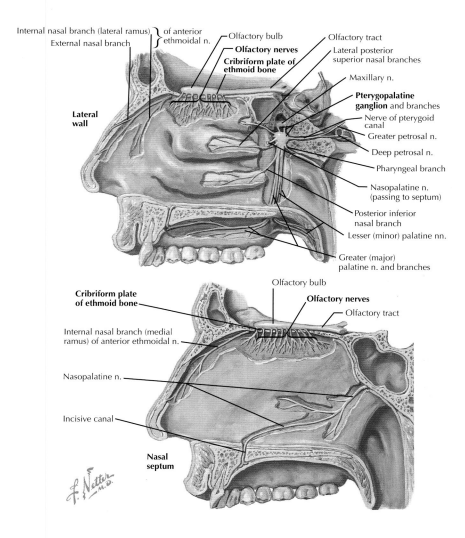

OLFACTORY NERVE (CN-I) *continued*

STRUCTURE	ANATOMIC NOTES	FUNCTIONAL SIGNIFICANCE
Rhinencephalon	"Nose brain"	Central nervous system (CNS) structures involved in olfaction
Olfactory cells	Sensory receptors	Transmit sensation via olfactory nerves to bulb
Olfactory bulb	Lies on the cribriform plate of ethmoid bone, near the rostral extent of the floor of anterior cranial fossa	Contains cell bodies of secondary sensory neurons for relay of olfaction
Mitral cells Tufted cells	Secondary sensory neurons whose axons form olfactory tract	Compression of olfactory tract can cause unilateral loss of smell (anosmia)
Olfactory trigone	Divergence of olfactory tract into medial and lateral stria just rostral to the anterior perforated substance	Prepyriform cortex and periamygdaloid area receive fibers from the lateral olfactory stria and constitute primary olfactory cortex

Meningioma in the floor of the anterior cranial fossa can compress the olfactory bulb or tract and cause unilateral loss of smell *(anosmia).*

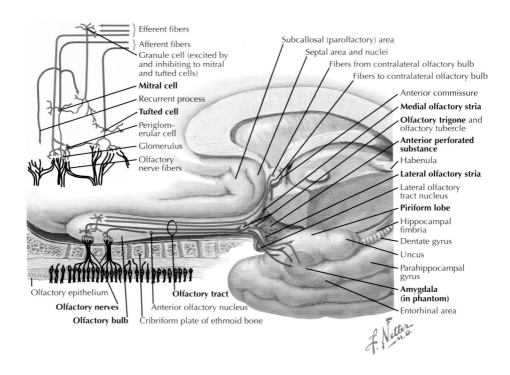

OLFACTORY NERVE (CN-I) *continued*

STRUCTURE	ANATOMIC NOTES	FUNCTIONAL SIGNIFICANCE
Olfactory tract	Most axons of the tract pass via the lateral olfactory stria to the lateral olfactory area: uncus, parahippocampal gyrus, amygdala	Uncus, parahippocampal gyrus, and amygdala are common sites for seizure focus, causing an aura of a sense of smell at onset
Lateral olfactory stria, uncus, and medial parahippocampal gyrus	Comprises the pyriform (pear-shaped) lobe	Olfactory "hallucinations" caused by irritation of the uncus, parahippocampal gyrus, or amygdala; called *uncinate fits* and may precede a generalized convulsion

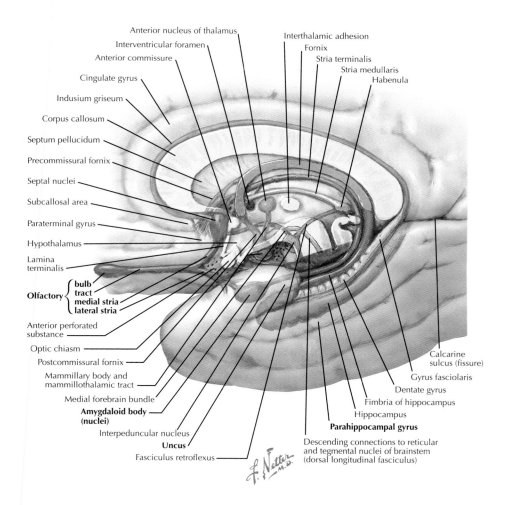

Anterior nucleus of thalamus
Interventricular foramen
Anterior commissure
Cingulate gyrus
Indusium griseum
Corpus callosum
Septum pellucidum
Precommissural fornix
Septal nuclei
Subcallosal area
Paraterminal gyrus
Hypothalamus
Lamina terminalis
Olfactory { bulb / tract / medial stria / lateral stria }
Anterior perforated substance
Optic chiasm
Postcommissural fornix
Mammillary body and mammillothalamic tract
Medial forebrain bundle
Amygdaloid body (nuclei)
Interpeduncular nucleus
Uncus
Fasciculus retroflexus

Interthalamic adhesion
Fornix
Stria terminalis
Stria medullaris
Habenula

Calcarine sulcus (fissure)
Gyrus fasciolaris
Dentate gyrus
Fimbria of hippocampus
Hippocampus
Parahippocampal gyrus
Descending connections to reticular and tegmental nuclei of brainstem (dorsal longitudinal fasciculus)

OPTIC NERVE (CN-II)

OPTIC NERVE (CN-II)		
Structure	**Anatomic notes**	**Functional Significance**
Optic nerve	Enters the cranial fossa through the optic foramen	Special sensory: vision from the contralateral visual field
	Four quadrants of nerve correspond to 4 quadrants of the retina; upper-quadrant retinal fibers remain superior; lower quadrant retinal fibers remain lower; macular fibers are in the center of CN II	Visual-field defects affecting only 1 eye indicate retinal or optic nerve pathology Optic nerve lesion causes central scotoma in the ipsilateral eye (central macular fibers) and contralateral temporal-field defect
Optic chiasm	Nasal retinal fibers cross in the chiasm, upper retinal fibers cross dorsally, lower retinal fibers cross ventrally	Chiasmal lesions, usually compressive, produce bitemporal visual-field defects (nasal retinal fiber involvement)
Optic tract	Superior retinal quadrant fibers occupy medial optic tract, inferior retinal quadrant fibers occupy lateral optic tract	Optic tract lesion produces homonymous hemianopia that is incongruous (not identical in both eyes)
Lateral geniculate body	Origin of geniculocalcarine tract, optic radiations; passes through the retrolenticular portion of the internal capsule to end in the striate cortex (area 17)	Lesions of the lateral geniculate body cause strikingly incongruous visual-field defects
Optic radiations: dorsal fibers	Pass almost directly back to the striate cortex (area 17) on the medial surface of occipital lobes on both banks of the calcarine fissure	Lesion in the retrolenticular portion of the internal capsule can produce motor and sensory impairment, with homonymous hemianopia
Optic radiations: ventral fibers	First turn forward and downward into temporal lobe, spread out over the rostral part of the inferior (temporal) horn of lateral ventricle, then loop backward, running close to the outer wall of the temporal horn of the lateral ventricle to occipital cortex (the Meyer loop)	Stroke or tumor involving the temporal lobe can affect the Meyer loop, resulting in contralateral upper quadrantanopia ("pie in the sky") visual-field deficit
Occipital pole	Macula projects here	Macular sparing, retention of central 5 degrees of visual field, occurs with occipital lobe infarction due to the middle cerebral artery's contribution to this cortical area

- Light from the upper half of the visual field falls on the lower half of the retina and vice versa.
- Light from the temporal half of the visual field falls on the nasal half of the retina and vice versa.

OPTIC NERVE (CN-II) *continued*

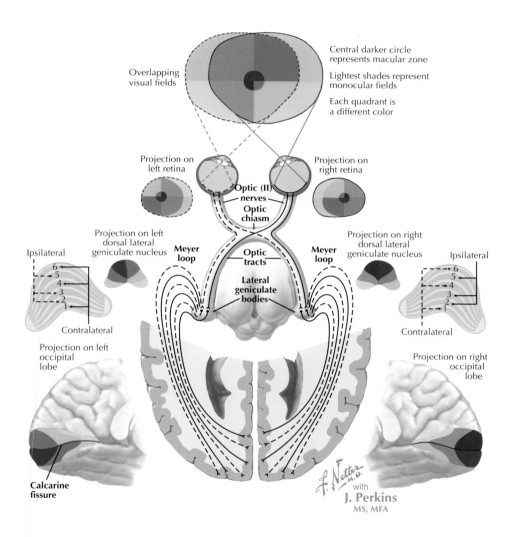

Central darker circle represents macular zone

Lightest shades represent monocular fields

Each quadrant is a different color

Overlapping visual fields

Projection on left retina

Projection on right retina

Optic (II) nerves

Optic chiasm

Projection on left dorsal lateral geniculate nucleus

Meyer loop

Optic tracts

Meyer loop

Projection on right dorsal lateral geniculate nucleus

Ipsilateral

Lateral geniculate bodies

Ipsilateral

Contralateral

Contralateral

Projection on left occipital lobe

Projection on right occipital lobe

Calcarine fissure

with
J. Perkins
MS, MFA

OPTIC TRACT (CN-II)

ANATOMIC NOTES	FUNCTIONAL SIGNIFICANCE
Sweeps out and back, around the hypothalamus and rostral crus cerebri	Pituitary tumor may compress the chiasm, resulting in bitemporal hemianopia
Most fibers terminate in the lateral geniculate body Small portion continue as brachium of the superior colliculus to the superior colliculi	Fibers from the upper retinal quadrants (lower visual field) terminate in the medial lateral geniculate, and those from the lower retinal quadrants (upper visual field) terminate in the lateral part of the lateral geniculate
Medial half of the lateral geniculate project to the superior lip of the calcarine fissure via the superior portion of the optic radiation	Transmits vision from the upper retinal quadrant (lower visual field)
Lateral half of the lateral geniculate project to the inferior lip of the calcarine fissure via the inferior portion of optic radiation (the Meyer loop)	Transmits vision from the lower retinal quadrant (upper visual field)

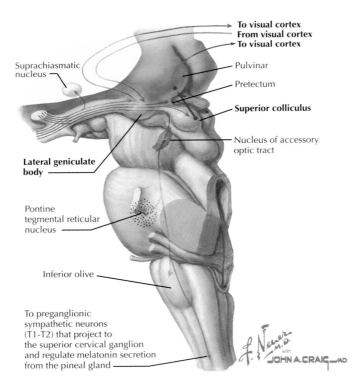

To visual cortex
From visual cortex
To visual cortex

Suprachiasmatic nucleus

Pulvinar

Pretectum

Superior colliculus

Nucleus of accessory optic tract

Lateral geniculate body

Pontine tegmental reticular nucleus

Inferior olive

To preganglionic sympathetic neurons (T1-T2) that project to the superior cervical ganglion and regulate melatonin secretion from the pineal gland

OCULOMOTOR NERVE (CN-III)

STRUCTURE	ANATOMIC NOTES	FUNCTIONAL SIGNIFICANCE
Oculomotor nucleus	Located at the level of superior colliculus	Somatic motor fibers from the oculomotor nucleus combine with parasympathetic fibers from the Edinger-Westphal nucleus to form CN-III.
Oculomotor nerve (CN-III)	Passes anteriorly between the posterior cerebral and superior cerebellar arteries, pierces the dura, and enters cavernous sinus

In sinus, CN-III runs along the lateral wall, superior to the trochlear nerve (CN-IV), enters the orbit through the superior orbital fissure, and splits into superior and inferior divisions | Superior division supplies the superior rectus and levator palpebrae superioris.

Inferior division supplies the inferior and medial recti and inferior oblique. |

Diabetic third-nerve palsy causes unilateral painful diplopia with weakness of the superior, inferior, and medial recti and the inferior oblique, but it spares the pupil because pupillary fibers run along the outer layer of the nerve and diabetes causes ischemia, which is most profound in the inner layers of the nerve. Compression of CN-III by a posterior cerebral artery aneurysm results in dilated pupil and ophthalmoplegia involving the superior, medial, and inferior recti and the inferior oblique. The pupil is affected because the nerve is compressed from the outside, which is where the pupillary fibers run.

OCULOMOTOR NERVE (CN-III) *continued*

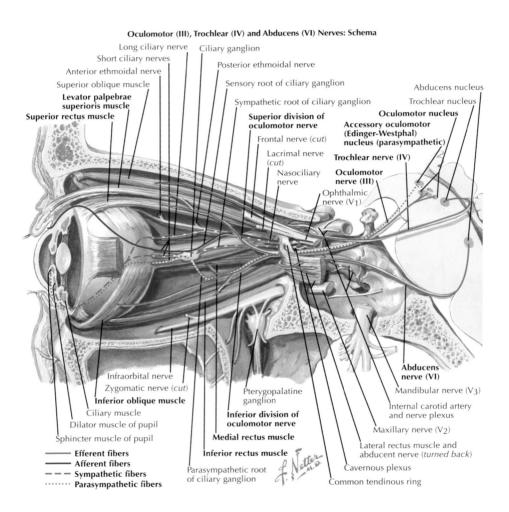

Oculomotor (III), Trochlear (IV) and Abducens (VI) Nerves: Schema

Long ciliary nerve
Short ciliary nerves
Anterior ethmoidal nerve
Superior oblique muscle
Levator palpebrae superioris muscle
Superior rectus muscle
Ciliary ganglion
Posterior ethmoidal nerve
Sensory root of ciliary ganglion
Sympathetic root of ciliary ganglion
Superior division of oculomotor nerve
Frontal nerve (*cut*)
Lacrimal nerve (*cut*)
Nasociliary nerve
Ophthalmic nerve (V₁)
Abducens nucleus
Trochlear nucleus
Oculomotor nucleus
Accessory oculomotor (Edinger-Westphal) nucleus (parasympathetic)
Trochlear nerve (IV)
Oculomotor nerve (III)

Infraorbital nerve
Zygomatic nerve (*cut*)
Inferior oblique muscle
Ciliary muscle
Dilator muscle of pupil
Sphincter muscle of pupil
Pterygopalatine ganglion
Inferior division of oculomotor nerve
Medial rectus muscle
Inferior rectus muscle
Parasympathetic root of ciliary ganglion
Abducens nerve (VI)
Mandibular nerve (V₃)
Internal carotid artery and nerve plexus
Maxillary nerve (V₂)
Lateral rectus muscle and abducent nerve (*turned back*)
Cavernous plexus
Common tendinous ring

Efferent fibers
Afferent fibers
Sympathetic fibers
Parasympathetic fibers

OCULOMOTOR NERVE (CN-III): PARASYMPATHETIC COMPONENT

STRUCTURE	ANATOMIC NOTES	FUNCTIONAL SIGNIFICANCE
Edinger-Westphal nucleus	Dorsal to oculomotor complex Innervates sphincter of pupil and ciliary muscles via ciliary ganglion Fibers run with CN-III to enter the orbit. There they leave the nerve and terminate in the ciliary ganglion near the apex of the cone of extraocular muscles	Visceral motor
Postganglionic axons	Leave ciliary ganglion as 6-10 short ciliary nerves and enter the eye along with sympathetic fibers In eyeball, fibers run forward between the choroid and sclera to terminate in sphincter muscle of the pupil (iris)	Iris sphincter muscle encircles the pupil and pulls toward the center, causing the pupil to constrict Ciliary muscles cause a change in the shape of the lens for additional refraction on near gaze

OCULOMOTOR NERVE (CN-III): PARASYMPATHETIC COMPONENT *continued*

Ciliary Ganglion: Schema

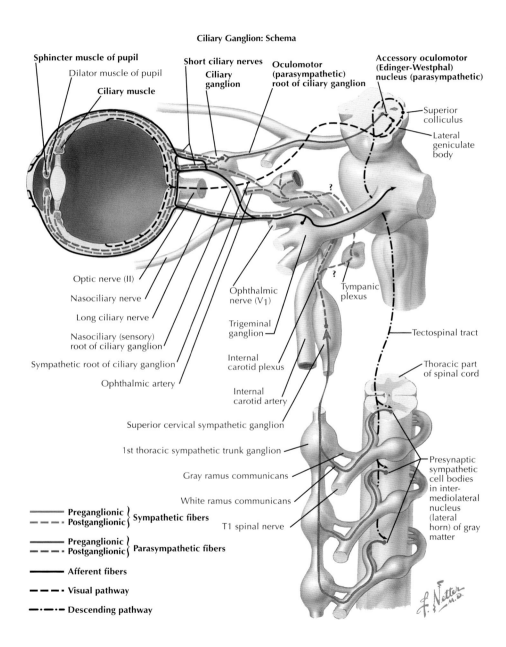

Sphincter muscle of pupil

Dilator muscle of pupil

Ciliary muscle

Short ciliary nerves

Ciliary ganglion

Oculomotor (parasympathetic) root of ciliary ganglion

Accessory oculomotor (Edinger-Westphal) nucleus (parasympathetic)

Superior colliculus

Lateral geniculate body

Optic nerve (II)

Nasociliary nerve

Long ciliary nerve

Nasociliary (sensory) root of ciliary ganglion

Sympathetic root of ciliary ganglion

Ophthalmic artery

Ophthalmic nerve (V₁)

Trigeminal ganglion

Internal carotid plexus

Internal carotid artery

Tympanic plexus

Tectospinal tract

Thoracic part of spinal cord

Superior cervical sympathetic ganglion

1st thoracic sympathetic trunk ganglion

Gray ramus communicans

White ramus communicans

T1 spinal nerve

Presynaptic sympathetic cell bodies in inter-mediolateral nucleus (lateral horn) of gray matter

——— Preganglionic ⎫
- - - - Postganglionic ⎬ Sympathetic fibers

——— Preganglionic ⎫
- - - - Postganglionic ⎬ Parasympathetic fibers

——— Afferent fibers

- - - - Visual pathway

—·—·— Descending pathway

TROCHLEAR NERVE (CN-IV)

STRUCTURE	ANATOMIC NOTES	FUNCTIONAL SIGNIFICANCE
Trochlear nucleus	In midbrain tegmentum, at the level of the inferior colliculus, ventral to the aqueduct	Somatic motor
Trochlear nerve	Axons leave the trochlear nucleus in the caudal midbrain Course dorsally and caudally around the aqueduct Decussate in the superior medullary velum Exit brainstem dorsally, caudal to the inferior colliculus Cross to the opposite side (the left trochlear nucleus gives rise to the right trochlear nerve and vice versa) Curve around the cerebral peduncle (crus) Pass between posterior cerebral and superior cerebellar arteries with CN-III Pierce the dura and enter the cavernous sinus with CN-III, -V_1, and -VI Run along the lateral wall, inferior to CN-III Continues through the superior orbital fissure, close to the roof of the orbit, to the superior oblique	Supplies the superior oblique Susceptible to injury following head trauma, resulting in vertical diplopia with head tilt to the opposite side to correct superior oblique weakness

See pages 223–4 for Oculomotor and Abducens Nerves: Schema.

TROCHLEAR NERVE (CN-IV) *continued*

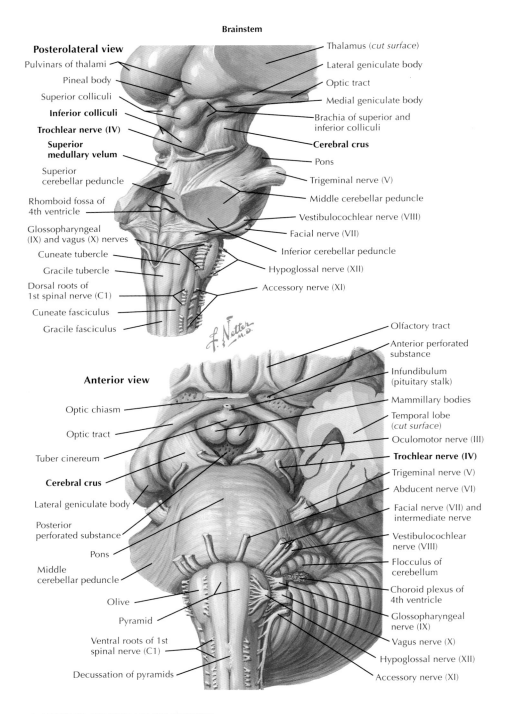

Brainstem

Posterolateral view
- Pulvinars of thalami
- Pineal body
- Superior colliculi
- **Inferior colliculi**
- **Trochlear nerve (IV)**
- **Superior medullary velum**
- Superior cerebellar peduncle
- Rhomboid fossa of 4th ventricle
- Glossopharyngeal (IX) and vagus (X) nerves
- Cuneate tubercle
- Gracile tubercle
- Dorsal roots of 1st spinal nerve (C1)
- Cuneate fasciculus
- Gracile fasciculus

- Thalamus (*cut surface*)
- Lateral geniculate body
- Optic tract
- Medial geniculate body
- Brachia of superior and inferior colliculi
- **Cerebral crus**
- Pons
- Trigeminal nerve (V)
- Middle cerebellar peduncle
- Vestibulocochlear nerve (VIII)
- Facial nerve (VII)
- Inferior cerebellar peduncle
- Hypoglossal nerve (XII)
- Accessory nerve (XI)

Anterior view
- Optic chiasm
- Optic tract
- Tuber cinereum
- **Cerebral crus**
- Lateral geniculate body
- Posterior perforated substance
- Pons
- Middle cerebellar peduncle
- Olive
- Pyramid
- Ventral roots of 1st spinal nerve (C1)
- Decussation of pyramids

- Olfactory tract
- Anterior perforated substance
- Infundibulum (pituitary stalk)
- Mammillary bodies
- Temporal lobe (*cut surface*)
- Oculomotor nerve (III)
- **Trochlear nerve (IV)**
- Trigeminal nerve (V)
- Abducent nerve (VI)
- Facial nerve (VII) and intermediate nerve
- Vestibulocochlear nerve (VIII)
- Flocculus of cerebellum
- Choroid plexus of 4th ventricle
- Glossopharyngeal nerve (IX)
- Vagus nerve (X)
- Hypoglossal nerve (XII)
- Accessory nerve (XI)

TROCHLEAR NERVE (CN-IV) *continued*

ANATOMIC NOTES	FUNCTIONAL SIGNIFICANCE
So-called because of the "trochlea" (pulley) through which the superior oblique muscle passes to reach the eyeball insertion site	Causes inward rotation (intortion) and downward and lateral movement of eye
Smallest nerve, 2400 axons, versus 1 million in the optic nerve Only cranial nerve to exit the dorsal brainstem Only nerve in which all lower motor axons decussate Nerve with longest intracranial course is 7.5 cm	In addition to vertical diplopia, when patient looks down, injury to the trochlear nerve results in a head tilt to the unaffected side as patients correct their (extorted) affected eye by intorting their good eye toward the affected side

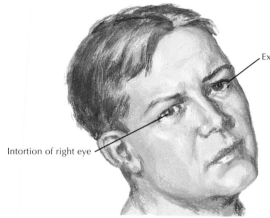

Extortion of left eye

Intortion of right eye

There is a left trochlear palsy, causing left eye extorsion, "clockwise" rotation as you look at the patient, and a rotational misalignment of the eyes causing diplopia. To compensate, the head tilts to the unaffected right side. This intorts the right eye resulting in rotational realignment of the (both) eyes.

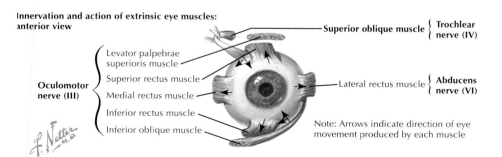

Innervation and action of extrinsic eye muscles: anterior view

Levator palpebrae superioris muscle

Oculomotor nerve (III)
Superior rectus muscle
Medial rectus muscle
Inferior rectus muscle
Inferior oblique muscle

Superior oblique muscle { **Trochlear nerve (IV)**

Lateral rectus muscle { **Abducens nerve (VI)**

Note: Arrows indicate direction of eye movement produced by each muscle

TROCHLEAR NERVE (CN-IV) *continued*

Right lateral view

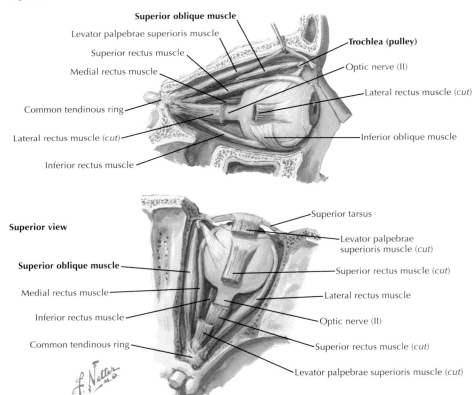

Superior oblique muscle

Levator palpebrae superioris muscle

Superior rectus muscle

Medial rectus muscle

Common tendinous ring

Lateral rectus muscle (*cut*)

Inferior rectus muscle

Trochlea (pulley)

Optic nerve (II)

Lateral rectus muscle (*cut*)

Inferior oblique muscle

Superior view

Superior oblique muscle

Medial rectus muscle

Inferior rectus muscle

Common tendinous ring

Superior tarsus

Levator palpebrae superioris muscle (*cut*)

Superior rectus muscle (*cut*)

Lateral rectus muscle

Optic nerve (II)

Superior rectus muscle (*cut*)

Levator palpebrae superioris muscle (*cut*)

TRIGEMINAL NERVE (CN-V)

STRUCTURE	ANATOMIC NOTES	FUNCTIONAL SIGNIFICANCE
Trigeminal nerve	Emerges from the midlateral pons as a large sensory root and a smaller motor root	Branchial motor to muscles of mastication, tensor tympani and palatini, mylohyoid, and anterior belly of digastric
Trigeminal sensory ganglion	Sits in a depression (Meckel's cave) in the floor of the middle cranial fossa	General sensory to the face, anterior scalp to the vertex of the skull, conjunctiva, globe of eye, mucous membranes of the paranasal, nasal, and oral cavities, anterior $^2/_3$ of the tongue, part of the external tympanic membrane, meninges of the anterior and middle cranial fossa
Trigeminal nerve	3 divisions exit the cranial fossa: • V_1 (ophthalmic division) through superior orbital fissure • V_2 (maxillary division) through foramen rotundum • V_3 (mandibular division) through foramen ovale	V_1 and V_2 run through the cavernous sinus before exiting the cranial fossa Motor root travels with V_3

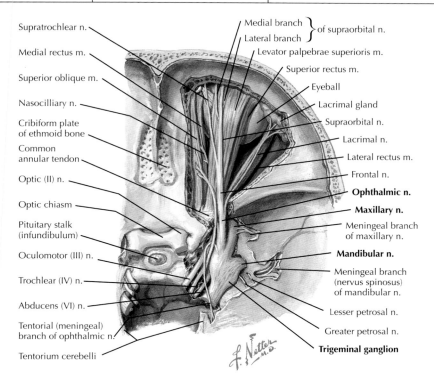

Supratrochlear n.

Medial branch ⎱ of supraorbital n.
Lateral branch ⎰

Medial rectus m.

Levator palpebrae superioris m.

Superior rectus m.

Superior oblique m.

Eyeball

Nasocilliary n.

Lacrimal gland

Cribiform plate of ethmoid bone

Supraorbital n.

Common annular tendon

Lacrimal n.

Optic (II) n.

Lateral rectus m.

Frontal n.

Optic chiasm

Ophthalmic n.

Pituitary stalk (infundibulum)

Maxillary n.

Meningeal branch of maxillary n.

Oculomotor (III) n.

Mandibular n.

Trochlear (IV) n.

Meningeal branch (nervus spinosus) of mandibular n.

Abducens (VI) n.

Lesser petrosal n.

Tentorial (meningeal) branch of ophthalmic n.

Greater petrosal n.

Tentorium cerebelli

Trigeminal ganglion

TRIGEMINAL NERVE NUCLEI

STRUCTURE	ANATOMIC NOTES	FUNCTIONAL SIGNIFICANCE
Motor (masticator) nucleus	Midpons, medial to the main sensory nucleus Input from corticobulbar fibers, reticular neurons, and collaterals from the mesencephalic root and other trigeminal afferents	Controls muscles of chewing, swallowing, and hearing
Sensory nucleus	Extends from midbrain to the spinal cord C2, largest grouping of cranial nerve nuclei, consisting of mesencephalic, principal sensory, and spinotrigeminal nuclei	Lesion involving this nucleus anywhere along its course (multiple sclerosis, stroke, tumor) impairs facial sensation
Mesencephalic nucleus	Column of primary sensory neurons Only primary sensory neurons in humans that reside within the central nervous system (CNS)	Carries proprioception from muscles of mastication and facial expression, for control of bite and facial movements
Principal sensory trigeminal nucleus	In pons near the entry point of the nerve	Carries fine touch, pressure, and vibration sensations from the face
Spinotrigeminal nucleus	Long cell column extending from the caudal pons to the upper cervical spinal cord, where it merges with the substantia gelatinosa of the dorsal gray matter	Carries pain and temperature mainly, also crude touch

TRIGEMINAL NERVE NUCLEI *continued*

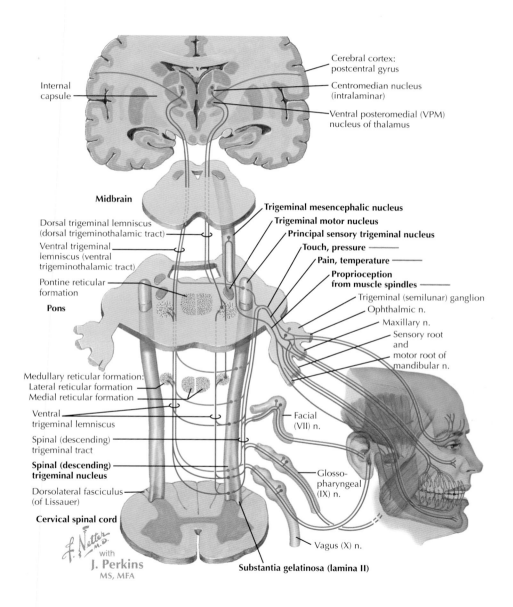

Cerebral cortex:
postcentral gyrus

Centromedian nucleus
(intralaminar)

Ventral posteromedial (VPM)
nucleus of thalamus

Internal
capsule

Midbrain

Trigeminal mesencephalic nucleus
Trigeminal motor nucleus
Principal sensory trigeminal nucleus
Touch, pressure
Pain, temperature
Proprioception
from muscle spindles

Dorsal trigeminal lemniscus
(dorsal trigeminothalamic tract)
Ventral trigeminal
lemniscus (ventral
trigeminothalamic tract)
Pontine reticular
formation

Trigeminal (semilunar) ganglion
Ophthalmic n.
Maxillary n.
Sensory root
and
motor root of
mandibular n.

Pons

Medullary reticular formation:
Lateral reticular formation
Medial reticular formation
Ventral
trigeminal lemniscus
Spinal (descending)
trigeminal tract
Spinal (descending)
trigeminal nucleus
Dorsolateral fasciculus
(of Lissauer)

Facial
(VII) n.

Glosso-
pharyngeal
(IX) n.

Cervical spinal cord

f. Netter
M.D.
with
J. Perkins
MS, MFA

Vagus (X) n.

Substantia gelatinosa (lamina II)

TRIGEMINAL NERVE MOTOR AND SENSORY BRANCHES

STRUCTURE	ANATOMIC NOTES	FUNCTIONAL SIGNIFICANCE
Efferent motor fibers	Exit the pons medial to sensory root to join sensory V_3 branches outside the cranium to form mandibular nerve	Mediates chewing, swallowing, and reflexive control of hearing
V_1 (ophthalmic division)	Exits through the superior orbital fissure	Mediates sensation from conjunctiva, cornea, orbit, dorsal aspect of the nose, upper eyelid, forehead to the vertex of skull, ethmoid, and frontal sinuses; proprioception from the extraocular and facial muscles of the eyelid and forehead
V_2 (maxillary division)	Exits through the foramen rotundum	Mediates sensation from maxilla and overlying skin, including the upper lip, side of nose, medial cheek, nasal cavity, palate, nasopharynx, and meninges of the anterior and middle cranial fossa
V_3 (mandibular division)	Exits through the foramen ovale	Mediates sensation from the buccal region, including the mucous membrane of the mouth, gums, the side of the head, scalp, entire lower jaw including teeth, gums, anterior $2/3$ of the tongue, chin, lower lip, and meninges of the anterior and middle cranial fossa

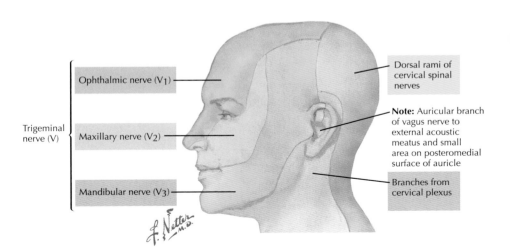

Ophthalmic nerve (V1)

Trigeminal nerve (V)

Maxillary nerve (V2)

Mandibular nerve (V3)

Dorsal rami of cervical spinal nerves

Note: Auricular branch of vagus nerve to external acoustic meatus and small area on posteromedial surface of auricle

Branches from cervical plexus

TRIGEMINAL NERVE MOTOR AND SENSORY BRANCHES *continued*

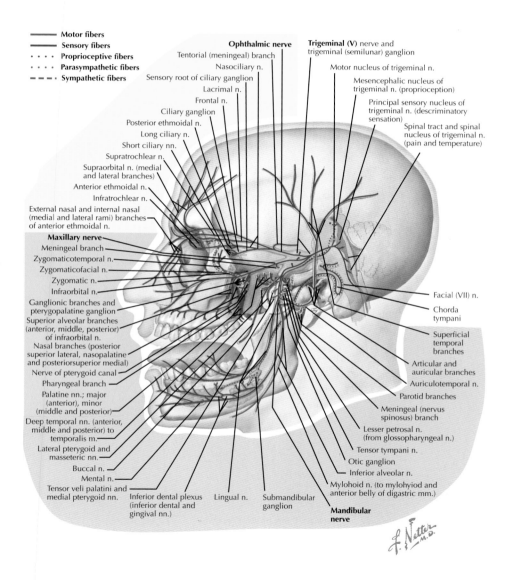

Motor fibers
Sensory fibers
• • • • Proprioceptive fibers
• • • • Parasympathetic fibers
– – – • Sympathetic fibers

Ophthalmic nerve
Tentorial (meningeal) branch
Nasociliary n.
Sensory root of ciliary ganglion
Lacrimal n.
Frontal n.
Ciliary ganglion
Posterior ethmoidal n.
Long ciliary n.
Short ciliary nn.
Supratrochlear n.
Supraorbital n. (medial and lateral branches)
Anterior ethmoidal n.
Infratrochlear n.
External nasal and internal nasal (medial and lateral rami) branches of anterior ethmoidal n.
Maxillary nerve
Meningeal branch
Zygomaticotemporal n.
Zygomaticofacial n.
Zygomatic n.
Infraorbital n.
Ganglionic branches and pterygopalatine ganglion
Superior alveolar branches (anterior, middle, posterior) of infraorbital n.
Nasal branches (posterior superior lateral, nasopalatine and posteriorsuperior medial)
Nerve of pterygoid canal
Pharyngeal branch
Palatine nn.; major (anterior), minor (middle and posterior)
Deep temporal nn. (anterior, middle and posterior) to temporalis m.
Lateral pterygoid and masseteric nn.
Buccal n.
Mental n.
Tensor veli palatini and medial pterygoid nn.
Inferior dental plexus (inferior dental and gingival nn.)
Lingual n.
Submandibular ganglion

Trigeminal (V) nerve and trigeminal (semilunar) ganglion
Motor nucleus of trigeminal n.
Mesencephalic nucleus of trigeminal n. (proprioception)
Principal sensory nucleus of trigeminal n. (descriminatory sensation)
Spinal tract and spinal nucleus of trigeminal n. (pain and temperature)

Facial (VII) n.
Chorda tympani
Superficial temporal branches
Articular and auricular branches
Auriculotemporal n.
Parotid branches
Meningeal (nervus spinosus) branch
Lesser petrosal n. (from glossopharyngeal n.)
Tensor tympani n.
Otic ganglion
Inferior alveolar n.
Mylohoid n. (to mylohyoid and anterior belly of digastric mm.)
Mandibular nerve

TRIGEMINAL NERVE MOTOR AND SENSORY BRANCHES *continued*

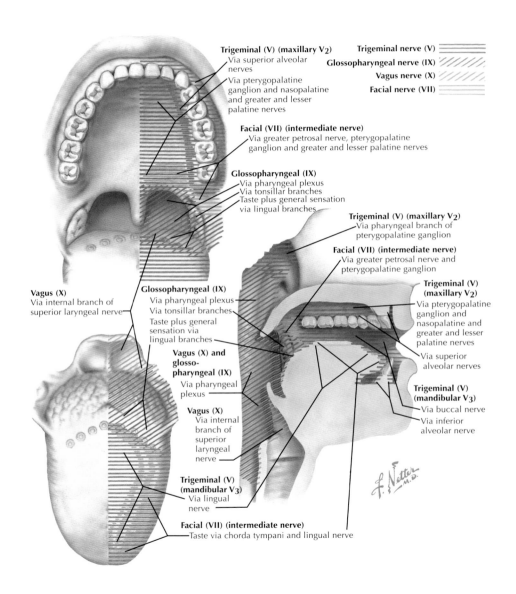

Trigeminal (V) (maxillary V2)
Via superior alveolar nerves
Via pterygopalatine ganglion and nasopalatine and greater and lesser palatine nerves

Trigeminal nerve (V)
Glossopharyngeal nerve (IX)
Vagus nerve (X)
Facial nerve (VII)

Facial (VII) (intermediate nerve)
Via greater petrosal nerve, pterygopalatine ganglion and greater and lesser palatine nerves

Glossopharyngeal (IX)
Via pharyngeal plexus
Via tonsillar branches
Taste plus general sensation via lingual branches

Trigeminal (V) (maxillary V2)
Via pharyngeal branch of pterygopalatine ganglion

Facial (VII) (intermediate nerve)
Via greater petrosal nerve and pterygopalatine ganglion

Trigeminal (V) (maxillary V2)
Via pterygopalatine ganglion and nasopalatine and greater and lesser palatine nerves
Via superior alveolar nerves

Vagus (X)
Via internal branch of superior laryngeal nerve

Glossopharyngeal (IX)
Via pharyngeal plexus
Via tonsillar branches
Taste plus general sensation via lingual branches

Vagus (X) and glosso-pharyngeal (IX)
Via pharyngeal plexus

Vagus (X)
Via internal branch of superior laryngeal nerve

Trigeminal (V) (mandibular V3)
Via lingual nerve

Trigeminal (V) (mandibular V3)
Via buccal nerve
Via inferior alveolar nerve

Facial (VII) (intermediate nerve)
Taste via chorda tympani and lingual nerve

TRIGEMINAL NEURALGIA (TIC DOULOUREUX)

- Stabbing pain in distribution of V_1 or V_2, rarely V_3
- Lasts seconds or a minute or two but so intense that the patient winces, hence called *tic*
- Paroxysms recur frequently, day or night, for weeks at a time
- No sensory or motor loss present on examination
- Aberrant vascular course of superior cerebellar artery, crossing the trigeminal branch, often cited as cause
- Most often, no lesion is identified, and etiology is labeled idiopathic

Trigeminal Neuralgia

Sensory distribution of trigeminal (V) nerve

Trigeminal (semilunar) ganglion
Ophthalmic n.
Frontal n.
Nasociliary n.
Lacrimal n.
Supraorbital nn.
Ant. and post. ethmoidal nn.
Int. nasal nn.
Ext. nasal n.
Maxillary n.
Zygomatico- temporal n.
Zygomaticofacial n.
Infraorbital n.
Sup. alveolar nn.
Sup. dental and gingival branches
Postnasal nn.
Palatine nn.
Pharyngeal branch

Mandibular n.
Auriculotemporal n.
Buccal n.
Lingual n.
Inf. alveolar n.
Inf. dental and gingival branches
Mental n.

Ophthalmic n. zone

Maxillary n. zone

Zones of skin innervation of trigeminal nerve divisions, where pain may occur in trigeminal neuralgia

Common trigger points

Mandibular n. zone

ABDUCENS NERVE (CN-VI)

STRUCTURE	ANATOMIC NOTES	FUNCTIONAL SIGNIFICANCE
Abducens nucleus	Located in the pontine tegmentum close to midline, just ventral to 4th ventricle	Somatic motor to lateral rectus Mediates eye abduction
Abducens nerve	Axons leave the nucleus, course ventrally through the tegmentum to exit at the junction of pons and medulla, near the midline In subarachnoid space of posterior fossa, runs anterolaterally, pierces the dura lateral to the dorsum sella, enters the cavernous sinus, lateral to carotid artery, medial to CN-III, -IV, -V₁, and -VI, continues through the medial portion of the superior orbital fissure, to the lateral rectus	With cavernous sinus thrombosis, headache, ptosis, ocular palsy, eye pain, and sensory loss over the forehead occur due to involvement of these nerves

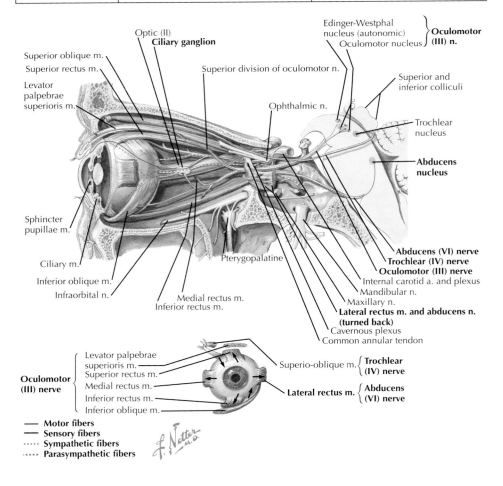

Optic (II)
Ciliary ganglion
Superior oblique m.
Superior rectus m.
Levator palpebrae superioris m.
Superior division of oculomotor n.
Ophthalmic n.
Edinger-Westphal nucleus (autonomic)
Oculomotor nucleus
Oculomotor (III) n.
Superior and inferior colliculi
Trochlear nucleus
Abducens nucleus
Sphincter pupillae m.
Ciliary m.
Inferior oblique m.
Infraorbital n.
Medial rectus m.
Inferior rectus m.
Pterygopalatine
Abducens (VI) nerve
Trochlear (IV) nerve
Oculomotor (III) nerve
Internal carotid a. and plexus
Mandibular n.
Maxillary n.
Lateral rectus m. and abducens n. (turned back)
Cavernous plexus
Common annular tendon

Oculomotor (III) nerve
Levator palpebrae superioris m.
Superior rectus m.
Medial rectus m.
Inferior rectus m.
Inferior oblique m.
Superio-oblique m. { Trochlear (IV) nerve
Lateral rectus m. { Abducens (VI) nerve

— Motor fibers
— Sensory fibers
····· Sympathetic fibers
····· Parasympathetic fibers

CONTROL OF EYE MOVEMENTS

STRUCTURE	ANATOMIC NOTES	FUNCTIONAL SIGNIFICANCE
Paramedian pontine reticular formation (PPRF)	Input: • Vestibular nuclei • Superior colliculus • Frontal eye fields • Interstitial nucleus of Cajal	Horizontal gaze center Because stimulation of the frontal eye field causes eye deviation to the opposite side by stimulating the contralateral PPRF, stroke involving frontal eye field results in conjugate eye deviation to same side of the lesion due to inability to look to opposite side
PPRF	Supplies: • Ipsilateral CN-VI to the lateral rectus • Contralateral CN-III via CN-VI nuclear interneurons and/or PPRF to the medial rectus, through the medial longitudinal fasciculus	Unilateral pontine stroke involving PPRF results in inability to move eyes ipsilaterally, to side of lesion Transiently, the eyes may be contralaterally deviated due to uninhibited action of the contralateral PPRF moving eyes to that side. Nystagmus occurs when the patient looks to intact field of movement, with quick phase directed toward that side
Interstitial nucleus of Cajal	Projects axons to spinal cord and contralateral interstitial nucleus of Cajal	Axial muscle control and coordinates vertical and oblique eye movements

CONTROL OF EYE MOVEMENTS *continued*

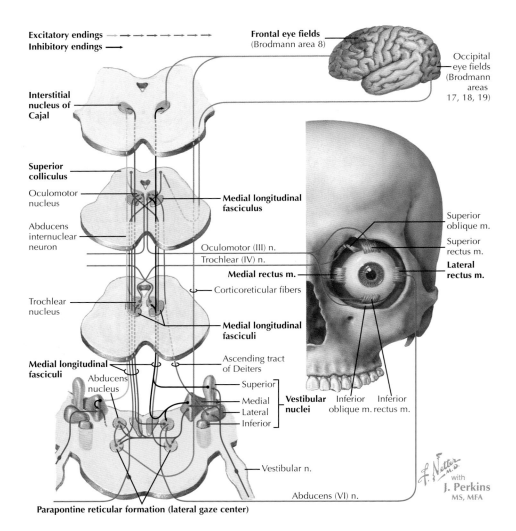

Excitatory endings
Inhibitory endings

Frontal eye fields
(Brodmann area 8)

Occipital
eye fields
(Brodmann
areas
17, 18, 19)

Interstitial
nucleus of
Cajal

Superior
colliculus

Oculomotor
nucleus

Medial longitudinal
fasciculus

Superior
oblique m.

Abducens
internuclear
neuron

Superior
rectus m.

Lateral
rectus m.

Oculomotor (III) n.
Trochlear (IV) n.

Medial rectus m.

Corticoreticular fibers

Trochlear
nucleus

Medial longitudinal
fasciculi

Medial longitudinal
fasciculi

Ascending tract
of Deiters

Abducens
nucleus

Superior

Medial

Lateral

Inferior

Vestibular
nuclei

Inferior
oblique m.

Inferior
rectus m.

Vestibular n.

Abducens (VI) n.

Parapontine reticular formation (lateral gaze center)

with
J. Perkins
MS, MFA

FACIAL NERVE (CN-VII)

STRUCTURE	ANATOMIC NOTES	FUNCTIONAL SIGNIFICANCE
Facial nerve	Emerges at the pontomedullary junction and enters the internal auditory meatus	Bell's palsy: acute facial muscle paralysis due to herpes simplex virus I infection of CN-VII
Branchial motor fibers	Emerge at the stylomastoid foramen, pass through the parotid gland	Innervates stapedius, stylohyoid, posterior digastric, and facial muscles
Visceral motor fibers	In petrous bone: preganglionic parasympathetic axons in the greater petrosal nerve, which branch off to pterygopalatine ganglion	Innervates lacrimal, submandibular, and sublingual glands and mucous membranes of the nose and palate
General sensory fibers	Accompany those of the auricular branch of vagus CN-X	Supply skin of the concha of the auricle and a small area behind the ear
Special sensory	As CN-VII courses through the petrous portion of the temporal bone, it displays a swelling, the geniculate ganglion (nerve cell bodies of taste fibers of tongue)	Taste from anterior $\frac{2}{3}$ of the tongue and the hard and soft palate (enter through chorda tympani), carrying taste from (and parasympathetic motor to) the tongue
Corticobulbar fibers	Project bilaterally to the portion of the facial nucleus that innervates forehead muscles but, to remaining (lower) facial muscles, projects only contralaterally	Lesion of cortical fibers thus causes contralateral weakness of facial muscles but spares the forehead; so-called upper motor neuron CN-VII or central CN-VII weakness

FACIAL NERVE (CN-VII) *continued*

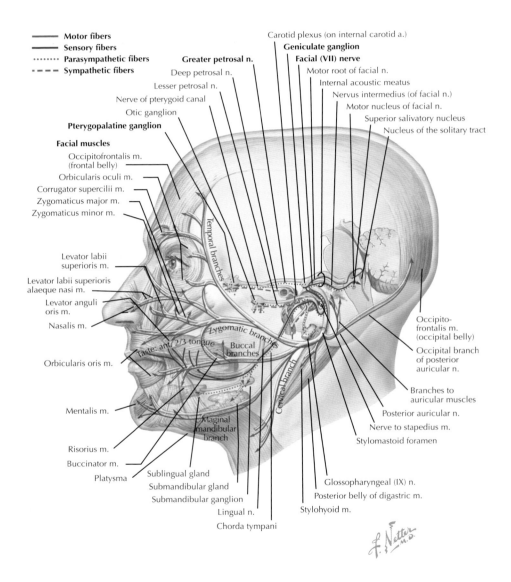

Motor fibers
Sensory fibers
Parasympathetic fibers
Sympathetic fibers

Carotid plexus (on internal carotid a.)
Geniculate ganglion
Facial (VII) nerve
Motor root of facial n.
Internal acoustic meatus
Nervus intermedius (of facial n.)
Motor nucleus of facial n.
Superior salivatory nucleus
Nucleus of the solitary tract

Greater petrosal n.
Deep petrosal n.
Lesser petrosal n.
Nerve of pterygoid canal
Otic ganglion
Pterygopalatine ganglion

Facial muscles
Occipitofrontalis m. (frontal belly)
Orbicularis oculi m.
Corrugator supercilii m.
Zygomaticus major m.
Zygomaticus minor m.

Levator labii superioris m.
Levator labii superioris alaeque nasi m.
Levator anguli oris m.
Nasalis m.

Orbicularis oris m.

Mentalis m.

Risorius m.
Buccinator m.
Platysma

Sublingual gland
Submandibular gland
Submandibular ganglion
Lingual n.
Chorda tympani

Temporal branches
Zygomatic branches
Taste: ant. 2/3 tongue
Buccal branches
Cervical branch
Maginal mandibular branch

Occipitofrontalis m. (occipital belly)
Occipital branch of posterior auricular n.
Branches to auricular muscles
Posterior auricular n.
Nerve to stapedius m.
Stylomastoid foramen

Glossopharyngeal (IX) n.
Posterior belly of digastric m.
Stylohyoid m.

FACIAL NERVE CRANIAL NERVE VII

STRUCTURE	ANATOMIC NOTES	FUNCTIONAL SIGNIFICANCE
Visceral motor	Cell bodies (preganglionic autonomic motor neurons) are scattered in the pontine tegmentum, called the superior salivatory nucleus, influenced by the hypothalamus	Parasympathetic to lacrimal, submandibular, and sublingual glands and the mucous membranes of the nose and palate
Superior salivatory nucleus (SSN)	Impulses from the limbic system enter the hypothalamus and are relayed via the dorsal longitudinal fasciculus to the SSN	Efferents from the SSN travel in the nervus intermedius and divide in the facial canal into the greater petrosal (to lacrimal and nasal glands) and chorda tympani (submandibular and sublingual glands)
Greater petrosal nerve	Exits the petrous bone via greater petrosal foramen to reach the foramen lacerum to reach the pterygoid canal to join deep petrosal nerve to become the nerve of the pterygoid canal, which opens into the pterygopalatine fossa from which the pterygopalatine ganglion is suspended from V_2	Preganglionic parasympathetic axons in the nerve of pterygoid canal synapse in pterygopalatine ganglion; postganglionic fibers go via V_2 branches to lacrimal and mucous glands
Chorda tympani	Joins the lingual branch of V_3 after V_3 passes through the foramen ovale Travels to the lateral floor of the mouth	Contains efferent preganglionic parasympathetic (secretomotor) fibers to the submandibular ganglion; relayed as postganglionic fibers to the submandibular and sublingual glands. Most fibers carry taste (see below)

FACIAL NERVE CRANIAL NERVE VII *continued*

Autonomic Innervation of Nasal Cavity

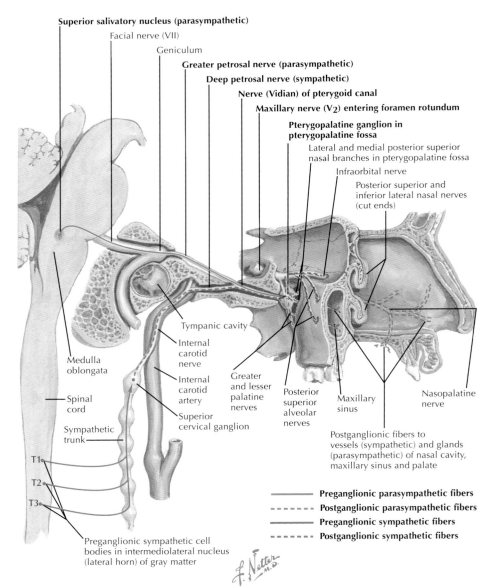

Superior salivatory nucleus (parasympathetic)

Facial nerve (VII)

Geniculum

Greater petrosal nerve (parasympathetic)

Deep petrosal nerve (sympathetic)

Nerve (Vidian) of pterygoid canal

Maxillary nerve (V₂) entering foramen rotundum

Pterygopalatine ganglion in pterygopalatine fossa

Lateral and medial posterior superior nasal branches in pterygopalatine fossa

Infraorbital nerve

Posterior superior and inferior lateral nasal nerves (cut ends)

Tympanic cavity

Internal carotid nerve

Medulla oblongata

Internal carotid artery

Greater and lesser palatine nerves

Posterior superior alveolar nerves

Maxillary sinus

Nasopalatine nerve

Spinal cord

Superior cervical ganglion

Sympathetic trunk

Postganglionic fibers to vessels (sympathetic) and glands (parasympathetic) of nasal cavity, maxillary sinus and palate

T1

T2

T3

——————— Preganglionic parasympathetic fibers

- - - - - - - Postganglionic parasympathetic fibers

——————— Preganglionic sympathetic fibers

- - - - - - - Postganglionic sympathetic fibers

Preganglionic sympathetic cell bodies in intermediolateral nucleus (lateral horn) of gray matter

FACIAL NERVE CRANIAL NERVE VII *continued*

Pterygopalatine and Submandibular Ganglia: Schema

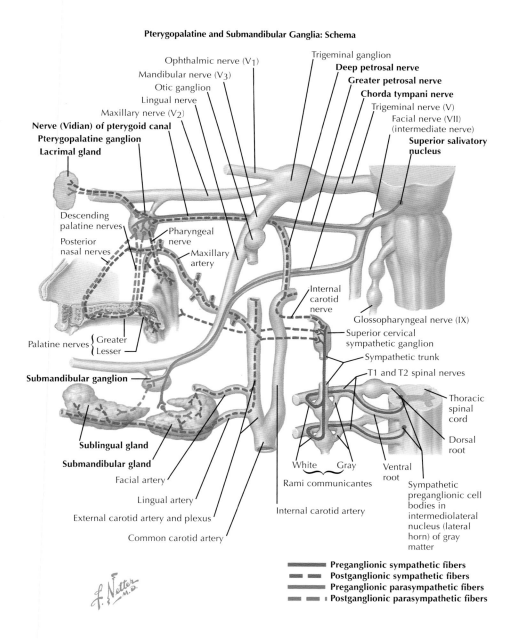

Ophthalmic nerve (V₁)
Mandibular nerve (V₃)
Otic ganglion
Lingual nerve
Maxillary nerve (V₂)
Nerve (Vidian) of pterygoid canal
Pterygopalatine ganglion
Lacrimal gland

Trigeminal ganglion
Deep petrosal nerve
Greater petrosal nerve
Chorda tympani nerve
Trigeminal nerve (V)
Facial nerve (VII)
(intermediate nerve)
Superior salivatory nucleus

Descending palatine nerves
Posterior nasal nerves
Pharyngeal nerve
Maxillary artery

Internal carotid nerve
Glossopharyngeal nerve (IX)
Superior cervical sympathetic ganglion
Sympathetic trunk
T1 and T2 spinal nerves

Palatine nerves { Greater / Lesser

Submandibular ganglion

Thoracic spinal cord

Dorsal root

Sublingual gland
Submandibular gland
Facial artery
Lingual artery
External carotid artery and plexus
Common carotid artery

White   Gray
Rami communicantes
Internal carotid artery

Ventral root
Sympathetic preganglionic cell bodies in intermediolateral nucleus (lateral horn) of gray matter

━━━ **Preganglionic sympathetic fibers**
■ ■ ■ **Postganglionic sympathetic fibers**
━━━ **Preganglionic parasympathetic fibers**
■ ■ ■ **Postganglionic parasympathetic fibers**

FACIAL NERVE SENSORY

STRUCTURE	ANATOMIC NOTES	FUNCTIONAL SIGNIFICANCE
General sensory fibers	Cell bodies of these fibers are in geniculate ganglion in temporal bone. Impulses enter the brainstem via the intermediate nerve (sensory root of CN-VII), synapse in the spinotrigeminal tract, project to contralateral ventroposterolateral (VPL) thalamus, then to sensory cortex.	For skin of the concha of the auricle and small area behind ear, supplements V_3
Special sensory fibers	Cell bodies of these fibers are in the geniculate ganglion in temporal bone Peripheral processes run with the lingual nerve, then separate to become chorda tympani, which joins the facial nerve in petrous temporal bone. Fibers enter the brainstem at the caudal pons with intermediate nerve (sensory root of CN-VII); enter the tractus solitarius, synapse in the rostal nucleus solitarius (gustatory nucleus), and ascend to the bilateral ventroposterior (VP) thalamus and then to the posterior internal capsule to the cortex.	Taste from anterior $2/3$ of the tongue and hard and soft palate

FACIAL NERVE SENSORY *continued*

Taste Pathways: Schema

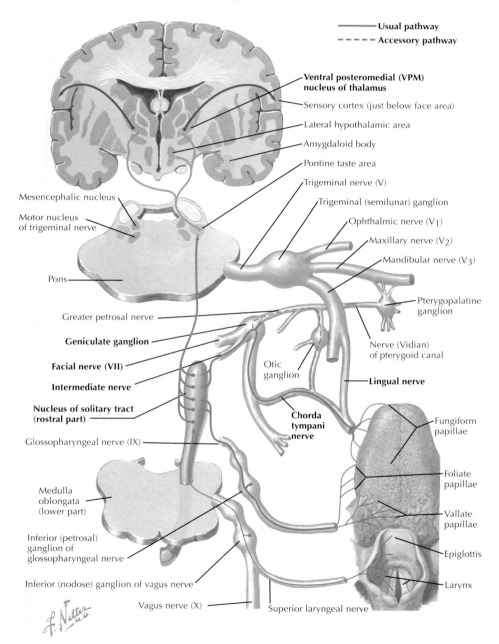

——— Usual pathway
- - - - Accessory pathway

Ventral posteromedial (VPM) nucleus of thalamus

Sensory cortex (just below face area)

Lateral hypothalamic area

Amygdaloid body

Pontine taste area

Trigeminal nerve (V)

Trigeminal (semilunar) ganglion

Ophthalmic nerve (V₁)

Maxillary nerve (V₂)

Mandibular nerve (V₃)

Mesencephalic nucleus

Motor nucleus of trigeminal nerve

Pons

Greater petrosal nerve

Geniculate ganglion

Facial nerve (VII)

Intermediate nerve

Nucleus of solitary tract (rostral part)

Glossopharyngeal nerve (IX)

Medulla oblongata (lower part)

Inferior (petrosal) ganglion of glossopharyngeal nerve

Inferior (nodose) ganglion of vagus nerve

Vagus nerve (X)

Pterygopalatine ganglion

Nerve (Vidian) of pterygoid canal

Otic ganglion

Lingual nerve

Chorda tympani nerve

Fungiform papillae

Foliate papillae

Vallate papillae

Epiglottis

Larynx

Superior laryngeal nerve

VESTIBULOCOCHLEAR NERVE (CN-VIII): AUDITORY COMPONENT

STRUCTURE	ANATOMIC NOTES	FUNCTIONAL SIGNIFICANCE
CN-VIII (vestibular and auditory components)	Enters the brainstem at the cerebellopontine angle	Special sensory nerve Auditory from the cochlea, balance from semicircular canals
CN-VIII (cochlear primary sensory neuron cell bodies)	Lie around modiolus (center) of the cochlea, where they constitute cochlear (spiral) ganglion	Their central processes form auditory component of CN-VIII
CN-VIII axons	Travel through the internal auditory meatus with CN-VII to enter pontomedullary junction, just lateral to CN-VII, and synapse in the cochlear nuclei	Peripheral lesion (e.g., compression by cerebellopontine angle tumor) produces ipsilateral deafness
Second-order cochlear neurons	Mostly cross via trapezoid body and ascend the contralateral lateral lemniscus to synapse in the inferior colliculus, then to medial geniculate (thalamus), and then through the internal capsule to the acoustic cortex (transverse temporal gyri of Heschl)	Because of the bilaterality of ascending pathways, central lesions (stroke, tumor) do not produce deafness but produce bilateral hearing reduction, which is worse on the contralateral side

VESTIBULOCOCHLEAR NERVE (CN-VIII): AUDITORY COMPONENT *continued*

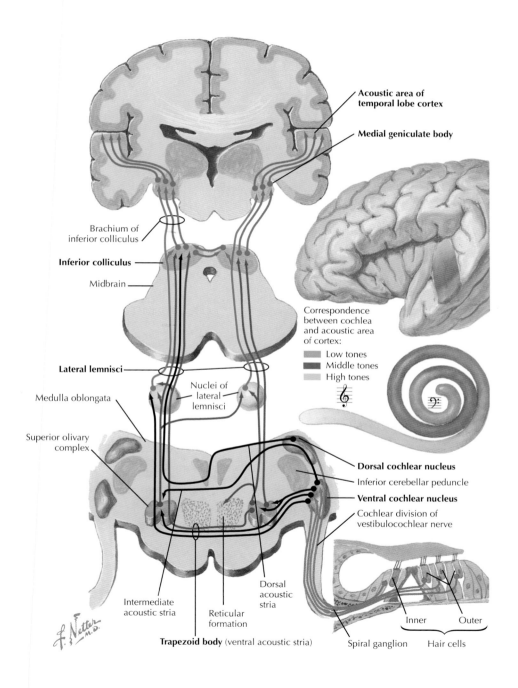

Acoustic area of temporal lobe cortex

Medial geniculate body

Brachium of inferior colliculus

Inferior colliculus

Midbrain

Lateral lemnisci

Medulla oblongata

Nuclei of lateral lemnisci

Superior olivary complex

Correspondence between cochlea and acoustic area of cortex:

- Low tones
- Middle tones
- High tones

Dorsal cochlear nucleus

Inferior cerebellar peduncle

Ventral cochlear nucleus

Cochlear division of vestibulocochlear nerve

Intermediate acoustic stria

Reticular formation

Dorsal acoustic stria

Trapezoid body (ventral acoustic stria)

Spiral ganglion

Inner   Outer

Hair cells

VESTIBULOCOCHLEAR NERVE (CN-VIII): VESTIBULAR

STRUCTURE	ANATOMIC NOTES	FUNCTIONAL SIGNIFICANCE
CN-VIII vestibular primary sensory neuron cell bodies	Lay in the vestibular ganglion	Central processes form the vestibular component of CN-VIII mediating balance
CN-VIII axons	Travel through the internal auditory meatus with cochlear division and CN-VII to enter the pontomedullary junction, just lateral to CN-VII, and synapse in the vestibular nuclear complex in the floor of the 4th ventricle	Second-order vestibular neurons send axons to: • The cerebellum (vestibulocerebellar tract) to coordinate balance • Lower motor neurons in the brainstem and spinal cord (vestibulospinal tract) to antigravity muscles • Medial longitudinal fasciculus (MLF) to maintain orientation in space
Second-order vestibular neurons	Send axons to: • Cerebellum via vestibulocerebellar tract • Lower motor neurons in the brainstem and spinal cord via vestibulospinal tract • Descending medial longitudinal fasciculus (MLF)	Vestibulocerebellar tract coordinates balance Vestibulospinal tract innervates antigravity muscles for balance MLF maintains orientation in space

VESTIBULOCOCHLEAR NERVE (CN-VIII): VESTIBULAR *continued*

Vestibulocochlear Nerve (VIII): Schema

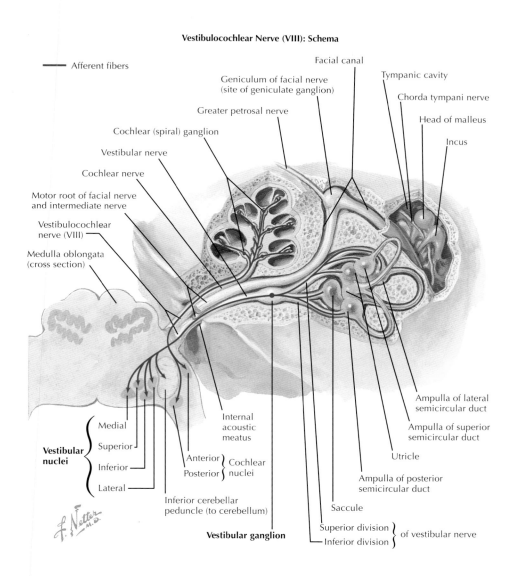

Afferent fibers

Facial canal

Geniculum of facial nerve
(site of geniculate ganglion)

Tympanic cavity

Chorda tympani nerve

Greater petrosal nerve

Head of malleus

Cochlear (spiral) ganglion

Incus

Vestibular nerve

Cochlear nerve

Motor root of facial nerve
and intermediate nerve

Vestibulocochlear
nerve (VIII)

Medulla oblongata
(cross section)

Ampulla of lateral
semicircular duct

Ampulla of superior
semicircular duct

Medial

Superior

Internal
acoustic
meatus

**Vestibular
nuclei**

Utricle

Inferior

Anterior } Cochlear
Posterior } nuclei

Lateral

Ampulla of posterior
semicircular duct

Inferior cerebellar
peduncle (to cerebellum)

Saccule

Vestibular ganglion

Superior division } of vestibular nerve
Inferior division }

CAUSES OF VERTIGO

STRUCTURE	ANATOMIC NOTES	FUNCTIONAL SIGNIFICANCE
Cerebellopontine angle	CN-VII and CN-VIII found here	Tumors (acoustic neuroma) can compress CN-VIII and CN-VII, causing vertigo, tinnitus, deafness, and facial asymmetry
Medulla	Lateral medulla co-localizes: • Vestibular nuclei • Spinothalamic tract • Sympathetic tract • CN-IX and-X fibers • Spinocerebellar fibers • Descending nucleus V • Nucleus solitarius	Lateral medullary infarction (Wallenberg's syndrome) include: • Nystagmus, vertigo, nausea, vomiting • Contralateral hemisensory loss of pain and temperature • Ipsilateral Horner's syndrome • Hoarseness, dysphagia • Ipsilateral ataxia • Ipsilateral pain, burning, and impaired sensation of the face • Loss of taste

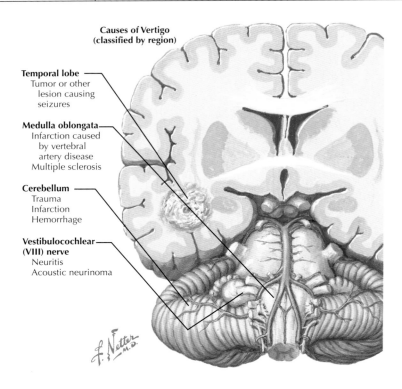

Causes of Vertigo
(classified by region)

Temporal lobe
Tumor or other
lesion causing
seizures

Medulla oblongata
Infarction caused
by vertebral
artery disease
Multiple sclerosis

Cerebellum
Trauma
Infarction
Hemorrhage

**Vestibulocochlear
(VIII) nerve**
Neuritis
Acoustic neurinoma

GLOSSOPHARYNGEAL NERVE (CN-IX)

STRUCTURE	ANATOMIC NOTES	FUNCTIONAL SIGNIFICANCE
CN-IX	Emerges from the medulla between the inferior olive and inferior cerebellar peduncle In jugular fossa, the tympanic nerve is given off Main trunk then exits the jugular foramen containing the superior and inferior glossopharyngeal ganglia (i.e., nerve cell bodies for general visceral and special visceral sensation)	Branchial motor—innervates the stylopharyngeus Visceral motor supplies preganglionic parasympathetic fibers to the otic ganglion, which sends fibers to the parotid gland General sensory—sensation posterior $\frac{1}{3}$ tongue, skin of external ear, internal surface of tympanic membrane Visceral sensory—mucous membranes of the pharynx, middle ear, unconscious sensory input from the carotid body and sinus Special sensory—taste posterior $\frac{1}{3}$ tongue
Inferior glosso-pharyngeal ganglion	Located in the jugular foramen, central fibers enter the brainstem and travel through the solitary tract to the rostral solitary tract nucleus (gustatory nucleus) in medulla	Mediates taste posterior $\frac{1}{3}$ tongue
Rostral solitary tract nucleus (gustatory nucleus)	Axons of these cells ascend central tegmental tract to the bilateral ventroposteromedial (VPM) nucleus of the thalamus. From thalamus they ascend through the posterior limb of the internal capsule to the postcentral gyrus	Central lesions do not affect taste
Corticobulbar fibers	Synapse *bilaterally* on lower motor neurons in the rostral nucleus ambiguus	Because of bilaterality, central lesions affecting the descending fibers do not affect the stylopharyngeus
CN-IX	Emerges from medulla between inferior olive and inferior cerebellar peduncle, passes laterally in the posterior fossa to exit the jugular foramen anterior to CN-X and CN-XI and descends in the neck to the stylopharyngeus	Elevates the pharynx during swallow and speech

GLOSSOPHARYNGEAL NERVE (CN-IX) *continued*

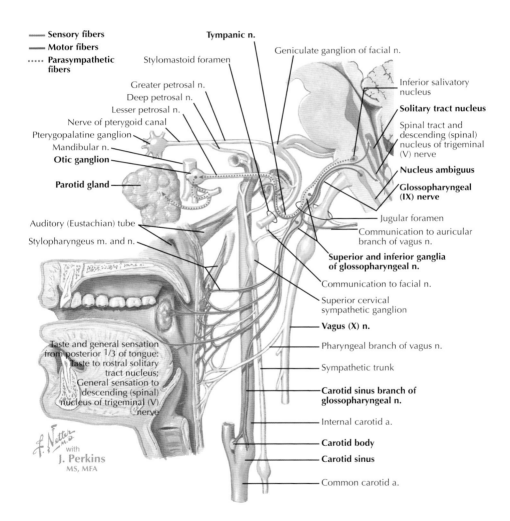

— Sensory fibers
— Motor fibers
..... Parasympathetic fibers

Tympanic n.

Geniculate ganglion of facial n.

Stylomastoid foramen

Greater petrosal n.
Deep petrosal n.
Lesser petrosal n.
Nerve of pterygoid canal
Pterygopalatine ganglion
Mandibular n.
Otic ganglion

Parotid gland

Auditory (Eustachian) tube

Stylopharyngeus m. and n.

Inferior salivatory nucleus
Solitary tract nucleus
Spinal tract and descending (spinal) nucleus of trigeminal (V) nerve
Nucleus ambiguus
Glossopharyngeal (IX) nerve
Jugular foramen
Communication to auricular branch of vagus n.
Superior and inferior ganglia of glossopharyngeal n.
Communication to facial n.
Superior cervical sympathetic ganglion
Vagus (X) n.
Pharyngeal branch of vagus n.
Sympathetic trunk
Carotid sinus branch of glossopharyngeal n.
Internal carotid a.
Carotid body
Carotid sinus
Common carotid a.

Taste and general sensation from posterior 1/3 of tongue: Taste to rostral solitary tract nucleus; General sensation to descending (spinal) nucleus of trigeminal (V) nerve

with
J. Perkins
MS, MFA

GLOSSOPHARYNGEAL NERVE (CN-IX): VISCERAL MOTOR

STRUCTURE	ANATOMIC NOTES	FUNCTIONAL SIGNIFICANCE
Intracranial CN-IX preganglionic parasympathetic neurons	Located in the inferior salivatory nucleus in medulla Axons join CN-IX and exit jugular foramen	Visceral motor: supplies otic ganglion, which sends postganglionic parasympathetic fibers to the parotid gland
Extracranial CN-IX preganglionic parasympathetic neurons	Branches to form the lesser petrosal nerve that travels back into the cranium through a small canal to reach the middle cranial fossa and descend through the foramen ovale to synapse in otic ganglion (immediately below foramen ovale) From otic ganglion, postganglionic fibers join auriculotemporal nerve	Supply the secretomotor fibers to the parotid gland

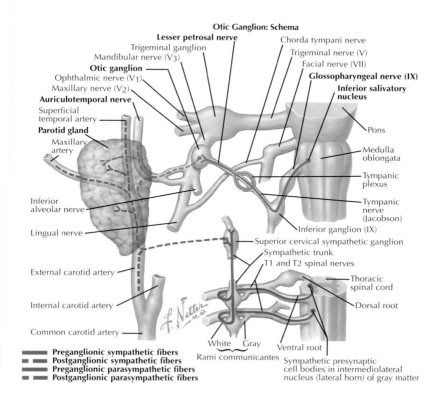

Otic Ganglion: Schema

GLOSSOPHARYNGEAL NERVE (CN-IX): VISCERAL SENSORY

STRUCTURE	ANATOMIC NOTES	FUNCTIONAL SIGNIFICANCE
CN-IX	Information is relayed from the carotid sinus nerve to the inferior ganglion of CN-IX, to the solitary tract, to the caudal solitary nucleus, to the reticular formation and hypothalamus for appropriate reflex responses	Chemoreceptors in the carotid body monitor blood oxygen Baroreceptors in the carotid sinus monitor arterial blood pressure

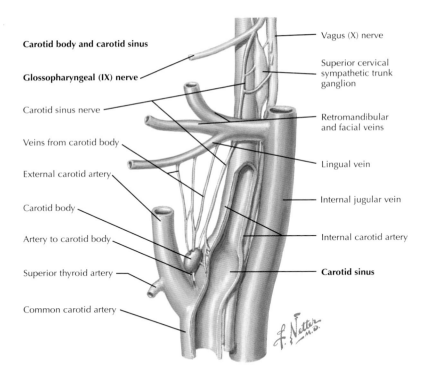

Carotid body and carotid sinus

Glossopharyngeal (IX) nerve

Carotid sinus nerve

Veins from carotid body

External carotid artery

Carotid body

Artery to carotid body

Superior thyroid artery

Common carotid artery

Vagus (X) nerve

Superior cervical sympathetic trunk ganglion

Retromandibular and facial veins

Lingual vein

Internal jugular vein

Internal carotid artery

Carotid sinus

GLOSSOPHARYNGEAL NERVE (CN-IX): GENERAL SENSORY

STRUCTURE	ANATOMIC NOTES	FUNCTIONAL SIGNIFICANCE
CN-IX	Cell bodies located in superior or inferior glossopharyngeal ganglion	Superior glossopharyngeal ganglion: contains primary sensory neurons mediating cutaneous sensation from area back of ear. central processes of these cells enter the spinal trigeminal tract and nucleus
		Inferior glossopharyngeal ganglion: contains cell bodies of visceral afferent fibers. Conveys touch, pain, and temperature from eustachian tube, posterior $\frac{1}{3}$ tongue, tonsil, and upper pharynx
CN-IX Secondary neurons	Cross the midline of the medulla and ascend to the VP nucleus of the thalamus	Same pathway is probably used for touch and pressure and is important for gag reflex
	Tertiary neurons thence project to the postcentral sensory gyrus	

GLOSSOPHARYNGEAL NERVE (CN-IX): GENERAL SENSORY *continued*

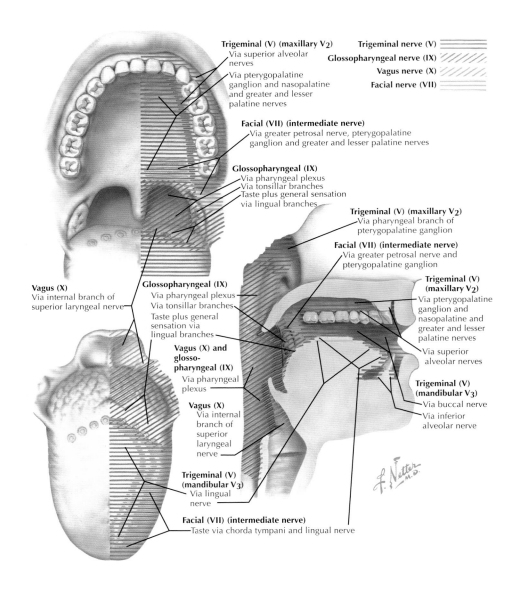

Trigeminal (V) (maxillary V2)
Via superior alveolar nerves
Via pterygopalatine ganglion and nasopalatine and greater and lesser palatine nerves

Trigeminal nerve (V)
Glossopharyngeal nerve (IX)
Vagus nerve (X)
Facial nerve (VII)

Facial (VII) (intermediate nerve)
Via greater petrosal nerve, pterygopalatine ganglion and greater and lesser palatine nerves

Glossopharyngeal (IX)
Via pharyngeal plexus
Via tonsillar branches
Taste plus general sensation via lingual branches

Trigeminal (V) (maxillary V2)
Via pharyngeal branch of pterygopalatine ganglion

Facial (VII) (intermediate nerve)
Via greater petrosal nerve and pterygopalatine ganglion

Trigeminal (V) (maxillary V2)
Via pterygopalatine ganglion and nasopalatine and greater and lesser palatine nerves
Via superior alveolar nerves

Vagus (X)
Via internal branch of superior laryngeal nerve

Glossopharyngeal (IX)
Via pharyngeal plexus
Via tonsillar branches
Taste plus general sensation via lingual branches

Vagus (X) and glosso-pharyngeal (IX)
Via pharyngeal plexus

Vagus (X)
Via internal branch of superior laryngeal nerve

Trigeminal (V) (mandibular V3)
Via lingual nerve

Trigeminal (V) (mandibular V3)
Via buccal nerve
Via inferior alveolar nerve

Facial (VII) (intermediate nerve)
Taste via chorda tympani and lingual nerve

VAGUS NERVE (CN-X)

STRUCTURE	ANATOMIC NOTES	FUNCTIONAL SIGNIFICANCE
CN-X	Emerges from the medulla as several rootlets, converge into 2 roots, exit cranial fossa through jugular foramen In the neck, the vagus nerve lies between the internal jugular vein and internal carotid artery	Branchial motor—striated muscle of pharynx (palatoglossus), larynx, and soft palate (except tensor veli palatini and stylopharyngeus) Visceral motor—smooth muscles and glands of pharynx, larynx, thoracic and abdominal viscera General sensory—skin of back of ear, external auditory meatus, external tympanic membrane General visceral sensory—input from viscera Special visceral sensory—input from periepiglottal taste buds
Superior (jugular) and inferior (nodosal) vagal ganglia	Two sensory ganglia of vagus, located on the nerve in the jugular foramen Inferior ganglion is joined by fibers from the nucleus ambiguus, which traveled with CN-XI	Superior (jugular) ganglion contains cells that give rise to general sensory afferents Inferior (nodosal) ganglion contains cells that give rise to both general and special visceral sensory afferents
Dorsal motor nucleus of X	Preganglionic parasympathetic nerve cell bodies of CN-X; gets input from hypothalamus, olfactory system, reticular formation, solitary tract nucleus	Secretomotor center (visceral motor) of CN-X sends preganglionic parasympathetic fibers to postganglionic cells that innervate all thoracic and abdominal viscera down to the left colic (splenic) flexure
Solitary tract nucleus	Visceral sensory input enters the nucleus and projects to the reticular formation, hypothalamus, and thalamus	Rostral part (gustatory nucleus) receives taste from CN-VII and CN-IX (special visceral sensory) Caudal part receives mainly general visceral afferents from CN-X
Recurrent and internal laryngeal nerves	Internal laryngeal unites with the external laryngeal to form the superior laryngeal nerve, which travels up CN-X to the inferior vagal ganglion	Internal laryngeal nerve—visceral sensory afferent from the larynx as far as the vocal cords External laryngeal—branchial motor to cricothyroid muscle Recurrent laryngeal nerve—branchial motor to all laryngeal muscles except cricothyroid, and visceral sensory afferent from larynx below vocal cords, and mucous membranes of the upper trachea
Auricular branch	Enters the superior vagal ganglion	Carries sensation from the ear

VAGUS NERVE (CN-X) *continued*

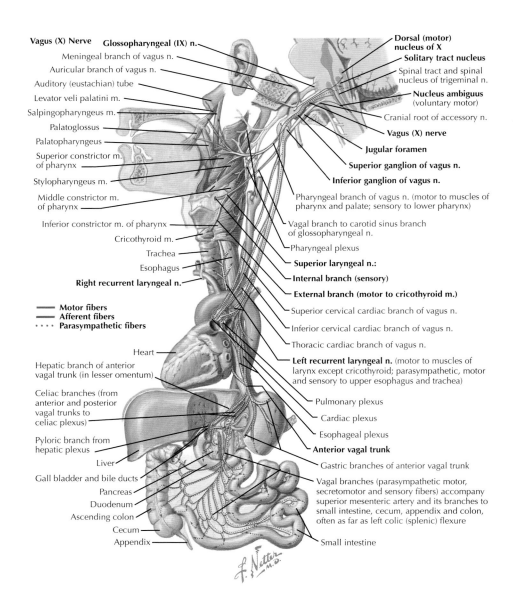

Vagus (X) Nerve
Glossopharyngeal (IX) n.
Meningeal branch of vagus n.
Auricular branch of vagus n.
Auditory (eustachian) tube
Levator veli palatini m.
Salpingopharyngeus m.
Palatoglossus
Palatopharyngeus
Superior constrictor m. of pharynx
Stylopharyngeus m.
Middle constrictor m. of pharynx
Inferior constrictor m. of pharynx
Cricothyroid m.
Trachea
Esophagus
Right recurrent laryngeal n.

—— **Motor fibers**
—— **Afferent fibers**
· · · · **Parasympathetic fibers**

Heart
Hepatic branch of anterior vagal trunk (in lesser omentum)
Celiac branches (from anterior and posterior vagal trunks to celiac plexus)
Pyloric branch from hepatic plexus
Liver
Gall bladder and bile ducts
Pancreas
Duodenum
Ascending colon
Cecum
Appendix

Dorsal (motor) nucleus of X
Solitary tract nucleus
Spinal tract and spinal nucleus of trigeminal n.
Nucleus ambiguus (voluntary motor)
Cranial root of accessory n.
Vagus (X) nerve
Jugular foramen
Superior ganglion of vagus n.
Inferior ganglion of vagus n.
Pharyngeal branch of vagus n. (motor to muscles of pharynx and palate; sensory to lower pharynx)
Vagal branch to carotid sinus branch of glossopharyngeal n.
Pharyngeal plexus
Superior laryngeal n.:
Internal branch (sensory)
External branch (motor to cricothyroid m.)
Superior cervical cardiac branch of vagus n.
Inferior cervical cardiac branch of vagus n.
Thoracic cardiac branch of vagus n.
Left recurrent laryngeal n. (motor to muscles of larynx except cricothyroid; parasympathetic, motor and sensory to upper esophagus and trachea)
Pulmonary plexus
Cardiac plexus
Esophageal plexus
Anterior vagal trunk
Gastric branches of anterior vagal trunk
Vagal branches (parasympathetic motor, secretomotor and sensory fibers) accompany superior mesenteric artery and its branches to small intestine, cecum, appendix and colon, often as far as left colic (splenic) flexure
Small intestine

ACCESSORY NERVE (CN-XI)

STRUCTURE	ANATOMIC NOTES	FUNCTIONAL SIGNIFICANCE
CN-XI	Accessory nerve has cranial root and spinal root (both motor) that briefly run together as they enter jugular foramen	Branchial motor to trapezius and sternocleidomastoid (SCM)
Spinal root	Lower motor neurons located in spinal cord segments C1-5 Axons ascend through the foramen magnum, exit the jugular foramen, and enter their muscles	Radical neck surgery for cancer often involves dissection of cervical lymph nodes. As they are closely associated with accessory nerve, injury to this nerve is common and results in shoulder droop (trapezius), and weakness of head turning to the contralateral side (SCM)
Cranial root	Cell bodies reside in the caudal part of nucleus ambiguus Axons from this nucleus briefly join the spinal root of CN-XI, pass through the jugular foramen, and join CN-X to form the motor component of recurrent laryngeal nerve	May be involved in motor-neuron disease, poliomyelitis, syringobulbia

ACCESSORY NERVE (CN-XI) *continued*

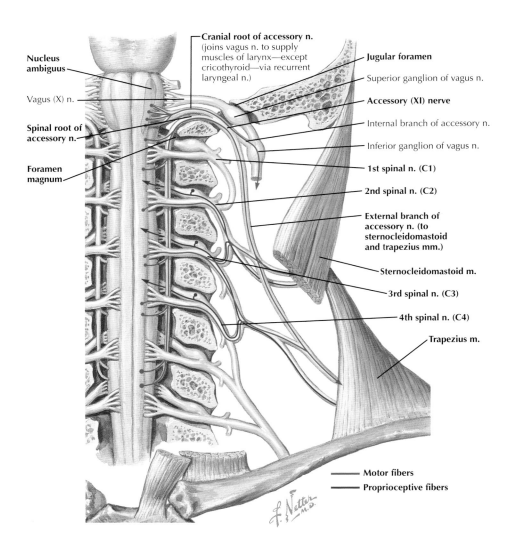

Nucleus ambiguus

Vagus (X) n.

Spinal root of accessory n.

Foramen magnum

Cranial root of accessory n. (joins vagus n. to supply muscles of larynx—except cricothyroid—via recurrent laryngeal n.)

Jugular foramen

Superior ganglion of vagus n.

Accessory (XI) nerve

Internal branch of accessory n.

Inferior ganglion of vagus n.

1st spinal n. (C1)

2nd spinal n. (C2)

External branch of accessory n. (to sternocleidomastoid and trapezius mm.)

Sternocleidomastoid m.

3rd spinal n. (C3)

4th spinal n. (C4)

Trapezius m.

Motor fibers

Proprioceptive fibers

HYPOGLOSSAL NERVE (CN-XII)

STRUCTURE	ANATOMIC NOTES	FUNCTIONAL SIGNIFICANCE
CN-XII	Corticobulbar fibers descend to the contralateral hypoglossal nucleus	Somatic motor to all tongue muscles except palatoglossus (CN-X)
CN-XII	Axons emerge between the olive and pyramid (preolivary sulcus) as a number of rootlets which converge and exit cranial fossa through the hypoglossal (anterior condylar) foramen	Complete interruption of the nerve results in paralysis of the ipsilateral side of the tongue with concomitant atrophy and muscle fasciculations (lower motor neuron lesion)
CN-XII	Passes laterally and downward to between the internal carotid artery and internal jugular vein, loops anteriorly above the hyoid, to innervate tongue	Occasionally damaged in neck surgery Rarely, carotid artery aneurysm may compress nerve

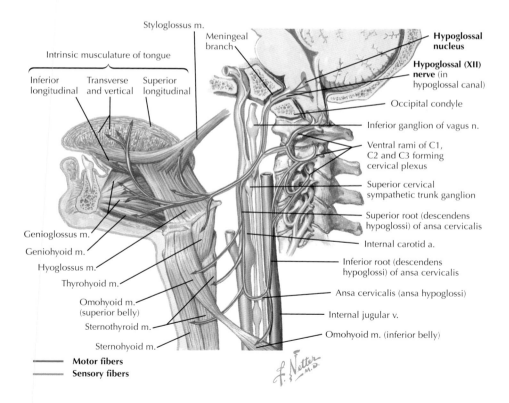

Styloglossus m.

Meningeal branch

Intrinsic musculature of tongue

Inferior longitudinal   Transverse and vertical   Superior longitudinal

Hypoglossal nucleus

Hypoglossal (XII) nerve (in hypoglossal canal)

Occipital condyle

Inferior ganglion of vagus n.

Ventral rami of C1, C2 and C3 forming cervical plexus

Superior cervical sympathetic trunk ganglion

Superior root (descendens hypoglossi) of ansa cervicalis

Internal carotid a.

Genioglossus m.

Geniohyoid m.

Hyoglossus m.

Thyrohyoid m.

Omohyoid m. (superior belly)

Sternothyroid m.

Sternohyoid m.

Inferior root (descendens hypoglossi) of ansa cervicalis

Ansa cervicalis (ansa hypoglossi)

Internal jugular v.

Omohyoid m. (inferior belly)

Motor fibers
Sensory fibers

CHAPTER 15

Major Sensory and Motor Pathways

SPINAL CORD PATHWAYS

White matter is divided into *dorsal* (top of each spinal cord cross-sectional drawing), *ventral* (bottom of each spinal cord cross-sectional drawing), and *lateral* (sides of each spinal cord cross-sectional drawing) columns (funiculi), each containing multiple fiber tracts.

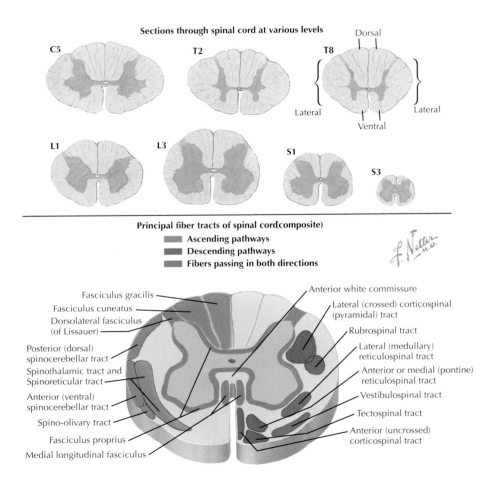

Sections through spinal cord at various levels

C5   T2   T8   Dorsal   Lateral   Ventral   Lateral

L1   L3   S1   S3

Principal fiber tracts of spinal cord (composite)
- Ascending pathways
- Descending pathways
- Fibers passing in both directions

Fasciculus gracilis
Fasciculus cuneatus
Dorsolateral fasciculus (of Lissauer)
Posterior (dorsal) spinocerebellar tract
Spinothalamic tract and Spinoreticular tract
Anterior (ventral) spinocerebellar tract
Spino-olivary tract
Fasciculus proprius
Medial longitudinal fasciculus

Anterior white commissure
Lateral (crossed) corticospinal (pyramidal) tract
Rubrospinal tract
Lateral (medullary) reticulospinal tract
Anterior or medial (pontine) reticulospinal tract
Vestibulospinal tract
Tectospinal tract
Anterior (uncrossed) corticospinal tract

SPINAL CORD CYTOARCHITECTURE

STRUCTURE	ANATOMIC NOTES	FUNCTIONAL SIGNIFICANCE
Gray matter	Butterfly-shaped pattern Divided into dorsal, intermediate, and ventral horns	Contains cell bodies of neurons (e.g., anterior horn cells of lower motor neurons) In amyotrophic lateral sclerosis, these cells degenerate
Dorsal horn	Larger at cervical and lumbosacral enlargements owing to innervation of arm and leg	Site of major sensory processing
Intermediolateral gray	Lateral horn seen from T1-L2 and S2-4	Preganglionic sympathetic (T1-L2) and parasympathetic (S2-4) neurons reside here
Ventral horn	Larger at cervical and lumbosacral enlargements owing to innervation of arm and leg	Anterior horn cells reside here
Laminae of Rexed	System of architectural classification	Most precise and widely used method for describing cell groups in the spinal cord
Nucleus dorsalis (of Clarke)	Cell column in the medial portion of lamina VII Begins to be well defined at the C8 level Gives rise to the uncrossed posterior spinocerebellar tract	Receives collaterals of dorsal roots from the entire body except the head and neck Functionally related primarily to the legs and lower trunk

SPINAL CORD CYTOARCHITECTURE *continued*

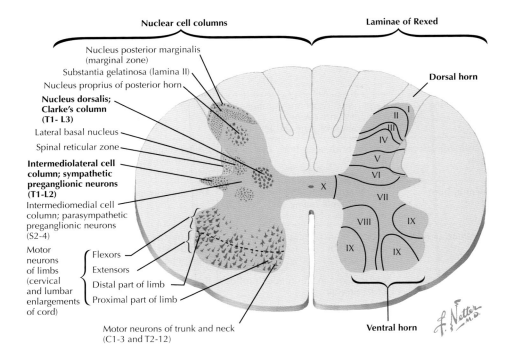

Nuclear cell columns

Laminae of Rexed

Nucleus posterior marginalis
(marginal zone)

Substantia gelatinosa (lamina II)

Nucleus proprius of posterior horn

**Nucleus dorsalis;
Clarke's column
(T1- L3)**

Lateral basal nucleus

Spinal reticular zone

**Intermediolateral cell
column; sympathetic
preganglionic neurons
(T1-L2)**

Intermediomedial cell
column; parasympathetic
preganglionic neurons
(S2-4)

Motor
neurons
of limbs
(cervical
and lumbar
enlargements
of cord)
- Flexors
- Extensors
- Distal part of limb
- Proximal part of limb

Motor neurons of trunk and neck
(C1-3 and T2-12)

Dorsal horn

I
II
III
IV
V
VI
X
VII
VIII
IX
IX
IX

Ventral horn

CORTICAL EFFERENT PATHWAYS

BRODMANN AREA	PROJECTS TO	ANATOMIC NOTES
4 and 6 (motor and premotor cortex)	Basal ganglia (caudate, putamen)	Corticostriate projections
	Thalamus: ventroanterior (VA), ventrolateral (VL)	Corticothalamic projections
	Red nucleus	Corticorubral projections
	Pontine nuclei	Corticopontine projections
	Motor cranial nuclei	Corticobulbar tract bilaterally
	Spinal cord ventral horn	Corticospinal tract, mainly contralaterally
3, 1, and 2 (sensory cortex)	Secondary sensory nuclei	Regulate incoming lemniscal projections
	Thalamus	
8 (frontal eye fields)	Superior colliculus	Coordinate voluntary eye and head movement
	Horizontal (paramedian pontine reticular formation [PPRF]) and vertical-gaze centers in the brainstem	
	Interstitial nucleus of Cajal	

CORTICAL EFFERENT PATHWAYS *continued*

Cerebral Cortex: Efferent Pathway

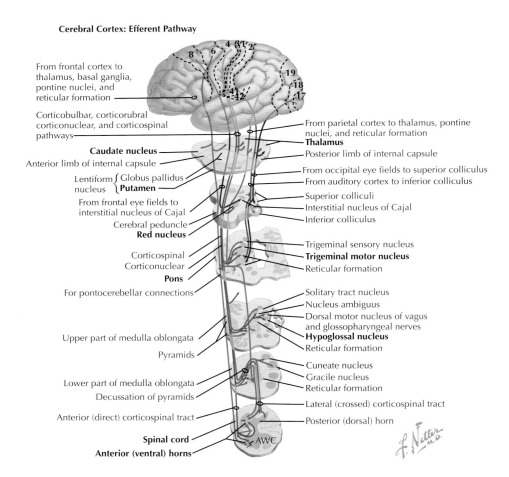

From frontal cortex to thalamus, basal ganglia, pontine nuclei, and reticular formation

Corticobulbar, corticorubral corticonuclear, and corticospinal pathways

Caudate nucleus

Anterior limb of internal capsule

Lentiform { Globus pallidus
nucleus { **Putamen**

From frontal eye fields to interstitial nucleus of Cajal

Cerebral peduncle

Red nucleus

Corticospinal
Corticonuclear

Pons

For pontocerebellar connections

Upper part of medulla oblongata

Pyramids

Lower part of medulla oblongata

Decussation of pyramids

Anterior (direct) corticospinal tract

Spinal cord

Anterior (ventral) horns

From parietal cortex to thalamus, pontine nuclei, and reticular formation
Thalamus
Posterior limb of internal capsule
From occipital eye fields to superior colliculus
From auditory cortex to inferior colliculus
Superior colliculi
Interstitial nucleus of Cajal
Inferior colliculus
Trigeminal sensory nucleus
Trigeminal motor nucleus
Reticular formation
Solitary tract nucleus
Nucleus ambiguus
Dorsal motor nucleus of vagus and glossopharyngeal nerves
Hypoglossal nucleus
Reticular formation
Cuneate nucleus
Gracile nucleus
Reticular formation
Lateral (crossed) corticospinal tract
Posterior (dorsal) horn

AWC

CORTICOBULBAR PATHWAYS

STRUCTURE	ANATOMIC NOTES	FUNCTIONAL SIGNIFICANCE
Corticobulbar pathways	Arise mainly from precentral and postcentral gyri	Project to sensory relay nuclei, reticular formation, and certain cranial motor nuclei
Sensory relay nuclei	Include: • Nucleus gracilis • Nucleus cuneatus • Sensory trigeminal nuclei • Solitary nucleus	Transmit sensory information from periphery to higher cortical centers
Corticoreticular fibers	Project bilaterally to: • Nucleus reticularis gigantocellularis in the medulla • Nucleus reticularis pontis oralis in the pons	Important in arousal and maintenance of the awake state
Corticobulbar pathways to the motor cranial nerve	Largely bilateral Include: • Laryngeal muscles • Pharyngeal muscles • Palatal muscles • Muscles of mastication • Extraocular muscles • Upper facial muscles (muscles that, as a rule, cannot be contracted voluntarily on one side)	Pseudobulbar palsy results from bilateral lesions of the corticobulbar system Characterized by weakness of chewing, swallowing, breathing, and speaking, without muscle atrophy

CORTICOBULBAR PATHWAYS *continued*

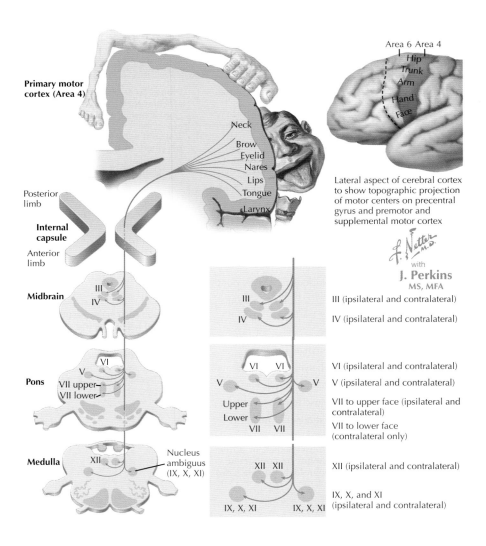

Primary motor cortex (Area 4)

Neck
Brow
Eyelid
Nares
Lips
Tongue
Larynx

Posterior limb

Internal capsule

Anterior limb

Midbrain
III
IV

Pons
VI
V
VII upper
VII lower

Medulla
XII
Nucleus ambiguus (IX, X, XI)

Area 6 Area 4
Hip
Trunk
Arm
Hand
Face

Lateral aspect of cerebral cortex to show topographic projection of motor centers on precentral gyrus and premotor and supplemental motor cortex

with
J. Perkins
MS, MFA

III (ipsilateral and contralateral)

IV (ipsilateral and contralateral)

VI (ipsilateral and contralateral)
V (ipsilateral and contralateral)

VII to upper face (ipsilateral and contralateral)

VII to lower face (contralateral only)

XII (ipsilateral and contralateral)

IX, X, and XI (ipsilateral and contralateral)

Upper
Lower

CORTICOSPINAL TRACT

ANATOMIC NOTES	FUNCTIONAL SIGNIFICANCE
Originates in the primary motor cortex (area 4), premotor cortex (area 6), postcentral gyrus (areas 3a, 3b,1, and 2), and parietal cortex (area 5)	Largest descending system in humans >1,000,000 fibers 70% myelinated
Descends through the corona radiata, internal capsule, cerebral peduncle, basis pontis, and medullary pyramid	Occlusion of small penetrating vessels in these areas results in lacunar infarction and causes contralateral hemiparesis
90% decussate in pyramid to descend in the lateral corticospinal tract of cord Synapse on anterior horn cells	Infarct or tumor in pyramid will cause ipsilateral tongue paralysis and contralateral hemiparesis
10% do not decussate in the pyramid Most of these descend in the anterior corticospinal tract, cross in the cervical spine, and synapse on the contralateral anterior horn cells to the arms and neck	It is not possible clinically to recognize lesions specifically involving anterior corticospinal tract

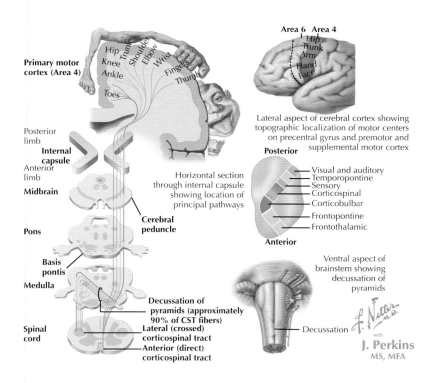

Primary motor cortex (Area 4)

Hip, Knee, Ankle, Toes, Trunk, Shoulder, Elbow, Wrist, Fingers, Thumb

Posterior limb
Internal capsule
Anterior limb
Midbrain

Pons

Basis pontis

Medulla

Spinal cord

Horizontal section through internal capsule showing location of principal pathways

Cerebral peduncle

Decussation of pyramids (approximately 90% of CST fibers)
Lateral (crossed) corticospinal tract
Anterior (direct) corticospinal tract

Area 6   Area 4

Hip, Trunk, Arm, Hand, Face

Lateral aspect of cerebral cortex showing topographic localization of motor centers on precentral gyrus and premotor and supplemental motor cortex

Posterior

Visual and auditory
Temporopontine
Sensory
Corticospinal
Corticobulbar
Frontopontine
Frontothalamic

Anterior

Ventral aspect of brainstem showing decussation of pyramids

Decussation

f. Netter
M.D.

with
J. Perkins
MS, MFA

RUBROSPINAL TRACT

ANATOMIC NOTES	FUNCTIONAL SIGNIFICANCE
Arises from cells in the red nucleus, and crosses the median raphe in the ventral tegmental decussation	Red nucleus lesion results in rubral (wing-beating) tremor
Descends to spinal levels anterior to the lateral corticospinal tract	Controls muscle tone in the flexor muscle groups
Terminates on the anterior horn cells	

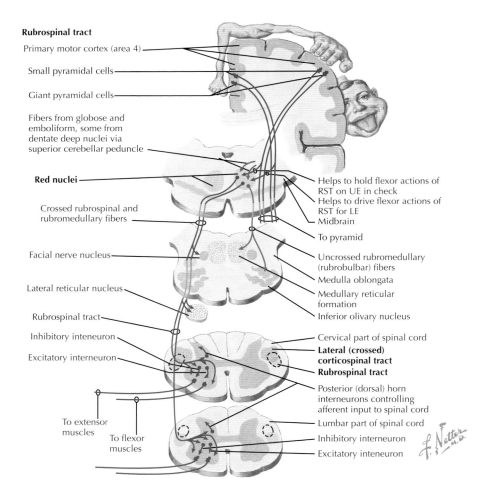

Rubrospinal tract

Primary motor cortex (area 4)

Small pyramidal cells

Giant pyramidal cells

Fibers from globose and emboliform, some from dentate deep nuclei via superior cerebellar peduncle

Red nuclei

Crossed rubrospinal and rubromedullary fibers

Facial nerve nucleus

Lateral reticular nucleus

Rubrospinal tract

Inhibitory interneuron

Excitatory interneuron

To extensor muscles

To flexor muscles

Helps to hold flexor actions of RST on UE in check
Helps to drive flexor actions of RST for LE
Midbrain

To pyramid

Uncrossed rubromedullary (rubrobulbar) fibers
Medulla oblongata
Medullary reticular formation
Inferior olivary nucleus

Cervical part of spinal cord
Lateral (crossed) corticospinal tract
Rubrospinal tract

Posterior (dorsal) horn interneurons controlling afferent input to spinal cord
Lumbar part of spinal cord
Inhibitory interneuron
Excitatory interneuron

VESTIBULOSPINAL TRACT

The vestibulospinal tracts work with the reticulospinal tracts to control tone and posture.

STRUCTURE	ANATOMIC NOTES	FUNCTIONAL SIGNIFICANCE
Lateral vestibulospinal tract	Arises from the lateral vestibular nucleus Descends the anterior part of the lateral funiculus of the spinal cord Terminates on the ipsilateral anterior horn cells	Associated with the extensor musculature to control tone and posture
Medial vestibulospinal tract	Arises from the medial vestibular nucleus	Inhibits the cervical spinal motor neurons controlling the neck and trunk

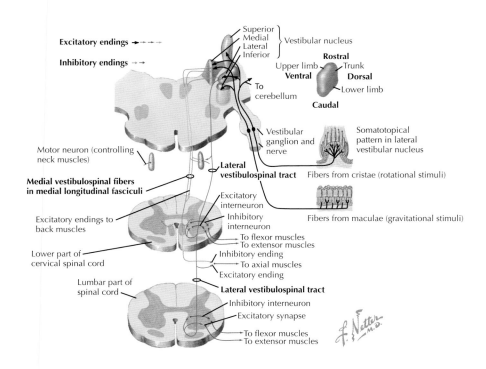

Excitatory endings ➞ ➞ ➞
Inhibitory endings ➞ ➞

Superior
Medial
Lateral
Inferior
} Vestibular nucleus

Rostral
Upper limb ↘ ↗ Trunk
Ventral   Dorsal
↘ Lower limb
Caudal

To cerebellum

Vestibular ganglion and nerve

Motor neuron (controlling neck muscles)

Somatotopical pattern in lateral vestibular nucleus

Medial vestibulospinal fibers in medial longitudinal fasciculi

Lateral vestibulospinal tract   Fibers from cristae (rotational stimuli)

Excitatory interneuron

Excitatory endings to back muscles

Inhibitory interneuron   Fibers from maculae (gravitational stimuli)

To flexor muscles
To extensor muscles

Lower part of cervical spinal cord

Inhibitory ending

To axial muscles
Excitatory ending

Lumbar part of spinal cord

Lateral vestibulospinal tract

Inhibitory interneuron

Excitatory synapse

To flexor muscles
To extensor muscles

RETICULOSPINAL AND CORTICORETICULAR PATHS

STRUCTURE	ANATOMIC NOTES	FUNCTIONAL SIGNIFICANCE
Pontine reticulospinal tract	Descends ipsilaterally Arises from nuclei in the medial pontine reticular formation (pontis caudalis and oralis)	Distinct extensor bias, reinforcing lateral vestibulospinal tract to regulate tone and posture
Medullary reticulospinal tract	Descends bilaterally Arises from nucleus gigantocellularis	Distinct flexor bias, reinforcing the corticospinal and reticulospinal tracts to regulate tone and posture

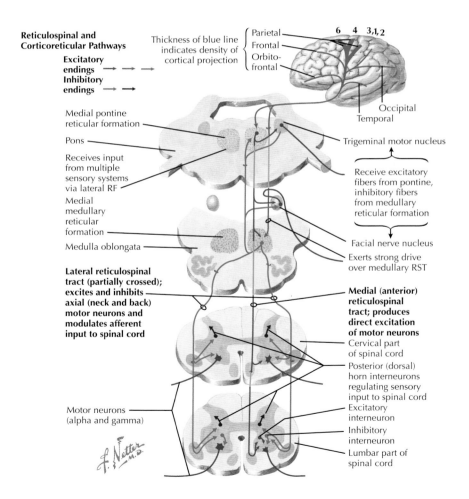

Reticulospinal and Corticoreticular Pathways

Excitatory endings → → →
Inhibitory endings → →

Thickness of blue line indicates density of cortical projection

{ Parietal, Frontal, Orbito-frontal

6 4 3,1,2

Medial pontine reticular formation

Pons

Receives input from multiple sensory systems via lateral RF

Medial medullary reticular formation

Medulla oblongata

Lateral reticulospinal tract (partially crossed); excites and inhibits axial (neck and back) motor neurons and modulates afferent input to spinal cord

Motor neurons (alpha and gamma)

Occipital
Temporal

Trigeminal motor nucleus

Receive excitatory fibers from pontine, inhibitory fibers from medullary reticular formation

Facial nerve nucleus

Exerts strong drive over medullary RST

Medial (anterior) reticulospinal tract; produces direct excitation of motor neurons

Cervical part of spinal cord

Posterior (dorsal) horn interneurons regulating sensory input to spinal cord

Excitatory interneuron

Inhibitory interneuron

Lumbar part of spinal cord

TECTOSPINAL TRACT AND MEDIAL LONGITUDINAL FASCICULUS (MLF)

STRUCTURE	ANATOMIC NOTES	FUNCTIONAL SIGNIFICANCE
Tectospinal tract	Arises from the superior colliculus	Mediates reflex and visual tracking for head and neck movement
	Descends contralaterally ventral to the MLF	
	Terminates mainly in upper 4 cervical spinal segments	
Interstitiospinal tract	Arises from the interstitial nucleus of Cajal	Terminates on spinal motor neurons associated with rotational trunk movement
	Descends in the ipsilateral MLF	

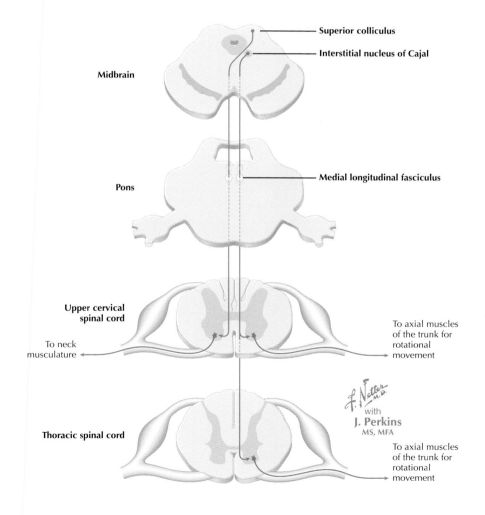

Superior colliculus

Interstitial nucleus of Cajal

Midbrain

Medial longitudinal fasciculus

Pons

Upper cervical spinal cord

To neck musculature

To axial muscles of the trunk for rotational movement

with
J. Perkins
MS, MFA

Thoracic spinal cord

To axial muscles of the trunk for rotational movement

ASCENDING SPINAL CORD PATHWAYS

STRUCTURE	ANATOMIC NOTES	FUNCTIONAL SIGNIFICANCE
Unmyelinated and small myelinated axons	Terminate in laminae I and V	Origin of the spinothalamic tract
Myelinated axons	Ascend the posterior columns	Mediate vibration and position

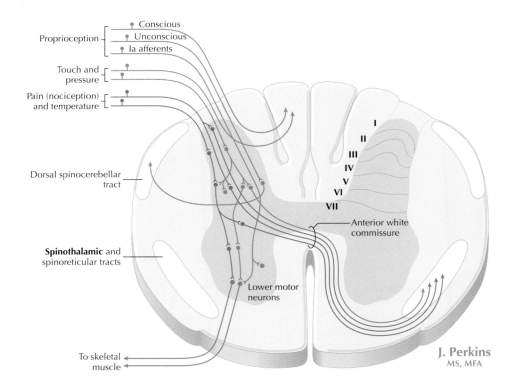

POSTERIOR WHITE COLUMNS

STRUCTURE	ANATOMIC NOTES	FUNCTIONAL SIGNIFICANCE
Myelinated axons	Enter the dorsal horn, ascend the fasciculus gracilis (medial, from leg) and cuneatus (lateral, from arm) to medullary nuclei	Mediate touch, vibration, position Posterior column lesion (B_{12} deficiency, demyelinating multiple sclerosis plaque) results in ataxia
Second-order neurons	Cross ventromedially as internal arcuate fibers Turn upward as medial lemniscus Medial lemniscus ascends to ventroposterolateral nucleus (VPL) of thalamus	Mediate touch, vibration, position Thalamic infarct results in contralateral numbness May cause contralateral pain syndrome
Third-order neurons	From the thalamus ascend the posterior limb internal capsule to terminate in the sensory cortex	Cortical infarction results in loss of cortical sensation, including graphesthesia, stereognosis

POSTERIOR WHITE COLUMNS *continued*

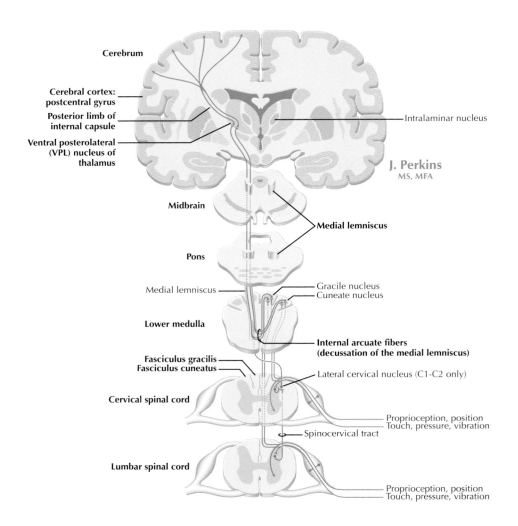

Cerebrum

Cerebral cortex:
postcentral gyrus

Posterior limb of
internal capsule

Ventral posterolateral
(VPL) nucleus of
thalamus

Intralaminar nucleus

J. Perkins
MS, MFA

Midbrain

Medial lemniscus

Pons

Medial lemniscus

Gracile nucleus
Cuneate nucleus

Lower medulla

Internal arcuate fibers
(decussation of the medial lemniscus)

Fasciculus gracilis
Fasciculus cuneatus

Lateral cervical nucleus (C1-C2 only)

Cervical spinal cord

Proprioception, position
Touch, pressure, vibration

Spinocervical tract

Lumbar spinal cord

Proprioception, position
Touch, pressure, vibration

SPINOTHALAMIC AND SPINORETICULAR TRACT

- Unilateral section of the spinothalamic tract produces contralateral sensory loss to a level 1 segment below the lesion owing to oblique crossing of fibers.
- Unilateral lesions do not markedly affect anogenital region.

STRUCTURE	ANATOMIC NOTES	FUNCTIONAL SIGNIFICANCE
Peripheral receptors for pain and temperature	Send central processes to the zone of Lissauer	Small-fiber neuropathy results in painful feet
Cells in laminae I, IV, and V	Give rise to axons that cross in anterior white commissure	Syrinx in the central canal interrupts these fibers with loss of pain and temperature in affected segments
Spinothalamic tract	Ascends in the contralateral lateral funiculus as the lateral spinothalamic tract Lateroposterior fibers represent the lower body; medial anterior fibers represent arms and neck	Compression of this tract affects pain and thermal sense below level of pathology
Spinoreticular tract	Ascends in the spinal cord with the spinothalamic tract Projects to the brainstem reticular formation, thalamus, and cortex	Processes information related to slow, excruciating pain

SPINOTHALAMIC AND SPINORETICULAR TRACT *continued*

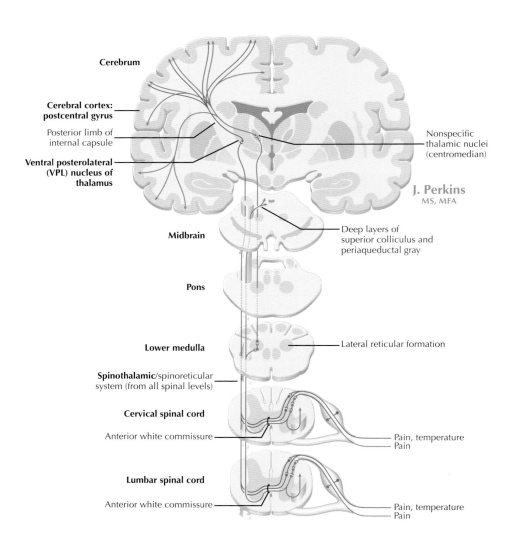

Cerebrum

Cerebral cortex: postcentral gyrus

Posterior limb of internal capsule

Ventral posterolateral (VPL) nucleus of thalamus

Nonspecific thalamic nuclei (centromedian)

J. Perkins
MS, MFA

Midbrain

Deep layers of superior colliculus and periaqueductal gray

Pons

Lower medulla

Lateral reticular formation

Spinothalamic/spinoreticular system (from all spinal levels)

Cervical spinal cord

Anterior white commissure

Pain, temperature
Pain

Lumbar spinal cord

Anterior white commissure

Pain, temperature
Pain

SPINOCEREBELLAR PATHWAYS

- Dorsal and cuneocerebellar tracts remain ipsilateral.
- Ventral spinocerebellar tract crosses twice, once in anterior commissure, again in cerebellum, thus remaining ultimately ipsilateral.

STRUCTURE	ANATOMIC NOTES	FUNCTIONAL SIGNIFICANCE
Ventral (anterior) spinocerebellar tract	Crosses in the anterior commissure, ascends to the superior cerebellar peduncle (brachium conjunctivum) Crosses again in cerebellum to contralateral cortex	Conveys impulses from the lower body Golgi tendon organ via Ib afferents Equivalent in the upper body is the rostral spinocerebellar tract
Dorsal (posterior) spinocerebellar tract	Projects to the ipsilateral nucleus dorsalis (Clarke column) and remains ipsilateral Nucleus dorsalis axons form the dorsal (posterior) spinocerebellar tract Ascends to the inferior cerebellar peduncle to the cerebellar cortex	Conveys impulses below T6 from muscle spindles and Golgi tendon organ via Ia, Ib, and II fibers Equivalent in the upper body is the cuneocerebellar tract
Cuneocerebellar tract	Cervical dorsal root fibers synapse in the accessory cuneate nucleus Second-order neurons form the cuneocerebellar tract Remains ipsilateral and travels with the dorsal spinocerebellar tract to the cerebellum	Clarke's column is not present above C8 but is replaced by accessory cuneate nucleus Equivalent in lower body is dorsal (posterior) spinocerebellar tract

SPINOCEREBELLAR PATHWAYS *continued*

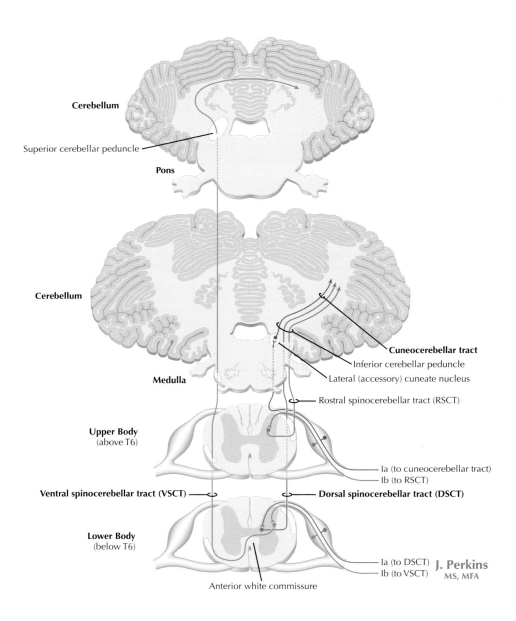

Cerebellum

Superior cerebellar peduncle

Pons

Cerebellum

Cuneocerebellar tract

Inferior cerebellar peduncle

Medulla

Lateral (accessory) cuneate nucleus

Rostral spinocerebellar tract (RSCT)

Upper Body
(above T6)

Ia (to cuneocerebellar tract)
Ib (to RSCT)

Ventral spinocerebellar tract (VSCT)

Dorsal spinocerebellar tract (DSCT)

Lower Body
(below T6)

Ia (to DSCT)
Ib (to VSCT)

Anterior white commissure

J. Perkins
MS, MFA

SPINOCEREBELLAR SYNAPTIC PATHWAY

Primary somatosensory axons transmit information from the following:
- Muscle spindles
- Golgi tendon organs
- Touch and pressure receptors

STRUCTURE	ANATOMIC NOTES	FUNCTIONAL SIGNIFICANCE
Dorsal and ventral spinocerebellar tract	Enter via the dorsal root Convey information to the ipsilateral cerebellum	Carry information from T6 and below
Rostral spinocerebellar tract and cuneocerebellar tract	Enter via the dorsal root Convey information to the ipsilateral cerebellum	Carry information from above T6

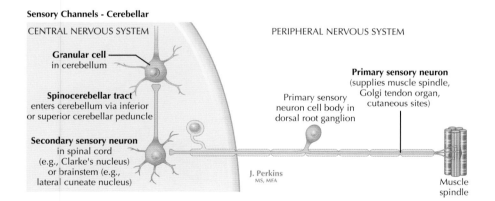

Sensory Channels - Cerebellar

CENTRAL NERVOUS SYSTEM

Granular cell
in cerebellum

Spinocerebellar tract
enters cerebellum via inferior
or superior cerebellar peduncle

Secondary sensory neuron
in spinal cord
(e.g., Clarke's nucleus)
or brainstem (e.g.,
lateral cuneate nucleus)

PERIPHERAL NERVOUS SYSTEM

Primary sensory neuron
(supplies muscle spindle,
Golgi tendon organ,
cutaneous sites)

Primary sensory
neuron cell body in
dorsal root ganglion

J. Perkins
MS, MFA

Muscle
spindle

RAPHE NUCLEI AND SEROTONERGIC PATHWAYS

- Main source of serotonin to central nervous system
- Important for wakefulness and sleep

STRUCTURE	ANATOMIC NOTES
Raphe dorsalis nucleus	Projects upward to the substantia nigra, lateral geniculate body, pyriform lobe (anteromedial temporal lobe), olfactory bulb, amygdaloid nuclear complex
	Projects downward to the locus ceruleus and parabrachial nucleus surrounding the superior cerebellar peduncle
Raphe pontis centralis superior (median raphe) nucleus	Projects upward to the interpeduncular nucleus, mammillary bodies, hippocampal formation
	Projects downward to the cerebellum (via middle cerebellar peduncle), locus ceruleus, pontine reticular formation
Nucleus raphe pontis	Projects to the brainstem and spinal cord
Nucleus raphe magnus	Projects, via the dorsal longitudinal fasciculus, to the dorsal motor nucleus of X, nucleus solitarius, spinal trigeminal nucleus, spinal cord (substantia gelatinosa)
Nucleus raphe pallidus and obscurus	Project to the spinal cord

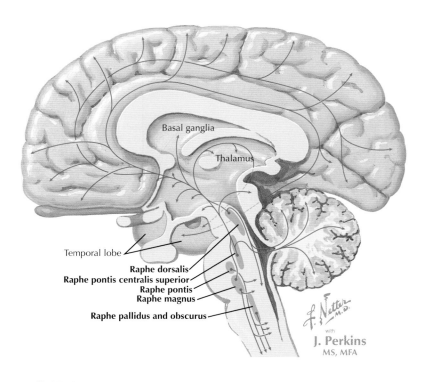

Basal ganglia

Thalamus

Temporal lobe

Raphe dorsalis
Raphe pontis centralis superior
Raphe pontis
Raphe magnus

Raphe pallidus and obscurus

J. Perkins
MS, MFA

LOCUS CERULEUS (NORADRENERGIC PATHWAYS)

- Provides noradrenergic innervation to most of central nervous system
- Believed to play role in regulation of respiration and in rapid eye movement (REM) sleep

STRUCTURE	ANATOMIC NOTES
Locus ceruleus (nucleus pigmentosus)	Small nucleus in the upper pons, near the periventricular gray of the upper 4th ventricle
Descending pathway	Fibers descend in the anterior and lateral funiculi, largely uncrossed, ending in the anterior horn, intermediate gray, and ventral half of the posterior horn
Ascending pathway	Fibers ascend through the midbrain, lateral to the MLF, and ventrolateral to central gray
	In caudal diencephalon, fibers enter the medial forebrain bundle, via the mammillary peduncle, to and through the lateral hypothalamus
	Fibers continue rostrally to the anterior commissure, divide, and innervate the diencephalon and telencephalon
	Stria medullaris component turns caudally to innervate the midline thalamus
	Stria terminalis component supplies the amygdaloid nuclear complex
	Most rostral fibers pass from the medial forebrain bundle to the external capsule to frontal cortex

LOCUS CERULEUS (NORADRENERGIC PATHWAYS) *continued*

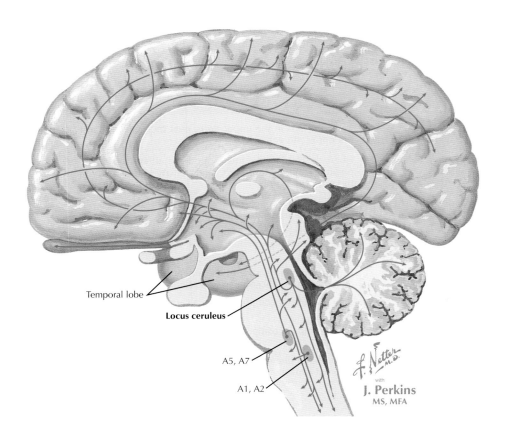

Temporal lobe

Locus ceruleus

A5, A7

A1, A2

Reticular Formation

16 Reticular Formation

RETICULAR FORMATION: OVERVIEW

- A somewhat diffuse collection of neurons and nerve fibers extending from the caudal medulla, beginning just above the pyramidal decussation, to the rostral midbrain, and continuous with the subthalamic zona incerta and thalamic nuclei
- Essentially a matrix within which nuclei and tracts are embedded
- Neurons within the reticular formation discharge in relation to multiple stimuli, including sensory input, pain and escape behavior, conditioning and habituation, arousal, complex motivational states, rapid eye movement (REM) sleep, eye movements, respiration, and locomotion

STRUCTURE	ANATOMIC NOTES	FUNCTIONAL SIGNIFICANCE
Lateral group nuclei	Includes: • Nucleus reticularis lateralis in the medulla • Nucleus reticularis parvocellularis in the pons and medulla • Parabrachial and pedunculopontine in the pons and midbrain • Cuneiform and subcuneiform in the midbrain	Relate to locomotion and autonomic regulation
Medial group nuclei	Includes: • Nucleus reticularis gigantocellularis in the medulla • Nucleus reticularis pontis caudalis and oralis in the pons	Descending connections play a role in motor control, ascending connections play a role in consciousness and alertness
Column of raphe nuclei	Includes: • Raphe obscurus and pallidus in medulla • Raphe magnus in pons and medulla • Dorsal raphe and superior central nuclei in midbrain	Caudal nuclei concerned with pain mechanisms; rostral nuclei relate to sleep, wakefulness, and alertness

OVERVIEW *continued*

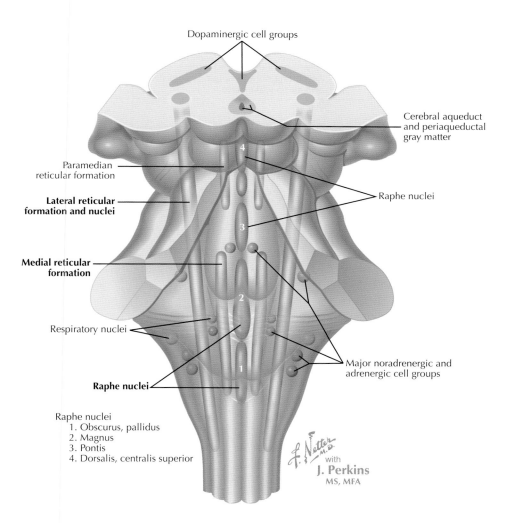

Dopaminergic cell groups

Cerebral aqueduct and periaqueductal gray matter

Paramedian reticular formation

Lateral reticular formation and nuclei

Raphe nuclei

Medial reticular formation

Respiratory nuclei

Major noradrenergic and adrenergic cell groups

Raphe nuclei

Raphe nuclei
1. Obscurus, pallidus
2. Magnus
3. Pontis
4. Dorsalis, centralis superior

with
J. Perkins
MS, MFA

RETICULAR NUCLEI

STRUCTURE	FUNCTIONAL SIGNIFICANCE
Nucleus reticularis gigantocellularis	Reticulospinal regulation of spinal cord lower motor neurons
Paramedian pontine reticular formation (PPRF)	Lateral gaze center
Raphe nuclei	Rostral nuclei are part of ascending reticular activating system concerned with sleep, wakefulness, and alertness
Locus ceruleus	Ascending noradrenergic system involved in attention, mood, and sleep-wake state

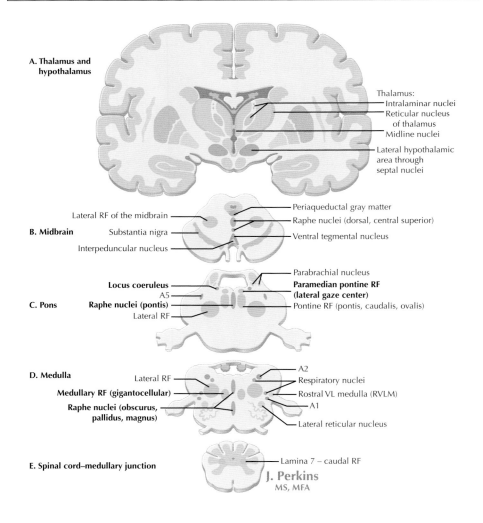

A. Thalamus and hypothalamus

Thalamus:
Intralaminar nuclei
Reticular nucleus of thalamus
Midline nuclei
Lateral hypothalamic area through septal nuclei

B. Midbrain

Lateral RF of the midbrain
Substantia nigra
Interpeduncular nucleus

Periaqueductal gray matter
Raphe nuclei (dorsal, central superior)
Ventral tegmental nucleus

C. Pons

Locus coeruleus
A5
Raphe nuclei (pontis)
Lateral RF

Parabrachial nucleus
Paramedian pontine RF (lateral gaze center)
Pontine RF (pontis, caudalis, ovalis)

D. Medulla

Lateral RF
Medullary RF (gigantocellular)
Raphe nuclei (obscurus, pallidus, magnus)

A2
Respiratory nuclei
Rostral VL medulla (RVLM)
A1
Lateral reticular nucleus

E. Spinal cord–medullary junction

Lamina 7 – caudal RF

J. Perkins
MS, MFA

MAJOR AFFERENT AND EFFERENT CONNECTIONS OF THE RETICULAR FORMATION

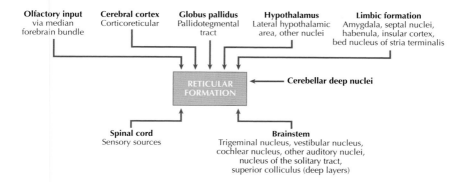

Olfactory input
via median forebrain bundle

Cerebral cortex
Corticoreticular

Globus pallidus
Pallidotegmental tract

Hypothalamus
Lateral hypothalamic area, other nuclei

Limbic formation
Amygdala, septal nuclei, habenula, insular cortex, bed nucleus of stria terminalis

RETICULAR FORMATION ← Cerebellar deep nuclei

Spinal cord
Sensory sources

Brainstem
Trigeminal nucleus, vestibular nucleus, cochlear nucleus, other auditory nuclei, nucleus of the solitary tract, superior colliculus (deep layers)

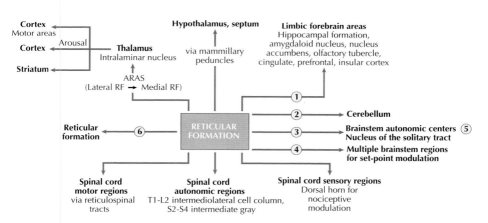

Cortex
Motor areas

Cortex

Striatum

Arousal

Thalamus
Intralaminar nucleus

ARAS
(Lateral RF → Medial RF)

Hypothalamus, septum

via mammillary peduncles

Limbic forebrain areas
Hippocampal formation, amygdaloid nucleus, nucleus accumbens, olfactory tubercle, cingulate, prefrontal, insular cortex

①

② → Cerebellum

Reticular formation ⑥ RETICULAR FORMATION ③ → Brainstem autonomic centers ⑤
Nucleus of the solitary tract

④ → Multiple brainstem regions for set-point modulation

Spinal cord motor regions
via reticulospinal tracts

Spinal cord autonomic regions
T1-L2 intermediolateral cell column, S2-S4 intermediate gray

Spinal cord sensory regions
Dorsal horn for nociceptive modulation

① From lateral reticular nucleus
Nucleus reticularis tegmenti pontis, paramedian reticular nucleus, locus ceruleus, raphe nuclei

② From locus ceruleus, raphe nuclei, ventral tegmental area

③ Via median forebrain bundle, dorsal longitudinal fasciculus, habenulopeduncular tract, mammillotegmental tract

④ From adrenergic, noradrenergic (tegmental and locus ceruleus), serotonergic (raphe) nuclei

⑤ Including ventrolateral and ventromedial tegmentum of caudal brain stem

⑥ Intrareticular connections

J. Perkins
MS, MFA

SLEEP WAKE CONTROL

STRUCTURE	ANATOMIC NOTES	FUNCTIONAL SIGNIFICANCE
Area postrema	Rostral to obex on each side of 4th ventricle	Associated with sleep induction. Also emetic chemoreceptor trigger zone
Suprachiasmatic nucleus of hypothalamus	Dorsal to the optic chiasm, close to the ventral part of the 3rd ventricle	Lesioning eliminates circadian rhythm of sleep-wake cycle
Preoptic hypothalamic area	Periventricular grey of most rostral part of 3rd ventricle	Receives fibers that carry sleep-inducing peptides enkephalin and endorphin
Nucleus basalis	Rostrally lies under cortex of anterior perforated substance	These cholinergic projection neurons are lost in Alzheimer's disease

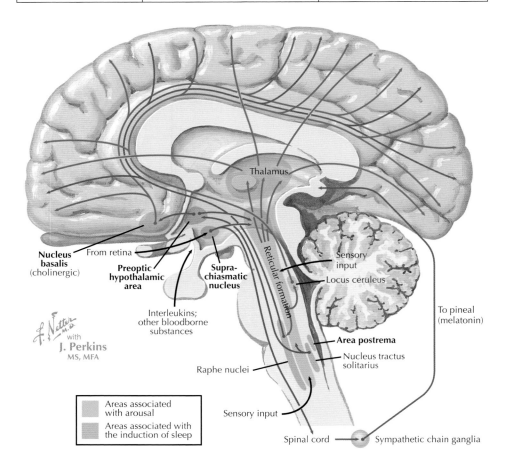

NORADRENERGIC PATHWAYS

STRUCTURE	ANATOMIC NOTES	FUNCTIONAL SIGNIFICANCE
Locus ceruleus	Gives rise to 3 major ascending tracts: • Central tegmental tract • Dorsal longitudinal fasciculus • Medial forebrain bundle	Ascending system involved in modulation of attention, sleep-wake state, and mood
Groups A1-A7 (lateral tegmental noradrenergic system)	Noradrenergic cell groups scattered in pons and medulla	Axons directed to the spinal cord/brainstem (modulate sympathetic function) and diencephalon/telencephalon (sleep-wake state)

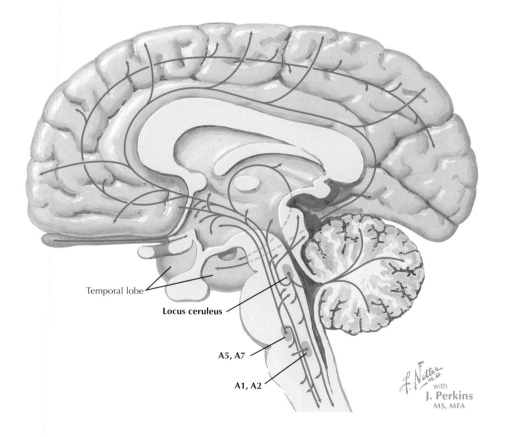

Temporal lobe

Locus ceruleus

A5, A7

A1, A2

SEROTONERGIC PATHWAYS

STRUCTURE	ANATOMIC NOTES	FUNCTIONAL SIGNIFICANCE
Groups B1-B7	Serotonergic neurons within the raphe nuclei of the medulla, pons, and midbrain	Regulate diverse physiologic processes including sleep, aggressive behavior, neuroendocrine function
Raphe dorsalis	Projects to the entire forebrain	Plays a role in psychiatric disorders: depression, anxiety, obsession-compulsion
Raphe pontis, magnus, pallidus, and obscurus	Project to the cerebellum, medulla, spinal cord	Inhibit dorsal horn neurons that give rise to the spinothalamic tract, modulating pain input

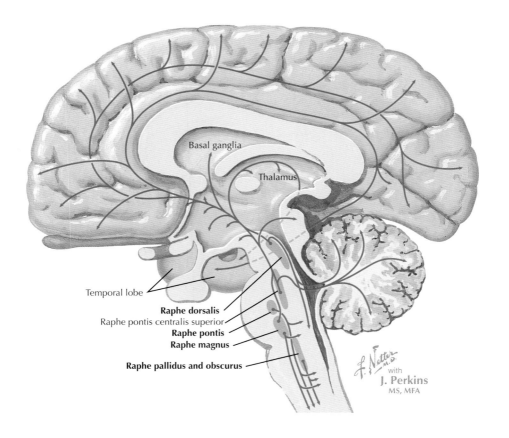

Basal ganglia

Thalamus

Temporal lobe

Raphe dorsalis

Raphe pontis centralis superior

Raphe pontis

Raphe magnus

Raphe pallidus and obscurus

with
J. Perkins
MS, MFA

CENTRAL CHOLINERGIC PATHWAYS

STRUCTURE	ANATOMIC NOTES	FUNCTIONAL SIGNIFICANCE
Brainstem tegmental group	Includes pedunculopontine reticular nucleus and adjacent lateral dorsal tegmental nucleus	Role in arousal and movement Pedunculopontine nucleus is affected in progressive supranuclear palsy
Nucleus basalis	Located in basal forebrain	Sends axons to almost the entire cerebral cortex
Medial septal nucleus	In subcallosal area, rostral to the anterior commissure	Provides interaction between the limbic and diencephalic structures Lesions in mice produce rage, hyperemotionality, heightened activity

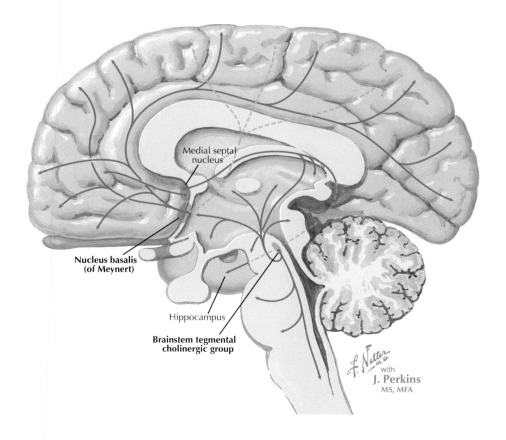

Medial septal nucleus

Nucleus basalis (of Meynert)

Hippocampus

Brainstem tegmental cholinergic group

with
J. Perkins
MS, MFA

CHAPTER 17

Anatomy of the Peripheral Nervous System: Upper Extremity

CERVICAL ROOT ANATOMY

- Filaments (rootlets) emerge from the spinal cord and combine to form the dorsal and ventral spinal nerve roots.
- Nerve roots fuse in the intervertebral foramen, distal to the dorsal root ganglion, to form short spinal nerves.
- C1 to C7 spinal nerves pass above the same-numbered cervical vertebrae to exit the spinal canal.
- C8 passes under C7 and above the T1 vertebra; T1 exits between T1 and T2 vertebrae.
- Spinal nerves divide into the dorsal and ventral ramus (plural, *rami*) on exiting foramen (except for C1, which has no dorsal ramus).
- Dorsal rami supply the skin and paraspinal muscles (except for C1, which has no cutaneous supply).
- The C2 dorsal ramus becomes the greater occipital nerve.
- Ventral rami of C1-4 form the cervical plexus.
- Ventral rami of C5-8 and T1 form the brachial plexus.

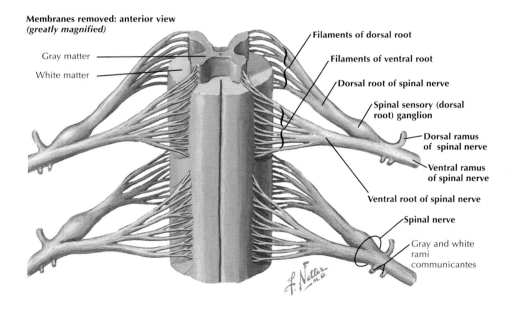

Membranes removed: anterior view
(greatly magnified)

Gray matter

White matter

Filaments of dorsal root

Filaments of ventral root

Dorsal root of spinal nerve

Spinal sensory (dorsal root) ganglion

Dorsal ramus of spinal nerve

Ventral ramus of spinal nerve

Ventral root of spinal nerve

Spinal nerve

Gray and white rami communicantes

CERVICAL ROOT ANATOMY *continued*

Spinal Nerve Origin: Cross Section

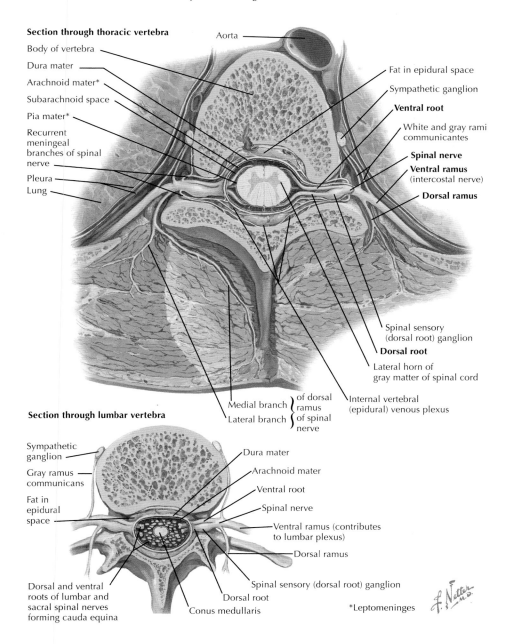

Section through thoracic vertebra

Body of vertebra

Dura mater

Arachnoid mater*

Subarachnoid space

Pia mater*

Recurrent meningeal branches of spinal nerve

Pleura

Lung

Aorta

Fat in epidural space

Sympathetic ganglion

Ventral root

White and gray rami communicantes

Spinal nerve

Ventral ramus (intercostal nerve)

Dorsal ramus

Spinal sensory (dorsal root) ganglion

Dorsal root

Lateral horn of gray matter of spinal cord

Internal vertebral (epidural) venous plexus

Medial branch } of dorsal ramus
Lateral branch } of spinal nerve

Section through lumbar vertebra

Sympathetic ganglion

Gray ramus communicans

Fat in epidural space

Dura mater

Arachnoid mater

Ventral root

Spinal nerve

Ventral ramus (contributes to lumbar plexus)

Dorsal ramus

Spinal sensory (dorsal root) ganglion

Dorsal and ventral roots of lumbar and sacral spinal nerves forming cauda equina

Dorsal root

Conus medullaris

*Leptomeninges

CERVICAL DISC HERNIATION SYNDROME

DISC LEVEL	ROOT AFFECTED	WEAKNESS	NUMBNESS	REFLEX AFFECTED
C3-4	C4	None	Epaulet	None
C4-5	C5	Rhomboid, supraspinatus, infraspinatus, deltoid, biceps, brachioradialis	Skin over deltoid muscle	Biceps, brachioradialis
C5-6	C6	C5 muscles above and extensor carpi radialis longus (ECRL), supinator, pronator teres	Thumb	Biceps, brachioradialis
C6-7	C7	Triceps, wrist and finger extensors, flexor carpi radialis (FCR), pronator teres	Middle (3rd) finger	Triceps
C7-T1	C8	C7 muscles above and finger flexors, flexor carpi ulnaris (FCU), intrinsic hand muscles	Fingers 4 and 5 and hypothenar eminence	Triceps, finger flexor reflex
T1-2	T1	Intrinsic hand muscles	Medial elbow region	Finger flexor reflex

Patients with radiculopathy infrequently lose sensation over the entire dermatome; rather, the sensory abnormality is confined to "signature areas."

CERVICAL DISC HERNIATION SYNDROME *continued*

Cervical disc herniation: clinical manifestations

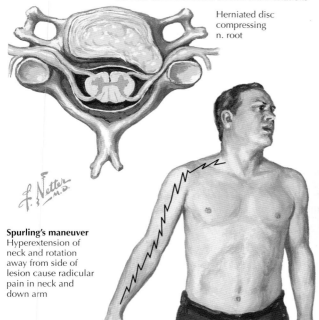

Herniated disc compressing n. root

Spurling's maneuver
Hyperextension of neck and rotation away from side of lesion cause radicular pain in neck and down arm

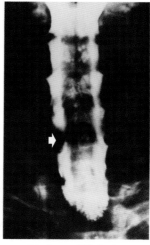

Myelogram (AP view) showing prominent (open arrow) at C6-7 extradural defect

Level	Motor signs (weakness)	Reflex signs	Sensory loss
C5	Deltoid	0	
C6	Biceps brachii	Biceps brachii — Weak or absent reflex	
C7	Triceps brachii	Triceps brachii — Weak or absent reflex	
C8	Interossei	Horner's syndrome	

CERVICAL PLEXUS

The cervical plexus has four cutaneous branches that emerge from the posterior border of the sternocleidomastoid.
- The great(er) auricular (C2-3) supplies skin over the angle of the mandible, parotid, mastoid, and auricle
- Lesser occipital (C2-3) supplies the lateral part of the occiput and medial surface of the auricle
- Supraclavicular (C3-4)
- The transverse cervical nerve (transverse cutaneous of neck) (C2-3) supplies skin over the anterior and lateral neck from the mandible to the sternum

The cervical plexus has several muscular branches:
- Phrenic nerve (C3-4-5 to diaphragm)
- Accessory nerve: receives branches from the cervical plexus; these branches ascend to enter the foramen magnum, join cranial nerve (CN)-XI, and exit through the jugular foramen with CN-IX and -X. This nerve supplies the trapezius and sternocleidomastoid
- The levator scapulae (C3-4) raises the medial border of the scapula and braces the shoulder backward
- Short, muscular branches to adjacent muscles

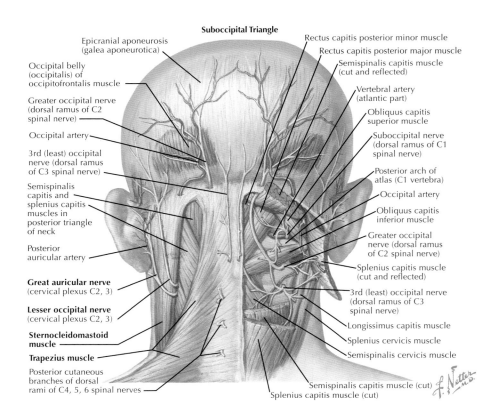

Suboccipital Triangle

Epicranial aponeurosis (galea aponeurotica)

Occipital belly (occipitalis) of occipitofrontalis muscle

Greater occipital nerve (dorsal ramus of C2 spinal nerve)

Occipital artery

3rd (least) occipital nerve (dorsal ramus of C3 spinal nerve)

Semispinalis capitis and splenius capitis muscles in posterior triangle of neck

Posterior auricular artery

Great auricular nerve (cervical plexus C2, 3)

Lesser occipital nerve (cervical plexus C2, 3)

Sternocleidomastoid muscle

Trapezius muscle

Posterior cutaneous branches of dorsal rami of C4, 5, 6 spinal nerves

Rectus capitis posterior minor muscle
Rectus capitis posterior major muscle
Semispinalis capitis muscle (cut and reflected)
Vertebral artery (atlantic part)
Obliquus capitis superior muscle
Suboccipital nerve (dorsal ramus of C1 spinal nerve)
Posterior arch of atlas (C1 vertebra)
Occipital artery
Obliquus capitis inferior muscle
Greater occipital nerve (dorsal ramus of C2 spinal nerve)
Splenius capitis muscle (cut and reflected)
3rd (least) occipital nerve (dorsal ramus of C3 spinal nerve)
Longissimus capitis muscle
Splenius cervicis muscle
Semispinalis cervicis muscle
Semispinalis capitis muscle (cut)
Splenius capitis muscle (cut)

CERVICAL PLEXUS *continued*

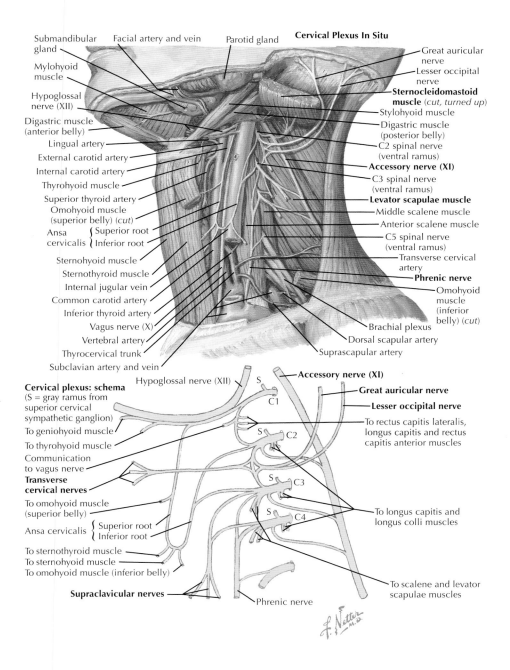

Cervical Plexus In Situ

Submandibular gland
Facial artery and vein
Parotid gland
Mylohyoid muscle
Hypoglossal nerve (XII)
Digastric muscle (anterior belly)
Lingual artery
External carotid artery
Internal carotid artery
Thyrohyoid muscle
Superior thyroid artery
Omohyoid muscle (superior belly) (cut)
Ansa cervicalis { Superior root / Inferior root }
Sternohyoid muscle
Sternothyroid muscle
Internal jugular vein
Common carotid artery
Inferior thyroid artery
Vagus nerve (X)
Vertebral artery
Thyrocervical trunk
Subclavian artery and vein

Great auricular nerve
Lesser occipital nerve
Sternocleidomastoid muscle (cut, turned up)
Stylohyoid muscle
Digastric muscle (posterior belly)
C2 spinal nerve (ventral ramus)
Accessory nerve (XI)
C3 spinal nerve (ventral ramus)
Levator scapulae muscle
Middle scalene muscle
Anterior scalene muscle
C5 spinal nerve (ventral ramus)
Transverse cervical artery
Phrenic nerve
Omohyoid muscle (inferior belly) (cut)
Brachial plexus
Dorsal scapular artery
Suprascapular artery

Cervical plexus: schema
(S = gray ramus from superior cervical sympathetic ganglion)

Hypoglossal nerve (XII)
S
C1

Accessory nerve (XI)
Great auricular nerve
Lesser occipital nerve

To geniohyoid muscle
To thyrohyoid muscle
Communication to vagus nerve
Transverse cervical nerves
To omohyoid muscle (superior belly)
Ansa cervicalis { Superior root / Inferior root }
To sternothyroid muscle
To sternohyoid muscle
To omohyoid muscle (inferior belly)
Supraclavicular nerves

S
C2
S
C3
S
C4

To rectus capitis lateralis, longus capitis and rectus capitis anterior muscles
To longus capitis and longus colli muscles
To scalene and levator scapulae muscles

Phrenic nerve

BRACHIAL PLEXUS COMPONENTS

NERVE	ROOT(S)	MUSCLE INNERVATED (ACTION)	SENSORY DERMATOME
Upper Trunk			
Suprascapular	C5-6	Supraspinatus (first 15 degrees of shoulder abduction), infraspinatus (external rotation)	None
To the subclavius	C5-6	Subclavius (depresses the clavicle and steadies it during shoulder movement)	None
Lateral Cord			
Lateral pectoral	C5-7	Upper part of the pectoralis major	None
Musculocutaneous	C5-6	Elbow flexors: biceps brachii, coracobrachialis, brachialis	Lateral aspect of forearm
Lateral component of median	C5-6 (C7 from middle trunk)	Pronator teres, flexor carpi radialis (FCR)	Median hand
Posterior Cord			
Thoracodorsal	C6-8	Latissimus dorsi	None
Upper subscapular	C5-6	Subscapularis	None
Lower subscapular	C5-6	Subscapularis, teres major	None
Axillary	C5-6	Deltoid, teres minor	Patch of skin over deltoid
Radial	C5-8	All radial muscles	Lateral 3 and $\frac{1}{2}$ dorsal hand
Medial Cord			
Medial pectoral	C8-T1	Lower part pectoralis major, pectoralis minor	None
Medial cutaneous nerve of the arm	C8-T1	None	Medial aspect of the arm
Medial cutaneous nerve of the forearm	C8-T1	None	Medial aspect of the forearm
Ulnar	C8-T1	All ulnar muscles	Medial 1 and $\frac{1}{2}$ hand
Medial component of median	C8-T1	Flexor digitorum superficialis (FDS), flexor pollicis longus (FPL), flexor digitorum profundus (FDP) I and II, lumbricals, opponens pollicis, abductor pollicis brevis, flexor pollicis brevis (superficial head) (LOAF)	None

BRACHIAL PLEXUS COMPONENTS *continued*

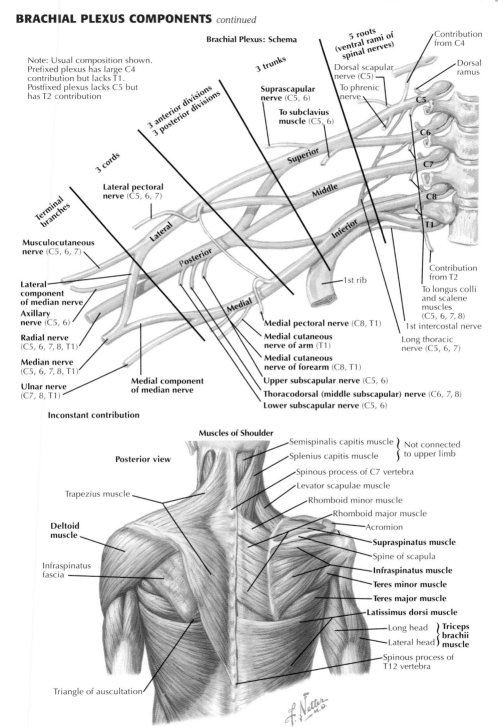

Brachial Plexus: Schema

Note: Usual composition shown.
Prefixed plexus has large C4
contribution but lacks T1.
Postfixed plexus lacks C5 but
has T2 contribution

5 roots
(ventral rami of
spinal nerves)

3 trunks

3 anterior divisions
3 posterior divisions

3 cords

Terminal
branches

Contribution
from C4

Dorsal scapular
nerve (C5)

Dorsal
ramus

Suprascapular
nerve (C5, 6)

To subclavius
muscle (C5, 6)

To phrenic
nerve

Superior

Middle

Inferior

Lateral

Posterior

Medial

Lateral pectoral
nerve (C5, 6, 7)

Musculocutaneous
nerve (C5, 6, 7)

Lateral
component
of median nerve

Axillary
nerve (C5, 6)

Radial nerve
(C5, 6, 7, 8, T1)

Median nerve
(C5, 6, 7, 8, T1)

Ulnar nerve
(C7, 8, T1)

Medial component
of median nerve

Inconstant contribution

1st rib

Medial pectoral nerve (C8, T1)

Medial cutaneous
nerve of arm (T1)

Medial cutaneous
nerve of forearm (C8, T1)

Upper subscapular nerve (C5, 6)

Thoracodorsal (middle subscapular) nerve (C6, 7, 8)

Lower subscapular nerve (C5, 6)

C5

C6

C7

C8

T1

Contribution
from T2

To longus colli
and scalene
muscles
(C5, 6, 7, 8)

1st intercostal nerve

Long thoracic
nerve (C5, 6, 7)

Muscles of Shoulder

Posterior view

Trapezius muscle

Deltoid
muscle

Infraspinatus
fascia

Triangle of auscultation

Semispinalis capitis muscle } Not connected
Splenius capitis muscle   } to upper limb

Spinous process of C7 vertebra

Levator scapulae muscle

Rhomboid minor muscle

Rhomboid major muscle

Acromion

Supraspinatus muscle

Spine of scapula

Infraspinatus muscle

Teres minor muscle

Teres major muscle

Latissimus dorsi muscle

Long head } **Triceps**
Lateral head } **brachii**
             } **muscle**

Spinous process of
T12 vertebra

BRACHIAL PLEXUS

The brachial plexus forms from the ventral rami of C5-8 and T1:
- C5 and C6 ventral rami join to form the superior (upper) trunk.
- C7 ventral ramus continues alone to form the middle trunk.
- C8 and T1 ventral rami join to form the inferior (lower) trunk.

Each trunk divides into an anterior and posterior division:
- All three posterior divisions join to form the posterior cord.
- Anterior divisions of the superior and middle trunks join to form the lateral cord.
- The anterior division of the inferior trunk continues as the medial cord.

In the neck, the brachial plexus lies between the anterior and medial scalene muscles and above the first rib:
- It emerges behind the lower part of the sternocleidomastoid.
- It passes under the clavicle, over the first rib, to reach the axilla.
- The T1 ramus and lower trunk lie on pleura over the lung apex, and the trunk curves over the first rib to reach the axilla.

The dorsal scapular nerve supplies the rhomboid (elevates the medial border of the scapula and pulls it medially); it arises from the C5 ventral ramus.
- The phrenic nerve supplies the diaphragm; it arises from the ventral rami of C3-5.
- The long thoracic nerve supplies the serratus anterior; it arises from the ventral rami of C5-7.

BRACHIAL PLEXUS *continued*

Axilla (Dissection): Anterior View

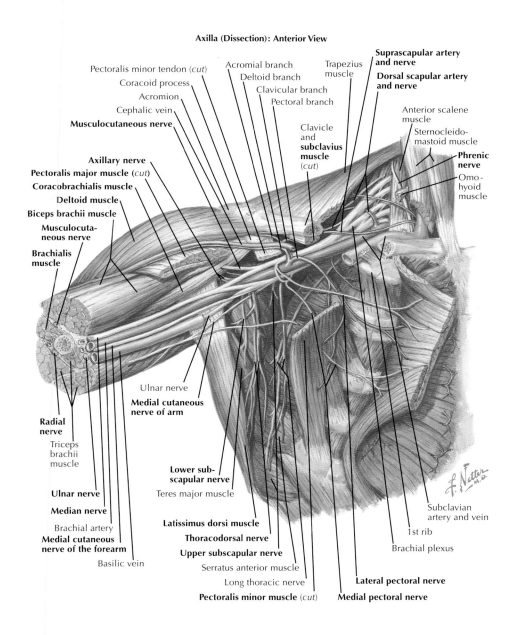

Pectoralis minor tendon (*cut*)
Coracoid process
Acromion
Cephalic vein
Musculocutaneous nerve

Acromial branch
Deltoid branch
Clavicular branch
Pectoral branch

Trapezius muscle

Suprascapular artery and nerve
Dorsal scapular artery and nerve

Clavicle and **subclavius muscle** (*cut*)

Anterior scalene muscle
Sternocleido-mastoid muscle
Phrenic nerve
Omo-hyoid muscle

Axillary nerve
Pectoralis major muscle (*cut*)
Coracobrachialis muscle
Deltoid muscle
Biceps brachii muscle
Musculocuta-neous nerve
Brachialis muscle

Ulnar nerve
Medial cutaneous nerve of arm

Radial nerve
Triceps brachii muscle

Ulnar nerve
Median nerve
Brachial artery
Medial cutaneous nerve of the forearm
Basilic vein

Lower sub-scapular nerve
Teres major muscle

Latissimus dorsi muscle
Thoracodorsal nerve
Upper subscapular nerve
Serratus anterior muscle
Long thoracic nerve
Pectoralis minor muscle (*cut*)

Subclavian artery and vein
1st rib
Brachial plexus

Lateral pectoral nerve
Medial pectoral nerve

BRACHIAL PLEXOPATHY

Causes of brachial plexopathy include the following:
- Trauma
- Tumor invasion
- Radiation-induced
- Acute brachial plexus neuropathy (brachial neuritis, neuralgic amyotrophy, Parsonage-Turner syndrome)
- Cervical rib (see Thoracic Outlet Syndrome to follow)
- Hereditary neuropathy with liability to pressure palsies

WEAKNESS PATTERN IN FOCAL BRACHIAL PLEXOPATHY	
Upper Trunk	Supraspinatus and infraspinatus, deltoid, biceps, brachioradialis (BR)
Middle Trunk	Latissimus dorsi, radial muscles (except BR), pronator teres, FCR
Lower Trunk	Intrinsic hand muscles, FCU, FDS, FPL, FDP
Lateral Cord	Biceps, FCR, pronator teres
Posterior Cord	Radial muscles, deltoid, latissimus dorsi
Medial Cord	Intrinsic hand muscles, FCU, FDP, FPL

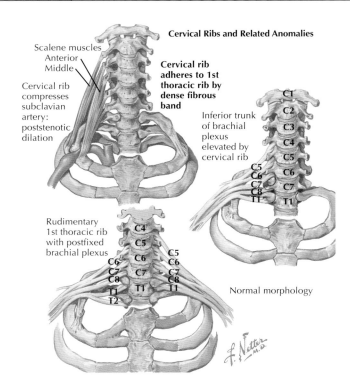

Scalene muscles
Anterior
Middle
Cervical rib compresses subclavian artery: poststenotic dilation

Cervical Ribs and Related Anomalies

Cervical rib adheres to 1st thoracic rib by dense fibrous band

Inferior trunk of brachial plexus elevated by cervical rib

Rudimentary 1st thoracic rib with postfixed brachial plexus

Normal morphology

THORACIC OUTLET

STRUCTURE	ANATOMIC NOTES	FUNCTIONAL SIGNIFICANCE
Thoracic outlet	This area contains the lower portions of the anterior and middle scalene muscles, the 1st rib, and the clavicle. The brachial plexus and subclavian artery and subclavian vein pass through it. The apex of the lung projects into it from below.	Thoracic outlet syndrome (TOS) denotes: • Arterial compromise of the subclavian artery (arterial TOS) • Venous compromise of the subclavian vein (venous TOS) • Neurologic compromise of the brachial plexus (neurologic TOS) with the lower trunk of the brachial plexus being stretched over a rudimentary cervical rib or fibrous band (lower trunk brachial plexopathy) • Combinations of the above Patients experience: • Wasting and weakness of the hand • Paresthesias over the medial forearm and hand • Aching of arm (pain is unusual)

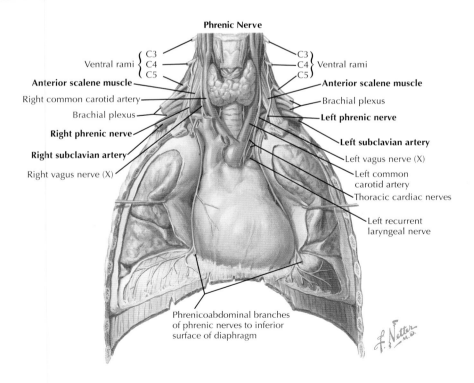

Phrenic Nerve

Ventral rami { C3 C4 C5 — C3 C4 C5 } Ventral rami

Anterior scalene muscle
Right common carotid artery
Brachial plexus
Right phrenic nerve
Right subclavian artery
Right vagus nerve (X)

Anterior scalene muscle
Brachial plexus
Left phrenic nerve
Left subclavian artery
Left vagus nerve (X)
Left common carotid artery
Thoracic cardiac nerves
Left recurrent laryngeal nerve

Phrenicoabdominal branches of phrenic nerves to inferior surface of diaphragm

NERVES OF THE BRACHIAL PLEXUS

NERVE	ROOTS	SUPPLIES	COURSE	INJURY
Long thoracic	C5-7 ventral rami directly	Serratus anterior	Down the anterolateral chest wall to digitations of serratus anterior	Results in winged scapula

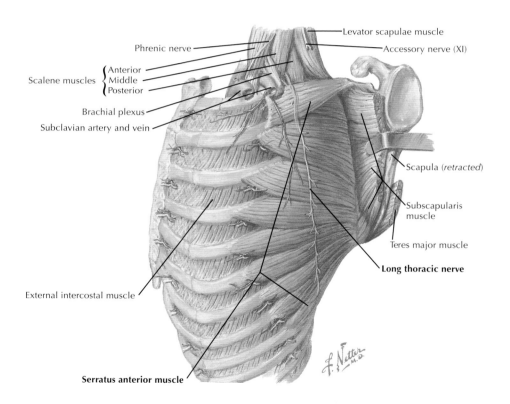

NERVES OF THE BRACHIAL PLEXUS *continued*

NERVE	ROOTS	SUPPLIES	COURSE	INJURY
Thoracodorsal	C6-8 ventral rami, posterior cord	Latissimus dorsi	Runs down on the subscapularis to reach latissimus dorsi muscle	Weakness of arm extension and adduction

Posterolateral Abdominal Wall

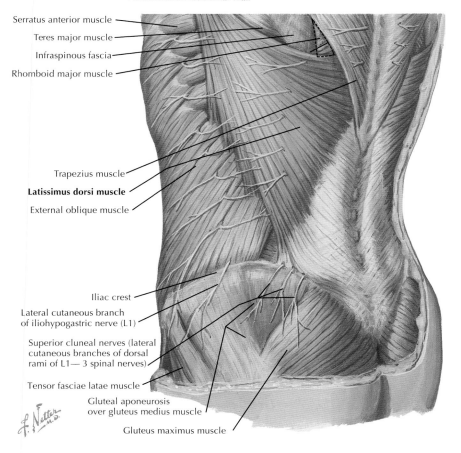

Serratus anterior muscle

Teres major muscle

Infraspinous fascia

Rhomboid major muscle

Trapezius muscle

Latissimus dorsi muscle

External oblique muscle

Iliac crest

Lateral cutaneous branch of iliohypogastric nerve (L1)

Superior cluneal nerves (lateral cutaneous branches of dorsal rami of L1— 3 spinal nerves)

Tensor fasciae latae muscle

Gluteal aponeurosis over gluteus medius muscle

Gluteus maximus muscle

NERVES OF THE BRACHIAL PLEXUS *continued*

NERVE	ROOTS	SUPPLIES	COURSE	INJURY
Suprascapular	C5-6 ventral rami, upper trunk	Supraspinatus and infraspinatus	Under the trapezius, through the suprascapular notch to the supraspinous fossa, and then around the spinoglenoid notch	Results in wasting and weakness of the supraspinatus (first 15 degrees of shoulder abduction) and infraspinatus (external [lateral] rotation of the shoulder)
Axillary nerve	C5-6 ventral rami, posterior cord	Deltoid muscle and skin over the deltoid muscle	Below the shoulder joint, around the posterior and lateral surface of the humerus, deep to the deltoid	Results in wasting and weakness of deltoid with weak shoulder abduction

NERVES OF THE BRACHIAL PLEXUS *continued*

Scapulohumeral Dissection

Anterior view

Coracoacromial ligament

Coracoid process

Acromion

Supraspinatus tendon

Suprascapular artery and nerve

Greater tubercle of humerus

Superior transverse scapular ligament and suprascapular notch

Subscapularis tendon

Pectoralis minor tendon (*cut*)

Biceps brachii tendon (short head) (cut) and coracobrachialis tendon (cut)

Biceps brachii tendon (long head) (*cut*)

Subscapularis muscle

Axillary nerve and posterior circumflex humeral artery

Lower subscapular nerve (to teres major muscle)

Radial nerve

Biceps brachii muscle { Long head / Short head

Thoracodorsal artery and nerve (to latissimus dorsi muscle)

Coracobrachialis muscle

Subscapularis muscle

Teres major muscle

Latissimus dorsi muscle

Suprascapular artery and nerve

Posterior view

Acromion

Infraspinatus tendon (*reflected*)

Joint capsule of shoulder

Superior transverse scapular ligament and suprascapular notch

Deltoid muscle (*reflected*)

Supraspinatus muscle (*cut*)

Teres minor muscle

Spine of scapula

Quadrangular space transmitting axillary nerve and posterior circumflex humeral artery

Infraspinatus muscle (*cut*)

Superior lateral cutaneous nerve of arm

Teres major muscle

Radial nerve shown between

Lateral head and

Long head of triceps brachii muscle

MEDIAN NERVE (TO WRIST)

Roots	C5-T1
Trunk of Brachial Plexus	Upper, middle, lower
Division of Brachial Plexus	Anterior division of the upper, middle, and lower trunk
Cord of Brachial Plexus	Lateral and medial
Course from Axilla to Hand	Union of the lateral and medial cord of the brachial plexus (See page 311)
	Lateral wall of axilla to the medial upper arm
	Crosses the antecubital fossa medial to the biceps tendon and brachial artery
	Passes beneath the bicipital aponeurosis (site of entrapment)
	Between the heads of the pronator teres (site of entrapment)
	Under the FDS sublimis bridge
	Descends the forearm between the FDS and FDP
	Enters the hand under the carpal ligament (the most common site of entrapment)
Muscles Innervated and Function	None above the elbow
	Pronator teres: pronates/flexes forearm
	FCR—flexes/abducts hand at wrist
	FDS—flexes the middle phalanx of fingers 2-5
	Anterior interosseous nerve
	FPL—flexes distal phalanx of thumb*
	FDP—2 and 3: flexes distal phalanx fingers 2-3*
	Pronator quadratus—pronates forearm*
Sensory Branches and Dermatome	No sensation above the wrist
	Palmar cutaneous branch (arises above the wrist): supplies the thenar eminence
Injury	May be injured at:
	• Axilla—compression by crutches, anterior shoulder dislocation
	• Upper arm—sleep palsy, knife wounds, tourniquet, humerus fracture
	• Elbow—supracondylar ligament, elbow dislocation, injection injury
	• Pronator teres—produces pronator teres syndrome with weakness of median innervated muscles distal to pronator teres
	• Anterior interosseous neuropathy—fibrous band, radius fracture
	• Carpal tunnel syndrome (below the wrist)
Clinical Notes	Anterior interosseous neuropathy results in "O" sign due to inability to flex DIP joint of index finger (FDP 2) and IP joint of thumb (FPL).
	Median neuropathy at elbow causes clumsy or weak fingers 1-4
	Tinel sign may be seen at site of lesion
	Median hand sensory symptoms occur with lesion at or above wrist

*The anterior interosseous nerve arises from the median nerve as it emerges between the two heads of the pronator teres. It supplies the FPL, FDP 2 and 3, and the pronator quadratus.

MEDIAN NERVE (TO WRIST) *continued*

Arteries and Nerves of Upper Limb

Anterior view

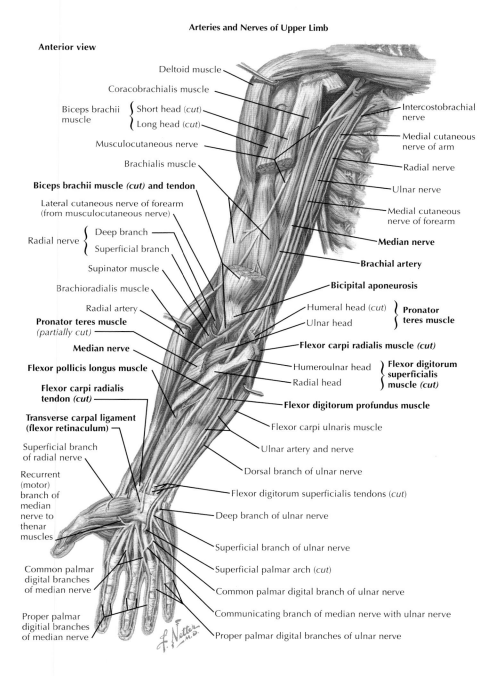

Deltoid muscle

Coracobrachialis muscle

Biceps brachii muscle { Short head *(cut)* / Long head *(cut)* }

Musculocutaneous nerve

Brachialis muscle

Biceps brachii muscle (cut) and tendon

Lateral cutaneous nerve of forearm (from musculocutaneous nerve)

Radial nerve { Deep branch / Superficial branch }

Supinator muscle

Brachioradialis muscle

Radial artery

Pronator teres muscle (partially cut)

Median nerve

Flexor pollicis longus muscle

Flexor carpi radialis tendon *(cut)*

Transverse carpal ligament (flexor retinaculum)

Superficial branch of radial nerve

Recurrent (motor) branch of median nerve to thenar muscles

Common palmar digital branches of median nerve

Proper palmar digitial branches of median nerve

Intercostobrachial nerve

Medial cutaneous nerve of arm

Radial nerve

Ulnar nerve

Medial cutaneous nerve of forearm

Median nerve

Brachial artery

Bicipital aponeurosis

Humeral head *(cut)* } **Pronator teres muscle**
Ulnar head

Flexor carpi radialis muscle *(cut)*

Humeroulnar head } **Flexor digitorum superficialis muscle *(cut)***
Radial head

Flexor digitorum profundus muscle

Flexor carpi ulnaris muscle

Ulnar artery and nerve

Dorsal branch of ulnar nerve

Flexor digitorum superficialis tendons *(cut)*

Deep branch of ulnar nerve

Superficial branch of ulnar nerve

Superficial palmar arch *(cut)*

Common palmar digital branch of ulnar nerve

Communicating branch of median nerve with ulnar nerve

Proper palmar digital branches of ulnar nerve

MEDIAN NERVE (TO WRIST) *continued*

Median Nerve

Anterior view

Note: Only muscles innervated by median nerve shown

Musculocutaneous nerve

Median nerve (C5, 6, 7, 8, T1)
Inconstant contribution

Pronator teres muscle (humeral head)

Articular branch

Flexor carpi radialis muscle

Palmaris longus muscle

Pronator teres muscle (ulnar head)

Flexor digitorum superficialis muscle *(turned up)*

Flexor digitorum profundus muscle (lateral part supplied by median [anterior interosseous] nerve; medial part supplied by ulnar nerve)

Anterior interosseous nerve

Flexor pollicis longus muscle

Pronator quadratus muscle

Palmar branch of median nerve

Abductor pollicis brevis

Opponens pollicis

Thenar muscles

Superficial head of flexor pollicis brevis (deep head supplied by ulnar nerve)

1st and 2nd lumbrical muscles

Dorsal branches to dorsum of middle and distal phalanges

Medial
Posterior
Lateral
} Cords of brachial plexus

Medial cutaneous nerve of arm

Medial cutaneous nerve of forearm

Axillary nerve

Radial nerve

Ulnar nerve

Cutaneous innervation

Palmar view

Communicating branch of median nerve with ulnar nerve

Common palmar digital nerves

Proper palmar digital nerves

Posterior (dorsal) view

MEDIAN NERVE (HAND)

Course in the Hand	Enters the hand through the carpal tunnel
	Distal to the tunnel, it divides into 2 major branches: lateral and medial terminal branches
	Lateral terminal branch divides into common digital nerves to supply thumb and lateral side of index finger through proper palmar digital nerves
	Medial terminal branch divides into common digital nerves to supply the medial index, finger 3, and lateral finger 4 through proper palmar digital nerves
Muscles Innervated and Function	Branch to thenar eminence
	Abductor pollicis brevis—abducts thumb at carpometacarpal and metacarpophalangeal (MCP) joints
	Opponens—pulls the thumb metacarpal (MC) medially and forward
	Flexor pollicis brevis—flexes MCP joint of thumb
	Lumbricals 1,2—flex MCP, extend IP joints
Sensory Branches and Dermatome	Digital branches: Palmar surface of thumb, fingers 2, 3, lateral half of finger 4 and associated palm and dorsal tips of lateral 3 and $\frac{1}{2}$ fingers
Disorders	Carpal tunnel syndrome
Clinical Notes	Paresthesiae and pain, particularly at night
	Relief by shaking hand
	Symptoms often worsen with hand activities
	Three times more common in women
	Dominant hand often first affected
	Often bilateral
Differential Diagnosis	C6 or C7 radiculopathy
	TOS

Mnemonic for median innervated intrinsic hand muscles is LOAF:

- **L**umbricals
- **O**pponens pollicis
- **A**bductor pollicis brevis
- **F**lexor pollicis brevis

MEDIAN NERVE (HAND) *continued*

Flexor Tendons, Arteries and Nerves at Wrist

Palmar view

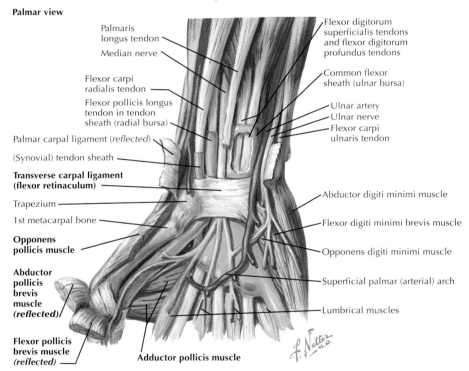

Palmaris longus tendon

Median nerve

Flexor carpi radialis tendon

Flexor pollicis longus tendon in tendon sheath (radial bursa)

Palmar carpal ligament (*reflected*)

(Synovial) tendon sheath

Transverse carpal ligament (flexor retinaculum)

Trapezium

1st metacarpal bone

Opponens pollicis muscle

Abductor pollicis brevis muscle (reflected)

Flexor pollicis brevis muscle (reflected)

Adductor pollicis muscle

Flexor digitorum superficialis tendons and flexor digitorum profundus tendons

Common flexor sheath (ulnar bursa)

Ulnar artery

Ulnar nerve

Flexor carpi ulnaris tendon

Abductor digiti minimi muscle

Flexor digiti minimi brevis muscle

Opponens digiti minimi muscle

Superficial palmar (arterial) arch

Lumbrical muscles

MEDIAN NERVE (HAND) *continued*

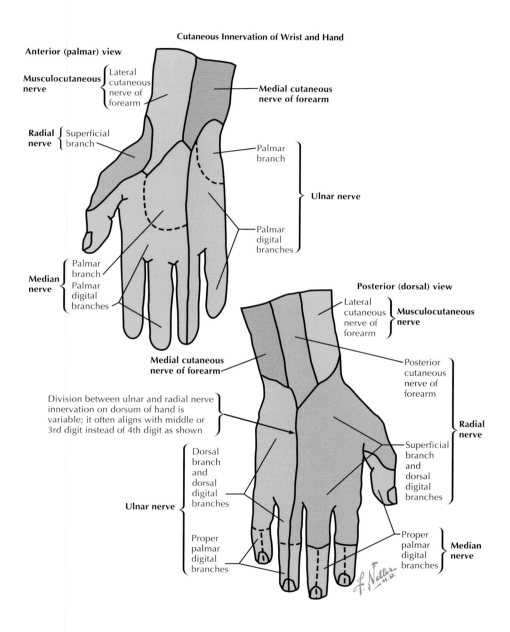

Cutaneous Innervation of Wrist and Hand

Anterior (palmar) view

Musculocutaneous nerve — Lateral cutaneous nerve of forearm

Medial cutaneous nerve of forearm

Radial nerve { Superficial branch

Palmar branch

Ulnar nerve

Palmar digital branches

Median nerve { Palmar branch — Palmar digital branches

Posterior (dorsal) view

Lateral cutaneous nerve of forearm — Musculocutaneous nerve

Medial cutaneous nerve of forearm

Posterior cutaneous nerve of forearm

Division between ulnar and radial nerve innervation on dorsum of hand is variable; it often aligns with middle or 3rd digit instead of 4th digit as shown

Radial nerve

Ulnar nerve { Dorsal branch and dorsal digital branches

Superficial branch and dorsal digital branches

Proper palmar digital branches

Proper palmar digital branches — Median nerve

ULNAR NERVE (TO WRIST)

Roots	C8-T1
Trunk of Brachial Plexus	Lower
Division of Brachial Plexus	Anterior division of the lower trunk
Cord of Brachial Plexus	Medial
Course from Axilla to Hand	Medial cord brachial plexus
	Lateral wall of axilla
	Medial upper arm
	Behind the medial epicondyle of humerus
	Under the FCU aponeurosis
	Runs down the forearm between the FDP (posterior) and FCU (anterior)
	Enters the hand through the Guyon canal (between pisiform and hook of hamate)
Muscles Innervated	Above the elbow, no branches
	Below the elbow, in forearm; only 2 branches:
	• FCU—flex/adduct hand at wrist • FDP—flex distal interphalangeal (DIP) joint of fingers 4 and 5
Sensory Branches and Dermatome	Palmar cutaneous (arises midforearm, crosses the wrist, not through the Guyon canal)—supplies proximal medial palm below wrist
	Dorsal cutaneous (arises 5 cm above the wrist, winds dorsally around wrist)—supplies the ulnar dorsum of the hand and dorsal fingers 5 and medial half of 4
Disorders	Old elbow fracture—tardy ulnar palsy
	Acute trauma—fracture, dislocation of elbow
	External pressure at elbow
	Soft tissue elbow masses—ganglia, lipoma, epidermoid cyst
Clinical Notes	Sensory symptoms in the ulnar innervated hand and fingers
	Pain at the elbow or ulnar innervated parts of hand or diffuse in the arm
	Clumsy or weak fingers
	Tinel sign over nerve at the region of injury
	Ulnar hand sensory loss
	Ulnar claw deformity
Anatomic Notes	Only 2 ulnar innervated muscles above the wrist: FCU and FDP 4 and 5
	All ulnar-innervated muscles have a C8-T1 root supply

ULNAR NERVE (TO WRIST) *continued*

Ulnar Nerve

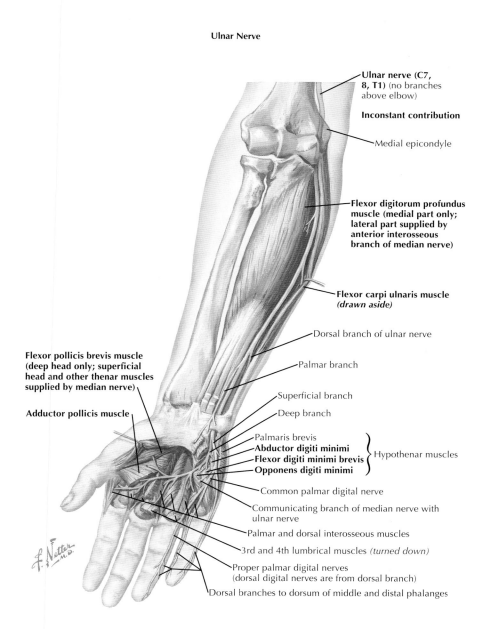

Ulnar nerve (C7,
8, T1) (no branches
above elbow)

Inconstant contribution

Medial epicondyle

Flexor digitorum profundus
muscle (medial part only;
lateral part supplied by
anterior interosseous
branch of median nerve)

Flexor carpi ulnaris muscle
(drawn aside)

Dorsal branch of ulnar nerve

Palmar branch

Flexor pollicis brevis muscle
(deep head only; superficial
head and other thenar muscles
supplied by median nerve)

Superficial branch

Deep branch

Adductor pollicis muscle

Palmaris brevis
Abductor digiti minimi   ⎫
Flexor digiti minimi brevis   ⎬ Hypothenar muscles
Opponens digiti minimi   ⎭

Common palmar digital nerve

Communicating branch of median nerve with
ulnar nerve

Palmar and dorsal interosseous muscles

3rd and 4th lumbrical muscles *(turned down)*

Proper palmar digital nerves
(dorsal digital nerves are from dorsal branch)

Dorsal branches to dorsum of middle and distal phalanges

ULNAR NERVE: HAND

Course in the Hand	Enters the hand through the Guyon canal (between the pisiform and the hook of hamate)
	Distal to the tunnel, gives branch to palmaris brevis
	Then divides into the superficial and deep terminal branches
	Superficial terminal branch (mainly sensory) supplies the distal ulnar border of the palm and then divides into 2 palmar digital nerves that innervate medial 1 and $\frac{1}{2}$ fingers
	Deep terminal branch (purely motor) supplies the opponens digiti minimi, then curves laterally deep to the flexor tendons, supplying the hypothenar muscles, interossei, lumbricals 3 and 4, and terminates in the thenar eminence, supplying the adductor pollicis and the ulnar head of the flexor pollicis brevis
Muscles Innervated and Function	Opponens digiti minimi rotates the 5th MC slightly
	Abductor digiti minimi abducts the 5th finger at MCP joint
	Flexor digiti minimi flexes 5th finger at MCP joint
	Dorsal interossei abduct fingers away from finger 3
	Palmar interossei adduct fingers toward finger 3
	Lumbricals 3 and 4 flex the MCP and extend IP joints
	Adductor pollicis adducts thumb at the carpometacarpal (CMC) and MCP joint
	Deep (ulnar head) of the flexor pollicis brevis (FPB) flexes the MCP of the thumb
Sensory Branches and Dermatome	Superficial terminal branch supplies distal ulnar border of the palm and then divides into 3 palmar digital branches to supply finger 5 and ulnar half of 4
Disorders	Compression in the Guyon canal
	Compression of the deep terminal branch distal to the hypothenar muscle innervation
Clinical Notes	Atrophy of intrinsic ulnar innervated muscles (varies with the precise site of lesion)
	Weakness of intrinsic ulnar innervated muscles (varies with the precise site of lesion)
	Ulnar distribution sensory loss (varies with the precise site of lesion)
Differential Diagnosis	Ulnar neuropathy at the elbow
	Amyotrophic lateral sclerosis
	C8-T1 radiculopathy

ULNAR NERVE: HAND *continued*

Intrinsic Muscles of Hand

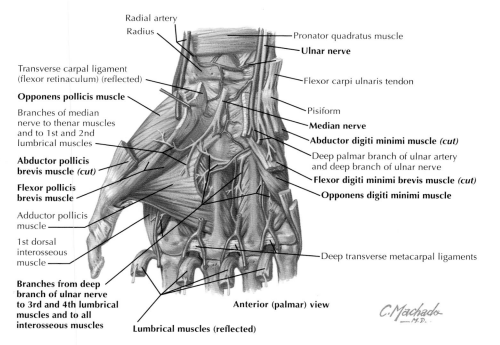

Radial artery

Radius

Transverse carpal ligament
(flexor retinaculum) (reflected)

Opponens pollicis muscle

Branches of median
nerve to thenar muscles
and to 1st and 2nd
lumbrical muscles

**Abductor pollicis
brevis muscle *(cut)***

**Flexor pollicis
brevis muscle**

Adductor pollicis
muscle

1st dorsal
interosseous
muscle

**Branches from deep
branch of ulnar nerve
to 3rd and 4th lumbrical
muscles and to all
interosseous muscles**

Pronator quadratus muscle

Ulnar nerve

Flexor carpi ulnaris tendon

Pisiform

Median nerve

Abductor digiti minimi muscle *(cut)*

Deep palmar branch of ulnar artery
and deep branch of ulnar nerve

Flexor digiti minimi brevis muscle *(cut)*

Opponens digiti minimi muscle

Deep transverse metacarpal ligaments

Anterior (palmar) view

Lumbrical muscles (reflected)

C. Machado
—M.D.

RADIAL NERVE

Roots	C5-T1
Trunk of Brachial Plexus	Upper, middle, lower
Division of Brachial Plexus	Posterior divisions of the upper, middle, and lower trunk
Cord of Brachial Plexus	Posterior
Course from Axilla to Elbow	Medial humerus Laterally around the spiral groove Lateral humerus below the deltoid insertion Enters the forearm between the biceps and the brachioradialis Divides into deep motor (posterior interosseous) and superficial radial sensory nerves

Muscles Innervated and Function	Above elbow branches:
	• Triceps extends the elbow
	• Brachioradialis flexes the elbow in neutral position
	• Extensor carpi radialis longus and brevis extend and abduct hand at the wrist
	
	At the level of the elbow joint, it divides into superficial sensory branch that supplies sensation to the dorsum of the hand and lateral 3 and $\frac{1}{2}$ fingers and a motor branch (posterior interosseous) to:
	  • Supinator supinates forearm
	  • Extensor digitorum extends fingers 2-5
	  • Extensor digiti minimi extends little finger
	  • Extensor carpi ulnaris extends and adducts hand at wrist
	  • Abductor pollicis longus abducts thumb at the CMC joint
	  • Extensor pollicis longus extends distal phalanx of thumb
	  • Extensor pollicis brevis extends MCP joint of thumb
	  • Extensor indicis extends index finger

Sensory Branches and Dermatome	Posterior cutaneous nerve of the arm arises in the upper spiral groove and supplies the posterior aspect of arm Lower lateral cutaneous nerve of the arm arises in the lower spiral groove and supplies lateral aspect of arm below deltoid mass Posterior cutaneous nerve of the forearm arises in the lower spiral groove and supplies posterior of forearm
Disorders	Axilla—crutch palsy Upper arm—humerus fracture, tourniquets, injections, muscular exertion "Saturday night palsy" Supinator syndrome—affects posterior interosseous nerve and causes fingerdrop

RADIAL NERVE *continued*

Clinical Notes	Wristdrop if the lesion is in the spiral groove
	Fingerdrop if the lesion affects the posterior interosseous nerve
Differential Diagnosis	C7 radiculopathy
	Posterior cord brachial plexopathy

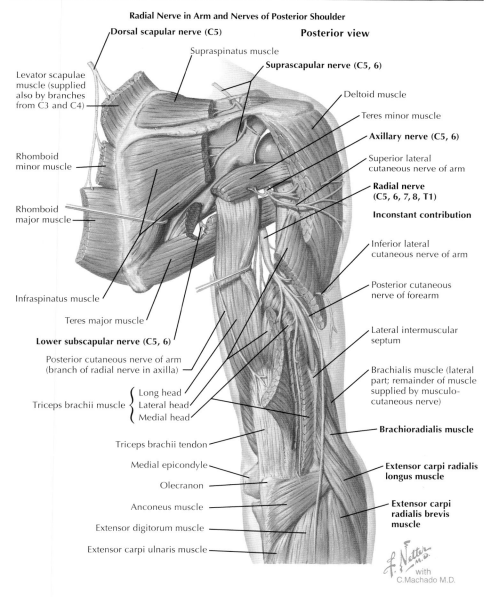

Radial Nerve in Arm and Nerves of Posterior Shoulder

Posterior view

Dorsal scapular nerve (C5)

Supraspinatus muscle

Suprascapular nerve (C5, 6)

Levator scapulae muscle (supplied also by branches from C3 and C4)

Deltoid muscle

Teres minor muscle

Axillary nerve (C5, 6)

Rhomboid minor muscle

Superior lateral cutaneous nerve of arm

Radial nerve (C5, 6, 7, 8, T1)

Inconstant contribution

Rhomboid major muscle

Inferior lateral cutaneous nerve of arm

Posterior cutaneous nerve of forearm

Infraspinatus muscle

Teres major muscle

Lateral intermuscular septum

Lower subscapular nerve (C5, 6)

Posterior cutaneous nerve of arm (branch of radial nerve in axilla)

Brachialis muscle (lateral part; remainder of muscle supplied by musculo-cutaneous nerve)

Triceps brachii muscle { Long head / Lateral head / Medial head }

Brachioradialis muscle

Triceps brachii tendon

Medial epicondyle

Extensor carpi radialis longus muscle

Olecranon

Anconeus muscle

Extensor carpi radialis brevis muscle

Extensor digitorum muscle

Extensor carpi ulnaris muscle

f. Netter M.D.
with
C.Machado M.D.

RADIAL NERVE *continued*

Radial Nerve in Forearm

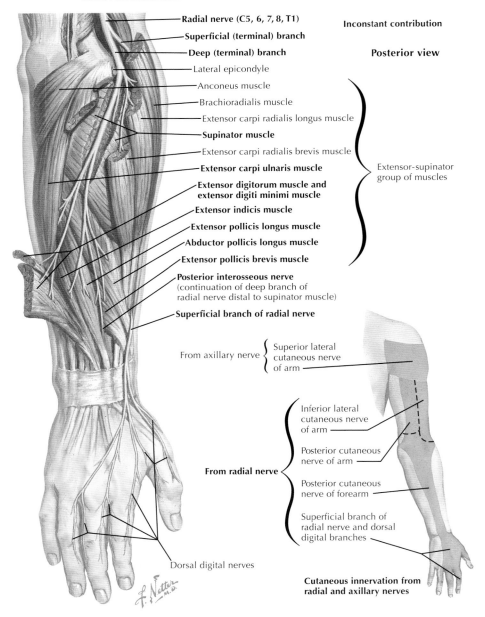

Radial nerve (C5, 6, 7, 8, T1)

Superficial (terminal) branch

Deep (terminal) branch

Lateral epicondyle

Anconeus muscle

Brachioradialis muscle

Extensor carpi radialis longus muscle

Supinator muscle

Extensor carpi radialis brevis muscle

Extensor carpi ulnaris muscle

Extensor digitorum muscle and extensor digiti minimi muscle

Extensor indicis muscle

Extensor pollicis longus muscle

Abductor pollicis longus muscle

Extensor pollicis brevis muscle

Posterior interosseous nerve
(continuation of deep branch of
radial nerve distal to supinator muscle)

Superficial branch of radial nerve

Inconstant contribution

Posterior view

Extensor-supinator
group of muscles

From axillary nerve {
Superior lateral
cutaneous nerve
of arm

Inferior lateral
cutaneous nerve
of arm

Posterior cutaneous
nerve of arm

From radial nerve {
Posterior cutaneous
nerve of forearm

Superficial branch of
radial nerve and dorsal
digital branches

Dorsal digital nerves

Cutaneous innervation from
radial and axillary nerves

POSTERIOR INTEROSSEOUS NERVE

Roots	C6-8
Trunk of Brachial Plexus	Upper, middle, lower
Division of Brachial Plexus	Posterior divisions of upper, middle, lower trunk
Cord of Brachial plexus	Posterior
Course in Arm	Dorsolaterally around the neck of radius through supinator
	Enters supinator through "arcade of Frohse"
	Runs between superficial and deep parts of supinator
	Runs between the deep and superficial extensor muscles
	Terminates at the dorsum of the wrist
Muscles Innervated and Function	Supinator supinates forearm
	Extensor digitorum extends fingers 2-5
	Extensor digiti minimi extends the little finger
	Extensor carpi ulnaris extends and adducts the hand at the wrist
	Abductor pollicis longus abducts thumb at the CMC joint
	Extensor pollicis longus extends the distal phalanx of the thumb
	Extensor pollicis brevis extends the MCP joint of the thumb
	Extensor indicis extends the index finger
Sensory Branches and Dermatome	None
Disorders	Radius fracture or dislocation
	Soft tissue masses
	Forearm laceration
	Idiopathic
Clinical Notes	Fingerdrop, no wristdrop
	Sensation normal
Differential Diagnosis	Extensor tendon rupture to the thumb and fingers (as in rheumatoid arthritis)
	Tennis elbow

POSTERIOR INTEROSSEOUS NERVE *continued*

Muscles of Forearm (Deep Layer): Posterior View

Ulnar nerve

Medial epicondyle of humerus

Triceps brachii tendon (*cut*)

Olecranon of ulna

Anconeus muscle

Flexor carpi ulnaris muscle

Ulna

Extensor pollicis longus muscle

Extensor indicis muscle

Extensor carpi ulnaris tendon *(cut)*
Extensor digiti minimi tendon *(cut)*
Extensor digitorum tendons *(cut)*

Extensor retinaculum
(compartments numbered)

5th metacarpal bone

Lateral intermuscular septum

Brachioradialis muscle

Extensor carpi radialis longus muscle

Lateral epicondyle of humerus

Common extensor tendon
(*partially cut*)

Extensor carpi radialis brevis muscle

Supinator muscle

Deep branch of radial nerve

Pronator teres muscle
(slip of insertion)

Radius

Posterior interosseous nerve

Abductor pollicis longus muscle

Extensor pollicis brevis muscle

Extensor carpi radialis brevis tendon
Extensor carpi radialis longus tendon

1st metacarpal bone

2nd metacarpal bone

1st dorsal
interosseous muscle

SUPERFICIAL RADIAL NERVE

Root	C6
Trunk of Brachial Plexus	Fibers pass through the upper trunk to reach the posterior division
Division of Brachial Plexus	Posterior
Cord of Brachial Plexus	Derives from the radial nerve, which comes off the posterior cord
Course from Elbow to Hand	Passes over the supinator
	Along the lateral radius in lower 3rd of the forearm
	Over the dorsolateral wrist
Muscles Innervated and Function	None
Sensory Branches and Dermatome	Terminal digital branches
	Dorsolateral hand and fingers 1-3
Disorders	Wrist—compression by handcuffs, tight cast
Clinical Notes	Sensory disturbance in distribution of nerve
	May be associated with causalgia

SUPERFICIAL RADIAL NERVE *continued*

Muscles of Forearm (Intermediate Layer): Anterior View

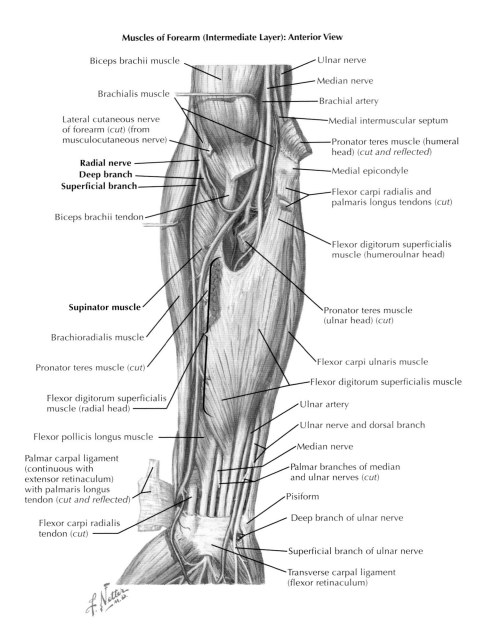

Biceps brachii muscle

Brachialis muscle

Lateral cutaneous nerve of forearm (*cut*) (from musculocutaneous nerve)

Radial nerve
Deep branch
Superficial branch

Biceps brachii tendon

Supinator muscle

Brachioradialis muscle

Pronator teres muscle (*cut*)

Flexor digitorum superficialis muscle (radial head)

Flexor pollicis longus muscle

Palmar carpal ligament (continuous with extensor retinaculum) with palmaris longus tendon (*cut and reflected*)

Flexor carpi radialis tendon (*cut*)

Ulnar nerve

Median nerve

Brachial artery

Medial intermuscular septum

Pronator teres muscle (humeral head) (*cut and reflected*)

Medial epicondyle

Flexor carpi radialis and palmaris longus tendons (*cut*)

Flexor digitorum superficialis muscle (humeroulnar head)

Pronator teres muscle (ulnar head) (*cut*)

Flexor carpi ulnaris muscle

Flexor digitorum superficialis muscle

Ulnar artery

Ulnar nerve and dorsal branch

Median nerve

Palmar branches of median and ulnar nerves (*cut*)

Pisiform

Deep branch of ulnar nerve

Superficial branch of ulnar nerve

Transverse carpal ligament (flexor retinaculum)

MUSCULOCUTANEOUS NERVE

Roots	C5-6
Trunk of Brachial Plexus	Upper
Division of Brachial Plexus	Anterior division of the upper trunk
Cord of Brachial Plexus	Lateral
Course from Axilla to Hand	Arises from lateral cord brachial plexus
	Pierces coracobrachialis
	Courses down anterior arm between biceps and brachialis
	Crosses anterior elbow lateral to biceps tendon
	Continues as lateral cutaneous nerve of forearm
Muscles Innervated and Function	Biceps brachii supinates forearm and flexes the elbow
	Coracobrachialis flexes the arm
	Brachialis flexes the elbow
Sensory Branches and Dermatome	Lateral cutaneous nerve of forearm
	Lateral forearm from elbow to wrist
Disorders	Shoulder dislocation
	Strenuous exercise
	Following general anesthesia
	Brachial neuritis (Parsonage-Turner syndrome)
Clinical Notes	Weak, wasted biceps with weak elbow flexion
	Numbness over the radial aspect of forearm
Differential Diagnosis	Biceps tendon rupture
	C6 radiculopathy

MUSCULOCUTANEOUS NERVE *continued*

Musculocutaneous Nerve

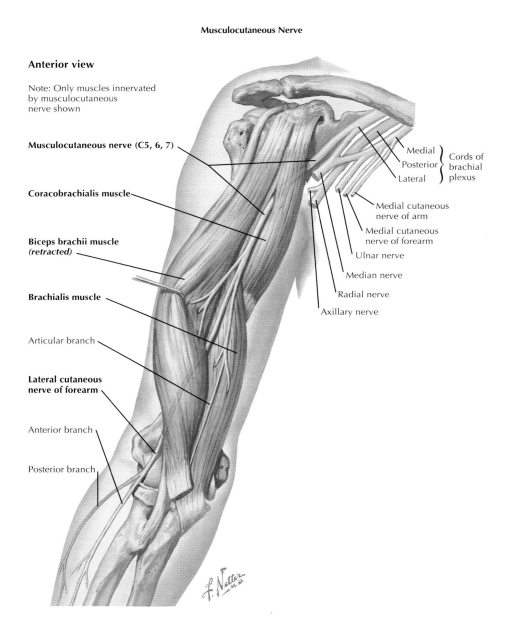

Anterior view

Note: Only muscles innervated
by musculocutaneous
nerve shown

Musculocutaneous nerve (C5, 6, 7)

Coracobrachialis muscle

Biceps brachii muscle
(retracted)

Brachialis muscle

Articular branch

**Lateral cutaneous
nerve of forearm**

Anterior branch

Posterior branch

Medial }
Posterior } Cords of
Lateral } brachial
plexus

Medial cutaneous
nerve of arm

Medial cutaneous
nerve of forearm

Ulnar nerve

Median nerve

Radial nerve

Axillary nerve

LATERAL CUTANEOUS NERVE OF FOREARM

Roots	C5 ventral ramus through the upper trunk, lateral cord
Supplies	Skin over the lateral forearm from elbow to wrist
Course	At the elbow lateral to the biceps tendon, crosses the cephalic vein, continues as the lateral cutaneous nerve of forearm (also called the *lateral antebrachial cutaneous nerve of forearm*)
Injury	May be injured during venipuncture
	Results in numbness over the radial aspect of the forearm

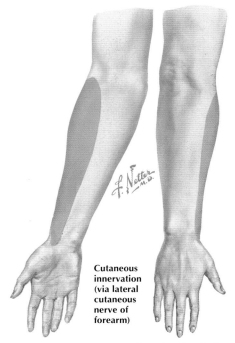

Cutaneous innervation (via lateral cutaneous nerve of forearm)

Anterior (palmar) view   Posterior (dorsal) view

CHAPTER 18

Anatomy of the Peripheral
Nervous System: Lower Extremity

LUMBAR AND SACRAL ROOT ANATOMY

- Lumbar and sacral nerve roots arise from the conus medullaris, then travel downward and laterally to intervertebral foramen from which they exit the spinal canal.
- Lumbar nerve roots fuse in the intervertebral foramen, distal to the dorsal root ganglion, and form spinal nerves.
- Lumbar nerve roots pass below the pedicle of same-numbered vertebra but above the level of the disc to exit the spinal canal (i.e., L4 root exits below L4 pedicle, above the level of the disc). Therefore, a herniated lumbar disc compresses the root which exits at the next lower level (i.e., L4 disc herniation compresses the L5 root).
- Lumbar spinal nerves divide into dorsal and ventral rami on exiting foramen.
- Ventral rami pass into the lumbar plexus, and dorsal rami supply the skin and paraspinal muscles.
- Sacral ventral and dorsal roots fuse within the spinal canal to form sacral spinal nerves.
- Sacral spinal nerves divide within the spinal canal into ventral and dorsal rami.
- Ventral rami exit through the ventral pelvic sacral foramina to join the sacral plexi.
- Dorsal rami exit through the dorsal sacral pelvic foramina to supply the lower paraspinal muscles and skin.

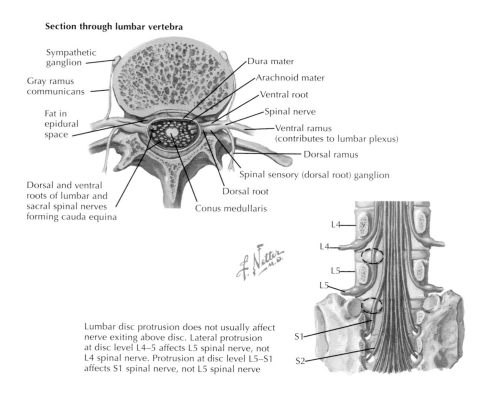

Section through lumbar vertebra

Sympathetic ganglion

Gray ramus communicans

Fat in epidural space

Dorsal and ventral roots of lumbar and sacral spinal nerves forming cauda equina

Dura mater

Arachnoid mater

Ventral root

Spinal nerve

Ventral ramus (contributes to lumbar plexus)

Dorsal ramus

Spinal sensory (dorsal root) ganglion

Dorsal root

Conus medullaris

L4

L4

L5

L5

S1

S2

Lumbar disc protrusion does not usually affect nerve exiting above disc. Lateral protrusion at disc level L4–5 affects L5 spinal nerve, not L4 spinal nerve. Protrusion at disc level L5–S1 affects S1 spinal nerve, not L5 spinal nerve

LUMBAR AND SACRAL ROOT ANATOMY *continued*

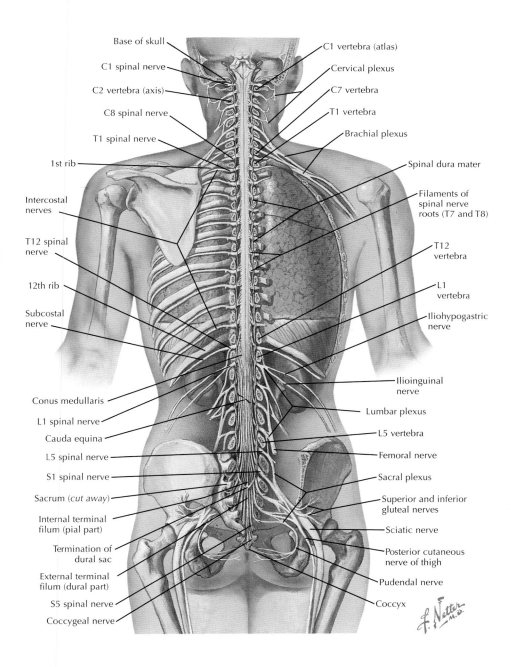

Base of skull

C1 spinal nerve

C2 vertebra (axis)

C8 spinal nerve

T1 spinal nerve

1st rib

Intercostal nerves

T12 spinal nerve

12th rib

Subcostal nerve

Conus medullaris

L1 spinal nerve

Cauda equina

L5 spinal nerve

S1 spinal nerve

Sacrum (*cut away*)

Internal terminal filum (pial part)

Termination of dural sac

External terminal filum (dural part)

S5 spinal nerve

Coccygeal nerve

C1 vertebra (atlas)

Cervical plexus

C7 vertebra

T1 vertebra

Brachial plexus

Spinal dura mater

Filaments of spinal nerve roots (T7 and T8)

T12 vertebra

L1 vertebra

Iliohypogastric nerve

Ilioinguinal nerve

Lumbar plexus

L5 vertebra

Femoral nerve

Sacral plexus

Superior and inferior gluteal nerves

Sciatic nerve

Posterior cutaneous nerve of thigh

Pudendal nerve

Coccyx

LUMBAR AND SACRAL ROOT ANATOMY *continued*

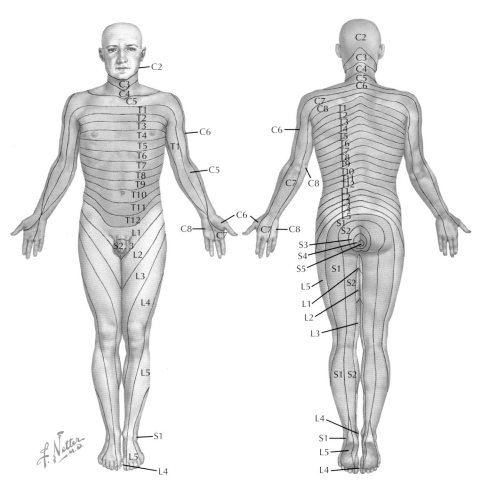

Levels of principal dermatomes

C5	Clavicles
C5, 6, 7	Lateral parts of upper limbs
C8, T1	Medial sides of upper limbs
C6	Thumb
C6, 7, 8	Hand
C8	Ring and little fingers
T4	Level of nipples

T10	Level of umbilicus
T12	Inguinal or groin regions
L1, 2, 3, 4	Anterior and inner surfaces of lower limbs
L4, 5, S1	Foot
L4	Medial side of great toe
S1, 2, L5	Posterior and outer surfaces of lower limbs
S1	Lateral margin of foot and little toe
S2, 3, 4	Perineum

**LUMBOSACRAL RADICULOPATHY
(DERMATOMES AND SEGMENTAL INNERVATION)**

ROOT	REFLEX LOSS	SENSORY LOSS	MAJOR WEAKNESS	PAIN	MAIN DIFFERENTIAL DIAGNOSES
L2	None	Upper anterior thigh	Hip flexion	Anterior thigh	Femoral neuropathy
L3	Patella	Anterior knee	Hip flexion Knee extension Hip adductors	Anterior knee	Femoral neuropathy Obturator neuropathy
L4	Patella	Medial calf	Knee extension Ankle dorsiflexion	Medial calf	Femoral neuropathy Obturator neuropathy Common peroneal neuropathy
L5	None	Dorsal and medial foot Lateral calf	Ankle inversion, dorsiflexion Large-toe dorsiflexion	Lateral calf, dorsomedial foot, buttocks/posterior thigh	Common peroneal neuropathy
S1	Achilles	Plantar and lateral foot	Ankle plantarflexion Hip extension Knee flexion	Plantar and lateral foot, buttocks/ posterior thigh	Tibial neuropathy

LUMBOSACRAL RADICULOPATHY
(DERMATOMES AND SEGMENTAL INNERVATION) *continued*

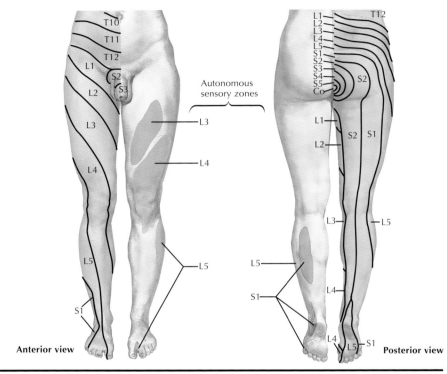

Anterior view

Posterior view

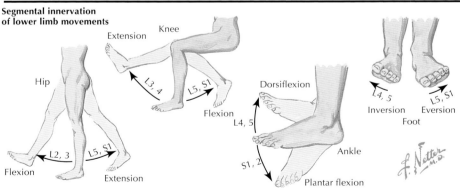

Segmental innervation
of lower limb movements

LUMBOSACRAL PLEXUS IN SITU

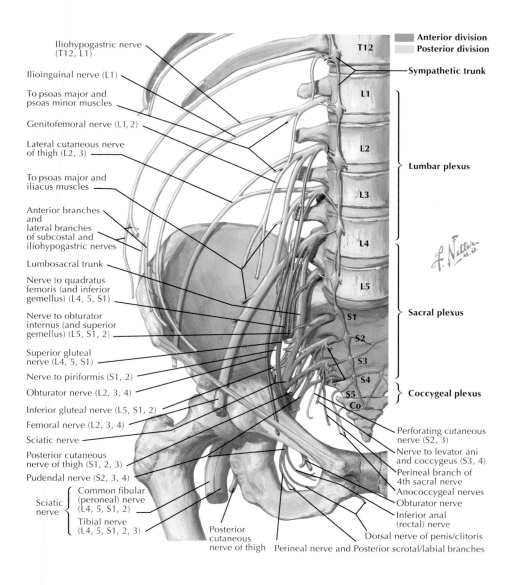

Iliohypogastric nerve (T12, L1)

Ilioinguinal nerve (L1)

To psoas major and psoas minor muscles

Genitofemoral nerve (L1, 2)

Lateral cutaneous nerve of thigh (L2, 3)

To psoas major and iliacus muscles

Anterior branches and lateral branches of subcostal and iliohypogastric nerves

Lumbosacral trunk

Nerve to quadratus femoris (and inferior gemellus) (L4, 5, S1)

Nerve to obturator internus (and superior gemellus) (L5, S1, 2)

Superior gluteal nerve (L4, 5, S1)

Nerve to piriformis (S1, 2)

Obturator nerve (L2, 3, 4)

Inferior gluteal nerve (L5, S1, 2)

Femoral nerve (L2, 3, 4)

Sciatic nerve

Posterior cutaneous nerve of thigh (S1, 2, 3)

Pudendal nerve (S2, 3, 4)

Sciatic nerve { Common fibular (peroneal) nerve (L4, 5, S1, 2) / Tibial nerve (L4, 5, S1, 2, 3) }

Posterior cutaneous nerve of thigh

Perineal nerve and Posterior scrotal/labial branches

Anterior division
Posterior division

T12
L1
L2
L3
L4
L5
S1
S2
S3
S4
S5
Co

Sympathetic trunk

Lumbar plexus

Sacral plexus

Coccygeal plexus

Perforating cutaneous nerve (S2, 3)

Nerve to levator ani and coccygeus (S3, 4)

Perineal branch of 4th sacral nerve

Anococcygeal nerves

Obturator nerve

Inferior anal (rectal) nerve

Dorsal nerve of penis/clitoris

LUMBAR PLEXUS

NERVE	ROOT(S)	MUSCLE(S) INNERVATED (ACTION)	SENSORY DISTRIBUTION
Iliohypogastric	L1	Transversus abdominus (supports the abdominal wall) Internal oblique (supports the abdominal wall)	Lateral gluteal Above the pubis
Ilioinguinal	L1	None	Superomedial thigh and genitalia
Genitofemoral	L1-L2	Cremaster	Genitalia and skin over the femoral triangle
Lateral cutaneous nerve of the thigh	L2-L3	None	Lateral thigh
Femoral	L2-L4	Psoas, pectineus (hip flexors) Iliacus (hip flexor and internal rotator) Quadriceps femoris (knee extensors) Sartorius (hip flexor, abductor and external rotator) Articularis genus (retracts bursa as knee extends)	Anteromedial thigh Terminal branch (saphenous) supplies the medial leg
Obturator	L2-L4	Adductors longus, brevis and magnus (hip adductors) Gracilis (hip adductor) Obturator externus (hip external rotator) External oblique (supports abdominal wall)	Inferomedial thigh
Accessory obturator (variable)	L2-L4	Psoas (hip flexor)	None
Lumbosacral trunk	L4-L5	Contributes to sacral plexus	

LUMBAR PLEXUS *continued*

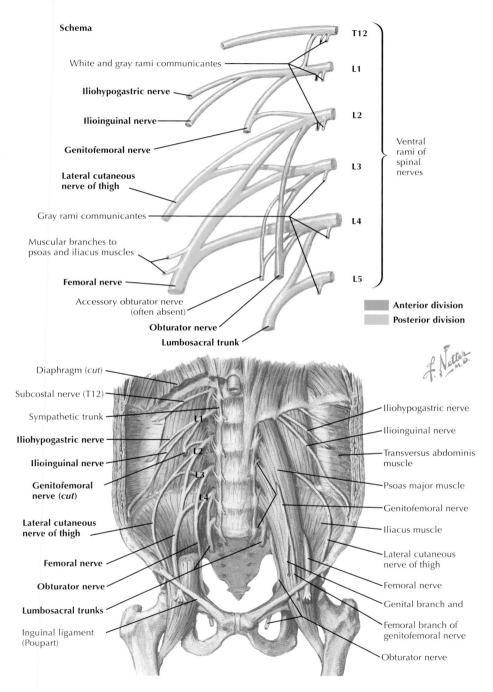

Schema

White and gray rami communicantes

Iliohypogastric nerve

Ilioinguinal nerve

Genitofemoral nerve

Lateral cutaneous nerve of thigh

Gray rami communicantes

Muscular branches to psoas and iliacus muscles

Femoral nerve

Accessory obturator nerve (often absent)

Obturator nerve

Lumbosacral trunk

T12
L1
L2
L3
L4
L5

Ventral rami of spinal nerves

Anterior division
Posterior division

Diaphragm (*cut*)

Subcostal nerve (T12)

Sympathetic trunk

Iliohypogastric nerve

Ilioinguinal nerve

Genitofemoral nerve (*cut*)

Lateral cutaneous nerve of thigh

Femoral nerve

Obturator nerve

Lumbosacral trunks

Inguinal ligament (Poupart)

L1
L2
L3
L4

Iliohypogastric nerve

Ilioinguinal nerve

Transversus abdominis muscle

Psoas major muscle

Genitofemoral nerve

Iliacus muscle

Lateral cutaneous nerve of thigh

Femoral nerve

Genital branch and

Femoral branch of genitofemoral nerve

Obturator nerve

SACRAL PLEXUS

NERVE	ROOT(S)	MUSCLE(S) INNERVATED (ACTION)	SENSORY DISTRIBUTION
Sciatic	L4-S3	Main trunk: hamstrings group (knee flexors) Tibial division (see page 362) Peroneal division (see page 360)	None from the main trunk Tibial and peroneal divisions supply the entire lower leg except the medial portion
Nerve to quadratus femoris	L4-S1	Quadratus femoris (hip external rotator) Inferior gemellus (hip external rotator)	None
Nerve to obturator internus	L5-S2	Obturator internus (hip external rotator) Superior gemellus (hip external rotator)	None
Pudendal	S2-4	Perineal branch: • Bulbospongiosis (controls urination, ejaculation) • Ischiocavernosus (controls urination, ejaculation) • Urethral sphincter (controls urination, ejaculation) • Urogenital diaphragm (supports pelvic floor)	Perineum
		Inferior rectal branch—external anal sphincter (controls defecation)	Perianal skin
		Dorsal nerve to the penis/clitoris—no muscles	Penis/Clitoris
Nerve to coccygeus	S3-S4	Coccygeus (supports pelvic floor) Levator ani (supports pelvic floor)	None
Superior gluteal	L4-S1	Gluteus medius (hip abductor) Gluteus minimus (hip abductor) Tensor fascia lata (hip abductor, external rotator)	None
Inferior gluteal	L5-S2	Gluteus maximus (hip extensor)	None
Nerve to piriformis	S2	Piriformis (hip external rotator)	None
Posterior femoral cutaneous	S1-S3	None	Posterior thigh

SACRAL PLEXUS *continued*

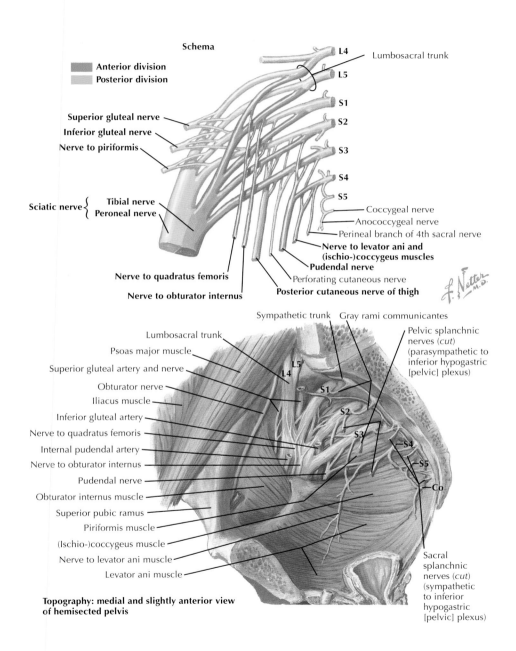

Schema

Anterior division
Posterior division

L4
Lumbosacral trunk
L5
S1
S2
S3
S4
S5

Superior gluteal nerve
Inferior gluteal nerve
Nerve to piriformis

Sciatic nerve { Tibial nerve
Peroneal nerve

Coccygeal nerve
Anococcygeal nerve
Perineal branch of 4th sacral nerve
Nerve to levator ani and (ischio-)coccygeus muscles
Pudendal nerve
Perforating cutaneous nerve
Posterior cutaneous nerve of thigh

Nerve to quadratus femoris
Nerve to obturator internus

Sympathetic trunk   Gray rami communicantes

Lumbosacral trunk
Psoas major muscle
Superior gluteal artery and nerve
Obturator nerve
Iliacus muscle
Inferior gluteal artery
Nerve to quadratus femoris
Internal pudendal artery
Nerve to obturator internus
Pudendal nerve
Obturator internus muscle
Superior pubic ramus
Piriformis muscle
(Ischio-)coccygeus muscle
Nerve to levator ani muscle
Levator ani muscle

L4
L5
S1
S2
S3
S4
S5
Co

Pelvic splanchnic nerves (*cut*) (parasympathetic to inferior hypogastric [pelvic] plexus)

Sacral splanchnic nerves (*cut*) (sympathetic to inferior hypogastric [pelvic] plexus)

Topography: medial and slightly anterior view of hemisected pelvis

OBTURATOR NERVE

Roots	L2, L3, L4
Course	Forms in psoas muscle
	Descends through psoas
	Enters thigh by passing through obturator foramen
Muscles Innervated	Adductor longus (*hip adductor*)
	Adductor brevis (*hip adductor*)
	Adductor magnus (*hip adductor component*)
	Gracilis (*hip adductor*)
	Obturator externus (*hip external rotator*)
	External oblique (*supports abdominal wall*)
Sensory Innervation	Small patch of skin on the inferomedial thigh
Selected Disorders	Rarely damaged, but damage can be caused by:
	• Pelvic fractures
	• Hip replacement surgery
	• Obturator hernias
	• Pelvic masses
	• Parturition
Clinical Notes	Hip adduction is weak
	Patch of parasthesias and/or numbness in medial thigh
Differential Diagnosis	Lumbar plexus or L3/L4 lesion also involves quadriceps group (*knee extension*) and patellar reflex

OBTURATOR NERVE *continued*

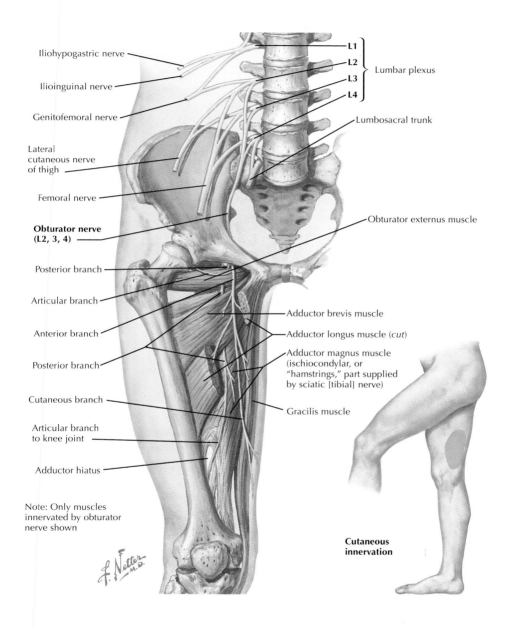

Iliohypogastric nerve

Ilioinguinal nerve

Genitofemoral nerve

Lateral cutaneous nerve of thigh

Femoral nerve

Obturator nerve (L2, 3, 4)

Posterior branch

Articular branch

Anterior branch

Posterior branch

Cutaneous branch

Articular branch to knee joint

Adductor hiatus

Note: Only muscles innervated by obturator nerve shown

L1
L2
L3
L4

Lumbar plexus

Lumbosacral trunk

Obturator externus muscle

Adductor brevis muscle

Adductor longus muscle (*cut*)

Adductor magnus muscle (ischiocondylar, or "hamstrings," part supplied by sciatic [tibial] nerve)

Gracilis muscle

Cutaneous innervation

FEMORAL NERVE

Roots	L2, L3, L4
Course	Forms in psoas muscle
	Descends between psoas and iliacus mucles
	Passes under the inguinal ligament, lateral to the femoral artery and vein
	Branches off to supply individual muscles
	Terminal branch (saphenous nerve) descends within quadriceps in the subsartorial canal emerging above the knee, then descends down the medial leg, crossing the medial malleolus and ending in inner foot
Muscles	Psoas, pectineus (hip flexors)
Innervated	Iliacus (hip flexor and internal rotator)
	Quadriceps group (knee extensors):
	• Rectus femoris
	• Vastus lateralis
	• Vastus intermedius
	• Vastus medialis
	• Sartorius (hip flexor, abductor and external rotator)
	• Articularis genus (retracts bursa as knee extends)
Sensory Innervation	Anteromedial thigh via anterior cutaneous branches
	Medial knee via infrapatellar branch of saphenous
	Medial leg and medial malleolus via saphenous
Selected Disorders	Can be damaged with:
	• Pelvic, inguinal hernia, and hip surgery
	• Femoral artery catheterization
	• Childbirth (from the lithotomy position)
	• Hematomas in iliacus muscle
	• Diabetes usually causes lumbar plexopathy, may involve only femoral nerve
	• Saphenous nerve can be damaged at the knee (arthroscopy) and in the leg (varicose vein procedures)
Clinical Notes	Weakness mainly noted in knee extension
	Patellar reflex hypoactive or absent
	Sensory involvement variably present but should involve anteromedial thigh and medial leg
Differential Diagnosis	L3-4 radiculopathy or lumbar plexopathy would involve hip adduction and hip flexion (iliopsoas mainly innervated by upper lumbar plexus branches).

FEMORAL NERVE *continued*

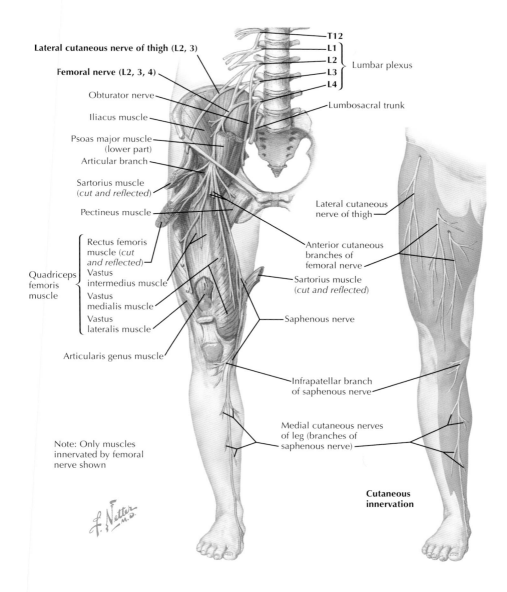

Lateral cutaneous nerve of thigh (L2, 3)

Femoral nerve (L2, 3, 4)

Obturator nerve

Iliacus muscle

Psoas major muscle (lower part)

Articular branch

Sartorius muscle (cut and reflected)

Pectineus muscle

Quadriceps femoris muscle
- Rectus femoris muscle (cut and reflected)
- Vastus intermedius muscle
- Vastus medialis muscle
- Vastus lateralis muscle

Articularis genus muscle

Note: Only muscles innervated by femoral nerve shown

T12
L1
L2
L3
L4
Lumbar plexus

Lumbosacral trunk

Lateral cutaneous nerve of thigh

Anterior cutaneous branches of femoral nerve

Sartorius muscle (cut and reflected)

Saphenous nerve

Infrapatellar branch of saphenous nerve

Medial cutaneous nerves of leg (branches of saphenous nerve)

Cutaneous innervation

LATERAL CUTANEOUS NERVE OF THE THIGH

Roots	L2, L3
Course	Variable course: • Emerges lateral to the psoas, crossing the iliacus • Passes under the lateral part of the inguinal ligament • May cross the anterior superior iliac spine or run in close proximity • Crosses over the upper part of the sartorius muscle • Terminates in the cutaneous branches
Muscles Innervated	None (purely sensory nerve)
Sensory Innervation	Lateral thigh
Selected Disorders	Can be damaged during surgery of retroperitoneum, iliac fossa, or inguinal region Compression by tight clothing or belts Usually no clear cause found
Clinical Notes	Syndrome known as *meralgia paresthetica* Pain and numbness in lateral thigh Usually numbness in smaller area than pain No weakness
Differential Diagnosis	L2 radiculopathy causes numbness in the lateral and anterior upper thigh L2 radiculopathy may cause weakness of hip flexion Lumbar plexopathy causes more extensive numbness with weakness Femoral neuropathy causes numbness in the anterior thigh and medial leg, knee extension weakness, and depressed patellar reflex

LATERAL CUTANEOUS NERVE OF THE THIGH *continued*

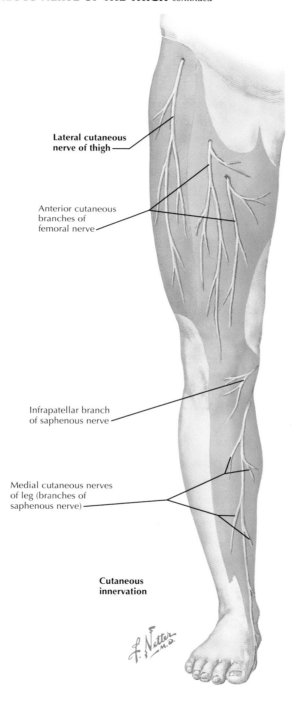

Lateral cutaneous
nerve of thigh

Anterior cutaneous
branches of
femoral nerve

Infrapatellar branch
of saphenous nerve

Medial cutaneous nerves
of leg (branches of
saphenous nerve)

**Cutaneous
innervation**

SCIATIC NERVE

Roots	L4-5 (lumbosacral trunk), S1, S2, S3
Course	Forms from the lumbosacral trunk and upper sacral plexus
	Travels down the inner wall of the pelvis
	Exits the pelvis through greater sciatic foramen
	Passes under the piriformis muscle
	Passes between the ischial tuberosity and greater trochanter of the femur
	Divides just above the popliteal fossa into the common peroneal (lateral trunk) and tibial nerve (medial trunk)
Muscles Innervated	Semitendinosus (medial trunk)
	Semimembranosus (medial trunk)
	Long head of the biceps femoris (medial trunk)
	Short head of the biceps femoris (lateral trunk)
	Adductor magnus (hip extensor component)
	Terminal branches of sciatic (tibial and common peroneal nerves) supply all muscles below the knee
Sensory Innervation	None from the sciatic trunk, although terminal branches (tibial and common peroneal nerves) supply much of the lower leg and foot
Selected Disorders	Hip trauma/fractures and hip surgeries
	Prolonged pressure against the nerve
	Gluteal hematomas
	Needle injury from injections into the buttock
	Thigh hematomas
	Femur fractures
Clinical Notes	Weakness of knee flexion if the lesion is proximal (gluteal region)
	Weakness of any muscles below the knee
	Usually weakness is variable below the knee and involves the common peroneal more than the tibial innervated muscles. Sciatic neuropathy may mimic common peroneal neuropathy
Differential Diagnosis	Difficult to differentiate from lumbosacral plexopathies
	Sacral plexopathies usually involve the pudendal nerve and posterior cutaneous nerve of the thigh
	Lumbosacral radiculopathies usually present with back pain
	Imaging pelvis/thigh with computed tomography (CT)/magnetic resonance imaging (MRI) helps to rule out hematomas
	Electromyography (EMG) is helpful in localization

SCIATIC NERVE *continued*

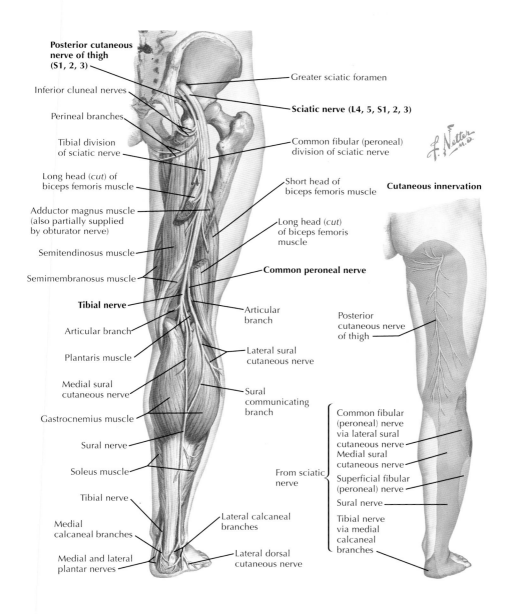

Posterior cutaneous
nerve of thigh
(S1, 2, 3)

Inferior cluneal nerves

Perineal branches

Tibial division
of sciatic nerve

Long head (*cut*) of
biceps femoris muscle

Adductor magnus muscle
(also partially supplied
by obturator nerve)

Semitendinosus muscle

Semimembranosus muscle

Tibial nerve

Articular branch

Plantaris muscle

Medial sural
cutaneous nerve

Gastrocnemius muscle

Sural nerve

Soleus muscle

Tibial nerve

Medial
calcaneal branches

Medial and lateral
plantar nerves

Greater sciatic foramen

Sciatic nerve (L4, 5, S1, 2, 3)

Common fibular (peroneal)
division of sciatic nerve

Short head of
biceps femoris muscle

Long head (*cut*)
of biceps femoris
muscle

Common peroneal nerve

Articular
branch

Lateral sural
cutaneous nerve

Sural
communicating
branch

From sciatic
nerve

Lateral calcaneal
branches

Lateral dorsal
cutaneous nerve

Cutaneous innervation

Posterior
cutaneous nerve
of thigh

Common fibular
(peroneal) nerve
via lateral sural
cutaneous nerve

Medial sural
cutaneous nerve

Superficial fibular
(peroneal) nerve

Sural nerve

Tibial nerve
via medial
calcaneal
branches

COMMON PERONEAL NERVE

Roots	L4, L5, S1, S2
Course	Formed from the lateral trunk of the sciatic nerve after its bifurcation in the distal thigh
	Passes anterolaterally around the neck of the fibula, close to the skin
	Pierces the peroneus longus and runs through the fibular tunnel formed by this muscle
	Divides in the upper leg into the superficial and deep peroneal nerves
	Superficial branch runs down the leg with the fibula
	Deep branch runs deeper in the leg between the tibialis anterior and toe extensors
Muscles Innervated	Deep peroneal nerve: • Tibialis anterior (foot dorsiflexion) • Extensor hallicus longus (first toe dorsiflexion) • Extensor digitorum longus (dorsiflexion of last four toes) • Peroneus tertius (foot dorsiflexion and eversion) • Extensor hallicus brevis (first toe dorsiflexion) • Extensor digitorum brevis (dorsiflexion of last 4 toes) • Superficial peroneal nerve: • Peroneus longus (foot eversion) • Peroneus brevis (foot eversion) • Peroneus tertius (foot eversion)
Sensory Innervation	Proximal lateral leg via the lateral sural nerve
	Distal lateral leg and dorsal foot via the superficial peroneal nerve
	Dorsal interdigital space between toes 1 and 2 via the deep peroneal nerve
Selected Disorders	Most commonly injured by external compression against the fibular head
	Frequent causes include: • Habitual leg crossing • Anesthesia, coma, positioning during sleep • Below knee casts • Prolonged squatting
Clinical Notes	"Footdrop" caused by weak foot dorsiflexion with high-stepping gait
	Weak foot eversion
	Sensory loss in the lateral leg and dorsal foot if complete
	Isolated lesion of the deep peroneal nerve causes footdrop with numbness only in the webspace between first 2 toes
Differential Diagnosis	L5 radiculopathy
	Lumbosacral trunk compression (difficult labor)
	Sciatic neuropathy

COMMON PERONEAL NERVE *continued*

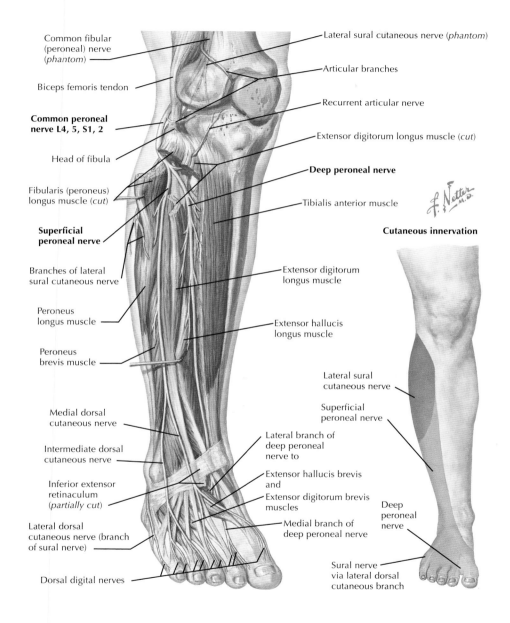

Common fibular (peroneal) nerve (*phantom*)

Biceps femoris tendon

Common peroneal nerve L4, 5, S1, 2

Head of fibula

Fibularis (peroneus) longus muscle (*cut*)

Superficial peroneal nerve

Branches of lateral sural cutaneous nerve

Peroneus longus muscle

Peroneus brevis muscle

Medial dorsal cutaneous nerve

Intermediate dorsal cutaneous nerve

Inferior extensor retinaculum (*partially cut*)

Lateral dorsal cutaneous nerve (branch of sural nerve)

Dorsal digital nerves

Lateral sural cutaneous nerve (*phantom*)

Articular branches

Recurrent articular nerve

Extensor digitorum longus muscle (*cut*)

Deep peroneal nerve

Tibialis anterior muscle

Cutaneous innervation

Extensor digitorum longus muscle

Extensor hallucis longus muscle

Lateral branch of deep peroneal nerve to

Extensor hallucis brevis and Extensor digitorum brevis muscles

Medial branch of deep peroneal nerve

Lateral sural cutaneous nerve

Superficial peroneal nerve

Deep peroneal nerve

Sural nerve via lateral dorsal cutaneous branch

TIBIAL NERVE

Roots	L5, S1, S2
Course	Formed from the medial trunk of the sciatic nerve after its bifurcation in the distal thigh
	Passes through the popliteal fossa between two heads of gastrocnemius
	Runs down the leg deep to the soleus
	Terminates in the tarsal tunnel as medial and lateral plantar nerves
Muscles Innervated	Soleus (ankle plantarflexor)
	Gastrocnemius (ankle plantarflexor)
	Plantaris (ankle plantarflexor)
	Popliteus (knee flexion)
	Tibialis posterior (foot inversion)
	Flexor hallicus longus (plantarflexor of the 1st toe)
	Flexor digitorum longus (plantarflexion of the lateral 4 toes)
	Via plantar divisions, supplies all foot muscles in the sole
	Medial plantar:
	• Abductor hallicus (*first toe abductor*)
	• Flexor digitorum brevis (*flexor of lateral 4 toes*)
	• First lumbrical (*flexes metatarsophalangeal joint, extends interphalangeal joint*)
	• Flexor hallicus brevis (*first toe plantarflexor*)
	Lateral plantar:
	• Abductor digiti minimi (*abducts 5th toe*)
	• Quadratus plantae (*flexes toes*)
	• Lumbricals 2-4 (*flexes metatarsophalangeal joint, extends interphalangeal joint*)
	• Abductor hallicus (*abuducts 1st toe*)
	• Flexor digiti minimi brevis (*flexes 5th toe*)
	• Dorsal interossei (*abduct toes*)
	• Plantar interossei (*adduct toes*)
Sensory Innervation	Posterolateral calf via medial sural and sural nerves
	Most of sole via calcaneal and plantar branches
Selected Disorders	Compression by Baker's cysts of knee
	Distal tibial nerve can be damaged by foot and ankle trauma
	Tarsal tunnel syndrome
Clinical Notes	Weakness of plantarflexion, foot inversion, toe flexion
	Hypoactive or absent Achilles tendon reflex
	Numbness/tingling in distribution of sural, calcaneal, or plantar nerves
Differential Diagnosis	S1 or S2 radiculopathy
	May be difficult to differentiate from partial sciatic neuropathy

TIBIAL NERVE *continued*

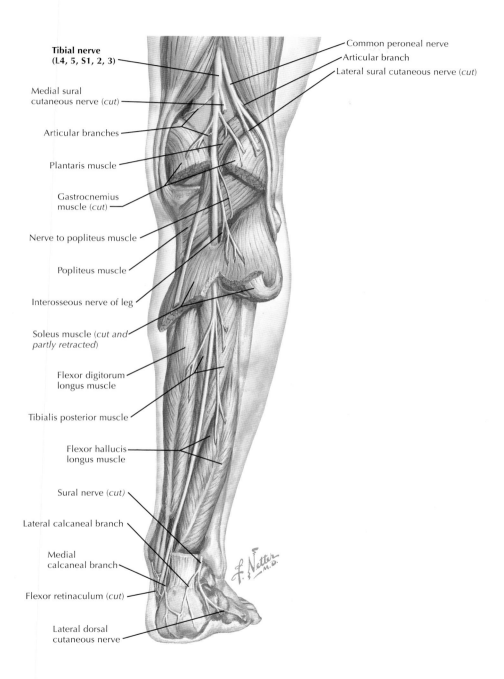

Tibial nerve
(L4, 5, S1, 2, 3)

Medial sural
cutaneous nerve (*cut*)

Articular branches

Plantaris muscle

Gastrocnemius
muscle (*cut*)

Nerve to popliteus muscle

Popliteus muscle

Interosseous nerve of leg

Soleus muscle (*cut and
partly retracted*)

Flexor digitorum
longus muscle

Tibialis posterior muscle

Flexor hallucis
longus muscle

Sural nerve (*cut*)

Lateral calcaneal branch

Medial
calcaneal branch

Flexor retinaculum (*cut*)

Lateral dorsal
cutaneous nerve

Common peroneal nerve
Articular branch
Lateral sural cutaneous nerve (*cut*)

PLANTAR NERVES AND FOOT SENSORY

Roots	L4, L5, S1, S2
Course	Two plantar nerves (medial and lateral) form from bifurcation of tibial nerve in tarsal tunnel medial to Achilles tendon
	Traverse sole of foot and end as interdigital branches
Muscles Innervated	Medial plantar nerve:
	• Abductor hallicus (1st-toe abductor)
	• Flexor digitorum brevis (flexor of lateral 4 toes)
	• First lumbrical (flexes metatarsophalangeal joint, extends interphalangeal joint)
	• Flexor hallicus brevis (1st-toe plantarflexor)
	Lateral plantar nerve:
	• Abductor digiti minimi (abducts 5th toe)
	• Quadratus plantae (flexes toes)
	• Lumbricals 2-4 (flexes metatarsophalangeal joint, extends interphalangeal joint)
	• Abductor hallicus (abuducts first toe)
	• Flexor digiti minimi brevis (flexes 5th toe)
	• Dorsal interossei (abduct toes)
	• Plantar interossei (adduct toes)
Sensory Innervation	Most of the anterior $\frac{2}{3}$ of the sole of the foot
	Calcaneal nerve supplies posterior $\frac{1}{3}$
Selected Disorders	Nerves can be damaged within tarsal tunnel by:
	• External compression by hard casts or tight shoes
	• Ankle trauma
	• Endocrinopathies (hypothyroidism, acromegaly)
Clinical Features	Tarsal tunnel syndrome: foot pain, paresthesias, sensory loss in distribution of one or both plantar nerves
	Weakness difficult to detect as short-toe flexors less clinically important than long-toe flexors

PLANTAR NERVES AND FOOT SENSORY *continued*

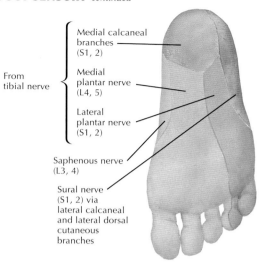

From tibial nerve
- Medial calcaneal branches (S1, 2)
- Medial plantar nerve (L4, 5)
- Lateral plantar nerve (S1, 2)

Saphenous nerve (L3, 4)

Sural nerve (S1, 2) via lateral calcaneal and lateral dorsal cutaneous branches

Cutaneous innervation of sole

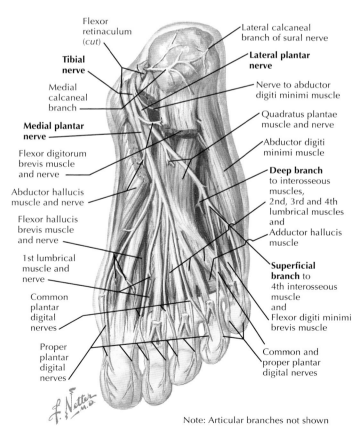

Flexor retinaculum (*cut*)

Tibial nerve

Medial calcaneal branch

Medial plantar nerve

Flexor digitorum brevis muscle and nerve

Abductor hallucis muscle and nerve

Flexor hallucis brevis muscle and nerve

1st lumbrical muscle and nerve

Common plantar digital nerves

Proper plantar digital nerves

Lateral calcaneal branch of sural nerve

Lateral plantar nerve

Nerve to abductor digiti minimi muscle

Quadratus plantae muscle and nerve

Abductor digiti minimi muscle

Deep branch to interosseous muscles, 2nd, 3rd and 4th lumbrical muscles and Adductor hallucis muscle

Superficial branch to 4th interosseous muscle and Flexor digiti minimi brevis muscle

Common and proper plantar digital nerves

Note: Articular branches not shown

AUTONOMIC NERVOUS SYSTEM SCHEMA

STRUCTURE	ANATOMIC NOTES	FUNCTIONAL SIGNIFICANCE
Peripheral autonomic nervous system	2-Neuron chain: • Preganglionic • Postganglionic	Responsible for visceral or vegetative functions
Preganglionic parasympathetic neurons	Arise in the brainstem (cranial nerve (CN)-III, -VII, -IX, -X) and spinal cord S2-4 (craniosacral)	Largest source of preganglionic parasympathetic fibers is the vagus nerve (CN-X)
Preganglionic sympathetic neurons	Arise in spinal cord T1-L2 Exiting fibers enter the sympathetic chain and terminate on the paravertebral and prevertebral ganglia	Cell bodies located in intermediolateral cell column give cord characteristic appearance in cross section
Postganglionic parasympathetic neurons	Cell body lies in intramural ganglion near the organ innervated	Neurotransmitter: acetylcholine
Postganglionic sympathetic neurons	Cell body lies in the sympathetic (paravertebral) chain and collateral (prevertebral) ganglia	Neurotransmitter: norepinephrine, except acetylcholine at the sweat glands

The neurotransmitter for all preganglionic autonomic fibers is acetylcholine.

AUTONOMIC NERVOUS SYSTEM SCHEMA *continued*

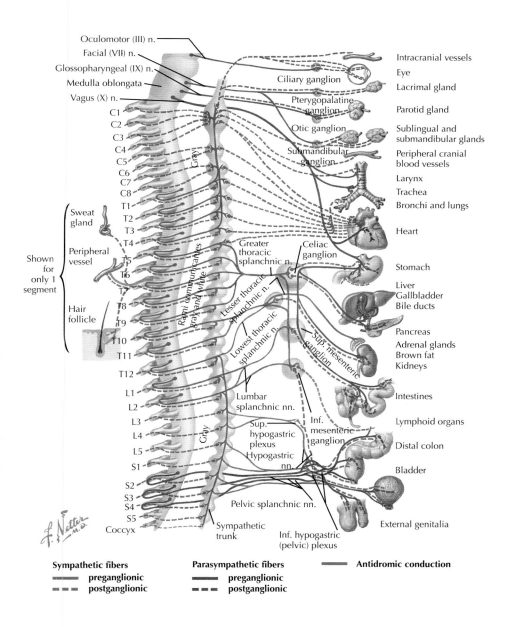

Oculomotor (III) n.
Facial (VII) n.
Glossopharyngeal (IX) n.
Medulla oblongata
Vagus (X) n.

C1
C2
C3
C4
C5
C6
C7
C8
T1
T2
T3
T4
T5
T6
T7
T8
T9
T10
T11
T12
L1
L2
L3
L4
L5
S1
S2
S3
S4
S5
Coccyx

Gray
Rami communicantes gray and white
Gray

Sweat gland
Peripheral vessel
Hair follicle

Shown for only 1 segment

Intracranial vessels
Eye
Lacrimal gland
Ciliary ganglion
Pterygopalatine ganglion
Parotid gland
Otic ganglion
Sublingual and submandibular glands
Submandibular ganglion
Peripheral cranial blood vessels
Larynx
Trachea
Bronchi and lungs
Heart

Greater thoracic splanchnic n.
Celiac ganglion
Lesser thoracic splanchnic n.
Stomach
Lowest thoracic splanchnic n.
Liver
Gallbladder
Bile ducts
Sup. mesenteric ganglion
Pancreas
Adrenal glands
Brown fat
Kidneys

Lumbar splanchnic nn.
Intestines
Inf. mesenteric ganglion
Lymphoid organs
Sup. hypogastric plexus
Distal colon
Hypogastric nn.
Bladder

Pelvic splanchnic nn.
External genitalia
Sympathetic trunk
Inf. hypogastric (pelvic) plexus

Sympathetic fibers
preganglionic
postganglionic

Parasympathetic fibers
preganglionic
postganglionic

Antidromic conduction

PARASYMPATHETIC AUTONOMIC CRANIAL NUCLEI: OVERVIEW

STRUCTURE	ANATOMIC NOTES	FUNCTIONAL SIGNIFICANCE
Nucleus of Edinger-Westphal	Preganglionic parasympathetic nucleus; fibers synapse in ciliary ganglion	Innervate ciliary muscle (accommodation) and iris sphincter (pupillary constriction)
Superior salivatory nucleus	Fibers exit with CN-VII, synapse on pterygopalatine and submandibular ganglia	Secretomotor innervation to lacrimal and nasal mucosal glands
Inferior salivatory nucleus	Exits with CN-IX, synapses on otic ganglion	Secretomotor innervation to parotid gland
Dorsal motor nucleus of CN-X	Fibers synapse on the terminal ganglia in thoracic and abdominal viscera	Innervates thoracic and abdominal viscera

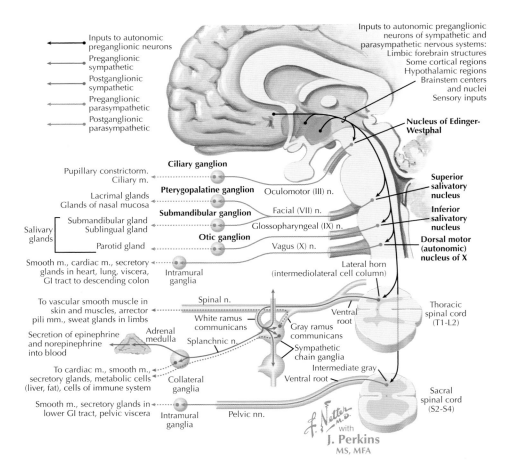

AUTONOMIC DISTRIBUTION TO THE EYE

STRUCTURE	ANATOMIC NOTES	FUNCTIONAL SIGNIFICANCE
Ciliary ganglion (parasympathetic)	Sends short ciliary nerves to the ciliary body and the iris of the eye	Accommodation for near vision Constriction of pupil
Superior cervical ganglion (sympathetic)	Innervated by preganglionic sympathetic fibers from T1-2 intermediolateral cell column (ciliospinal center of Budge) Postganglionic fibers follow the internal carotid artery to the eye, and external carotid artery to sweat glands of face	Dilates pupil Innervates Muller's muscle in upper and lower eyelid Sweating on ipsilateral face

- Pupillary light reflex: light shined into one eye activates CN-II. CN-II fibers synapse in the superior colliculus, thence to the nucleus of Edinger-Westphal bilaterally via the posterior commissure. Efferent limb travels through CN-III bilaterally to constrict pupils.
- Horner's syndrome: ptosis, miosis, and anhydrosis resulting from interruption of sympathetic pupillomotor pathway. Anhydrosis occurs only with lesions proximal to the carotid artery bifurcation because the external carotid carries the sudomotor axons.

AUTONOMIC DISTRIBUTION TO THE EYE *continued*

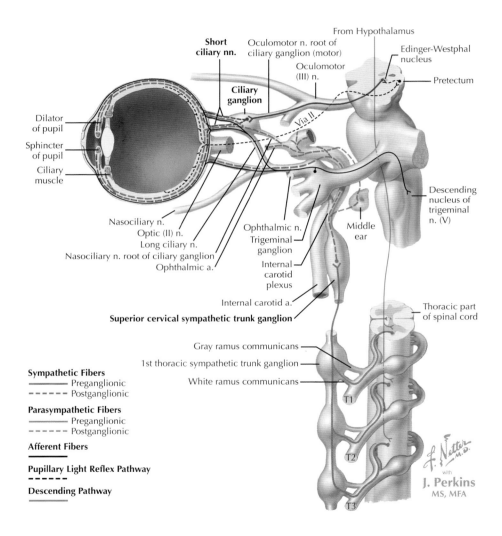

From Hypothalamus

Short ciliary nn.

Oculomotor n. root of ciliary ganglion (motor)

Edinger-Westphal nucleus

Oculomotor (III) n.

Pretectum

Ciliary ganglion

Via II

Dilator of pupil

Sphincter of pupil

Ciliary muscle

Nasociliary n.

Optic (II) n.

Long ciliary n.

Nasociliary n. root of ciliary ganglion

Ophthalmic a.

Ophthalmic n.

Trigeminal ganglion

Middle ear

Descending nucleus of trigeminal n. (V)

Internal carotid plexus

Internal carotid a.

Superior cervical sympathetic trunk ganglion

Gray ramus communicans

1st thoracic sympathetic trunk ganglion

White ramus communicans

Thoracic part of spinal cord

Sympathetic Fibers
——————— Preganglionic
- - - - - - Postganglionic

Parasympathetic Fibers
——————— Preganglionic
- - - - - - Postganglionic

Afferent Fibers
———————

Pupillary Light Reflex Pathway
- - - - - -

Descending Pathway
———————

T1

T2

T3

J. Netter M.D.

with

J. Perkins
MS, MFA

PTERYGOPALATINE AND SUBMANDIBULAR GANGLIA

STRUCTURE	ANATOMIC NOTES	FUNCTIONAL SIGNIFICANCE
Pterygopalatine ganglion (parasympathetic)	Supplied by the superior salivatory nucleus	Lacrimal and nasal mucosal gland secretion
Submandibular ganglion (parasympathetic)	Supplied by the superior salivatory nucleus	Sublingual and submandibular gland secretion
Superior cervical ganglion (sympathetic)	Innervated by preganglionic sympathetic fibers from T1-2 intermediolateral cell column	Innervates blood vessels in, and causes low level secretion of, lacrimal and nasal mucosal glands, sublingual and submandibular glands

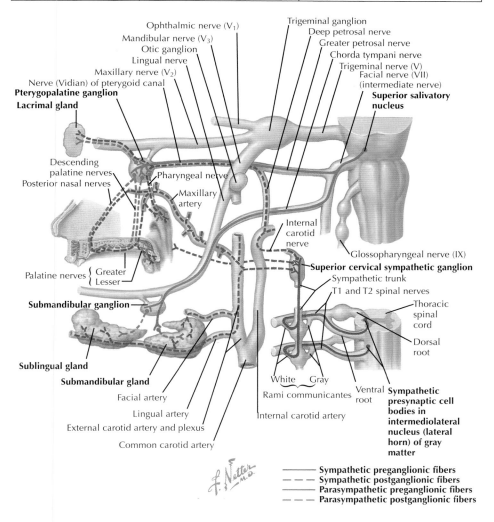

Ophthalmic nerve (V₁)
Mandibular nerve (V₃)
Otic ganglion
Lingual nerve
Maxillary nerve (V₂)
Nerve (Vidian) of pterygoid canal
Pterygopalatine ganglion
Lacrimal gland

Trigeminal ganglion
Deep petrosal nerve
Greater petrosal nerve
Chorda tympani nerve
Trigeminal nerve (V)
Facial nerve (VII) (intermediate nerve)
Superior salivatory nucleus

Descending palatine nerves
Posterior nasal nerves
Pharyngeal nerve
Maxillary artery

Internal carotid nerve

Glossopharyngeal nerve (IX)
Superior cervical sympathetic ganglion
Sympathetic trunk
T1 and T2 spinal nerves
Thoracic spinal cord
Dorsal root

Palatine nerves { Greater / Lesser

Submandibular ganglion

Sublingual gland
Submandibular gland
Facial artery
Lingual artery
External carotid artery and plexus
Common carotid artery

White   Gray
Rami communicantes
Internal carotid artery

Ventral root
Sympathetic presynaptic cell bodies in intermediolateral nucleus (lateral horn) of gray matter

——— Sympathetic preganglionic fibers
– – – Sympathetic postganglionic fibers
——— Parasympathetic preganglionic fibers
– – – Parasympathetic postganglionic fibers

PAROTID GLAND INNERVATION

STRUCTURE	ANATOMIC NOTES	FUNCTIONAL SIGNIFICANCE
Otic ganglion (parasympathetic)	Supplied by inferior salivatory nucleus	Parasympathetic secretomotor innervation to parotid gland
Superior cervical ganglion (sympathetic)	Innervated by preganglionic sympathetic fibers from T1-2 intermediolateral cell column Third-order neuron ascends external carotid artery to parotid	Sympathetic innervation to blood vessels in, and low level secretion of, the parotid gland

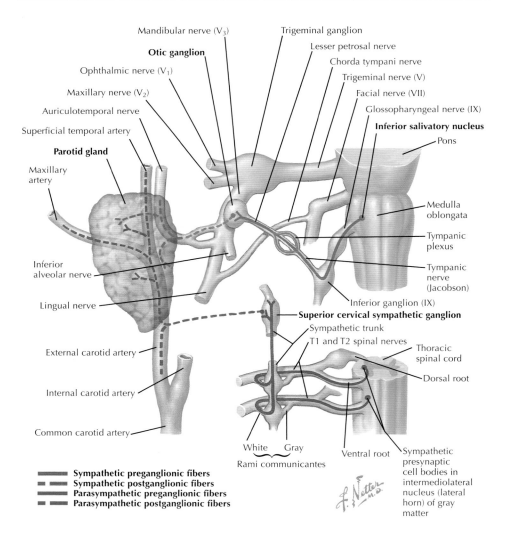

DORSAL MOTOR NUCLEUS OF CN-X

STRUCTURE	ANATOMIC NOTES	FUNCTIONAL SIGNIFICANCE
Dorsal motor nucleus of CN-X (parasympathetic)	Fibers synapse on the terminal ganglia in thoracic and abdominal viscera	Parasympathetic innervation to the thoracic and abdominal viscera
Lungs and bronchi	Postganglionic cell bodies in the pulmonary plexus ganglia	Constriction of air passages
Heart	Postganglionic cell bodies in the intracardiac atrial ganglia	Decreased pulse and myocardial activity
Esophagus	Postganglionic cell bodies in the myenteric plexus	Increased peristalsis and motility
Stomach to transverse colon	Postganglionic cell bodies in the myenteric plexus	Increased peristalsis and motility

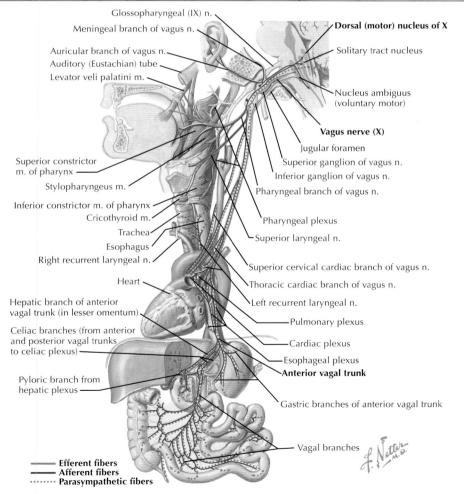

Glossopharyngeal (IX) n.
Meningeal branch of vagus n.
Auricular branch of vagus n.
Auditory (Eustachian) tube
Levator veli palatini m.
Superior constrictor m. of pharynx
Stylopharyngeus m.
Inferior constrictor m. of pharynx
Cricothyroid m.
Trachea
Esophagus
Right recurrent laryngeal n.
Heart
Hepatic branch of anterior vagal trunk (in lesser omentum)
Celiac branches (from anterior and posterior vagal trunks to celiac plexus)
Pyloric branch from hepatic plexus

Dorsal (motor) nucleus of X
Solitary tract nucleus
Nucleus ambiguus (voluntary motor)
Vagus nerve (X)
Jugular foramen
Superior ganglion of vagus n.
Inferior ganglion of vagus n.
Pharyngeal branch of vagus n.
Pharyngeal plexus
Superior laryngeal n.
Superior cervical cardiac branch of vagus n.
Thoracic cardiac branch of vagus n.
Left recurrent laryngeal n.
Pulmonary plexus
Cardiac plexus
Esophageal plexus
Anterior vagal trunk
Gastric branches of anterior vagal trunk
Vagal branches

Efferent fibers
Afferent fibers
Parasympathetic fibers

PARASYMPATHETIC AUTONOMIC SACRAL NUCLEI

STRUCTURE	ANATOMIC NOTES	FUNCTIONAL SIGNIFICANCE
Autonomic nuclei of intermediate gray in S2-4 spinal cord segments (parasympathetic)	Fibers synapse in: • Hemorrhoidal and myenteric ganglia • Ganglia along aorta and internal iliac arteries • Ganglia along vesical branches of internal iliac artery	Innervates: • Descending colon and rectum (peristalsis) • Sex organs (erection) • Urinary bladder (sphincter relaxation and bladder wall contraction)

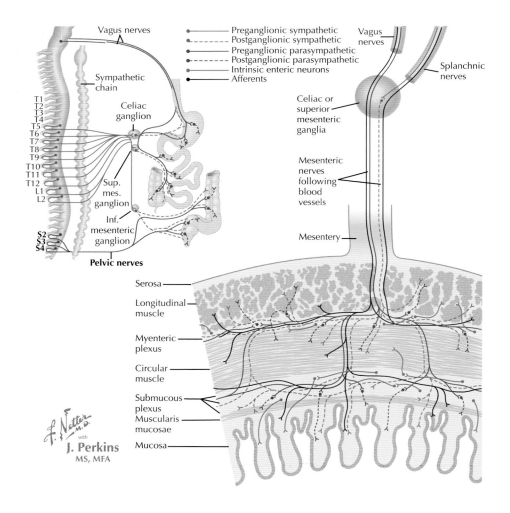

SYMPATHETIC SYSTEM

STRUCTURE	ANATOMIC NOTES	FUNCTIONAL SIGNIFICANCE
Sympathetic trunks (paravertebral ganglia)	2 symmetrical, ganglionated cords along the anterolateral vertebral column, running from the base of the skull to the coccyx	Second-order neuron runs from the intermediolateral cell column (ILCC) to sympathetic prevertebral or paravertebral ganglia
Prevertebral ganglia	Irregular ganglionic masses surrounding visceral branches of aorta	Third-order neuron runs from paravertebral and prevertebral ganglia to end organ
White ramus communicans	Myelinated, 2nd-order, preganglionic fibers from the ILCC enter sympathetic trunk to terminate on the paravertebral or prevertebral ganglia	Limited to T1-L2
Gray ramus communicans	Every spinal nerve receives 1 from the sympathetic trunk	Unmyelinated, 3rd-order, postganglionic fibers. Innervate blood vessels, arrector pili muscles, and glands of body wall

First-order neuron begins in the posterolateral hypothalamus, descends the reticular formation dorsolateral to the red nuclei, through the lateral pons and medulla and synapses on intermediolateral cell column (ILCC) from T1-L2.

SYMPATHETIC SYSTEM *continued*

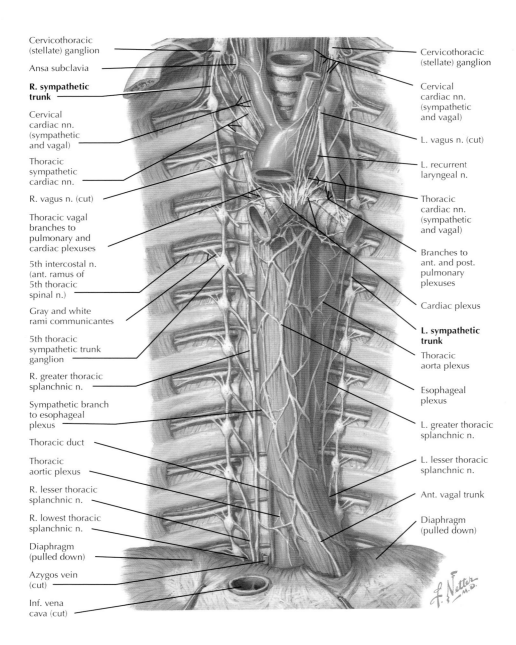

Cervicothoracic (stellate) ganglion

Ansa subclavia

R. sympathetic trunk

Cervical cardiac nn. (sympathetic and vagal)

Thoracic sympathetic cardiac nn.

R. vagus n. (cut)

Thoracic vagal branches to pulmonary and cardiac plexuses

5th intercostal n. (ant. ramus of 5th thoracic spinal n.)

Gray and white rami communicantes

5th thoracic sympathetic trunk ganglion

R. greater thoracic splanchnic n.

Sympathetic branch to esophageal plexus

Thoracic duct

Thoracic aortic plexus

R. lesser thoracic splanchnic n.

R. lowest thoracic splanchnic n.

Diaphragm (pulled down)

Azygos vein (cut)

Inf. vena cava (cut)

Cervicothoracic (stellate) ganglion

Cervical cardiac nn. (sympathetic and vagal)

L. vagus n. (cut)

L. recurrent laryngeal n.

Thoracic cardiac nn. (sympathetic and vagal)

Branches to ant. and post. pulmonary plexuses

Cardiac plexus

L. sympathetic trunk

Thoracic aorta plexus

Esophageal plexus

L. greater thoracic splanchnic n.

L. lesser thoracic splanchnic n.

Ant. vagal trunk

Diaphragm (pulled down)

SYMPATHETIC INNERVATION OF THORACO-ABDOMINAL-PELVIC VISCERA

STRUCTURE	ANATOMIC NOTES	FUNCTIONAL SIGNIFICANCE
C8-T2 (3) intermediolateral cell column	Superior cervical sympathetic ganglia	Iris: pupillary dilation
T1-2 intermediolateral cell column	Superior and middle cervical sympathetic ganglia	Lacrimal gland: vasomotor to blood vessels and low level glandular secretion
T1-3 (4) intermediolateral cell column	Superior and middle cervical sympathetic ganglia	Submandibular and sublingual gland: vasomotor to blood vessels, and low level glandular secretion
T1-3 (4) intermediolateral cell column	Superior and middle cervical sympathetic ganglia	Parotid gland: vasomotor to blood vessels, and low level glandular secretion
T1-3 intermediolateral cell column	3 cervical sympathetic ganglia	Sweat glands in head and neck: secretion
T1-5 intermediolateral cell column	Inferior cervical and thoracic T1-5 sympathetic ganglia	Lungs and bronchi: dilation
T1-5 (6,7) intermediolateral cell column	3 cervical and thoracic T1-6 sympathetic ganglia	Cardiac: increased pulse rate and myocardial activity
T1-6 intermediolateral cell column	Thoracic T(1-3) 4-6 sympathetic ganglia	Esophagus: decreased motility
T5-T11 intermediolateral cell column	Celiac and superior mesenteric plexus	Stomach to transverse colon: decreased motility
T12-L3 intermediolateral cell column	Lumbar and inferior mesenteric plexus	Descending colon and rectum: decreased motility
T10-L2 intermediolateral cell column	Lumbar, sacral, and inferior mesenteric plexus	Sex organs: ejaculation
T12-L2 intermediolateral cell column	Lumbar and inferior mesenteric plexus	Urinary bladder: sphincter contraction and bladder wall relaxation
L1-2 intermediolateral cell column	Lumbar and sacral sympathetic ganglia	Sweat glands: secretion Leg blood vessels: arteriolar constriction (generally)

SYMPATHETIC INNERVATION OF THORACO-ABDOMINAL-PELVIC VISCERA *continued*

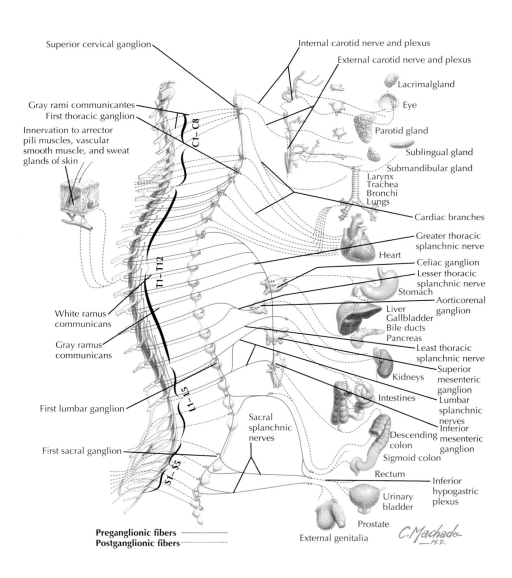

Superior cervical ganglion

Internal carotid nerve and plexus

External carotid nerve and plexus

Lacrimalgland

Eye

Gray rami communicantes

First thoracic ganglion

Parotid gland

Innervation to arrector pili muscles, vascular smooth muscle, and sweat glands of skin

Sublingual gland

Submandibular gland

Larynx
Trachea
Bronchi
Lungs

Cardiac branches

Greater thoracic splanchnic nerve

Heart

Celiac ganglion

Lesser thoracic splanchnic nerve

Stomach

White ramus communicans

Aorticorenal ganglion

Liver
Gallbladder
Bile ducts
Pancreas

Gray ramus communicans

Least thoracic splanchnic nerve

Kidneys

Superior mesenteric ganglion

Intestines

Lumbar splanchnic nerves

First lumbar ganglion

Inferior mesenteric ganglion

Sacral splanchnic nerves

Descending colon

Sigmoid colon

First sacral ganglion

Rectum

Inferior hypogastric plexus

Urinary bladder

Prostate

Preganglionic fibers
Postganglionic fibers

External genitalia

C. *Machado*
—M.D.

C1–C8

T1–T12

L1–L5

S1–S5

ABDOMINAL SYMPATHETIC AUTONOMIC NERVES AND GANGLIA

STRUCTURE	ANATOMIC NOTES	FUNCTIONAL SIGNIFICANCE
Greater splanchnic nerve	Arises from T5-9 Correspond to the white ramus communicans	Preganglionic fibers that innervate the celiac plexus
Lesser splanchnic nerve	Arises from T10-11 Correspond to white ramus communicans	Preganglionic fibers that innervate the celiac plexus
Celiac plexus	Surrounds celiac and superior mesenteric arteries	Largest autonomic plexus Contains celiac and superior mesenteric ganglia
Hypogastric plexus	Unpaired	Innervates pelvic viscera

White ramus communicans: Preganglionic sympathetic fibers that arise from the intermediolateral cell column T1-L2, leave the spinal cord via ventral roots of T1-L2, then leave the spinal nerve as the white ramus communicans, enter the sympathetic trunk, and terminate on cells in the prevertebral and paravertebral ganglia.

ABDOMINAL SYMPATHETIC AUTONOMIC NERVES AND GANGLIA *continued*

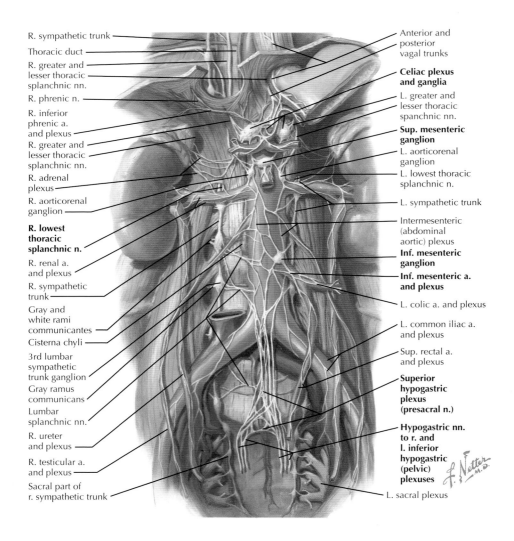

R. sympathetic trunk

Thoracic duct

R. greater and lesser thoracic splanchnic nn.

R. phrenic n.

R. inferior phrenic a. and plexus

R. greater and lesser thoracic splanchnic nn.

R. adrenal plexus

R. aorticorenal ganglion

R. lowest thoracic splanchnic n.

R. renal a. and plexus

R. sympathetic trunk

Gray and white rami communicantes

Cisterna chyli

3rd lumbar sympathetic trunk ganglion

Gray ramus communicans

Lumbar splanchnic nn.

R. ureter and plexus

R. testicular a. and plexus

Sacral part of r. sympathetic trunk

Anterior and posterior vagal trunks

Celiac plexus and ganglia

L. greater and lesser thoracic spanchnic nn.

Sup. mesenteric ganglion

L. aorticorenal ganglion

L. lowest thoracic splanchnic n.

L. sympathetic trunk

Intermesenteric (abdominal aortic) plexus

Inf. mesenteric ganglion

Inf. mesenteric a. and plexus

L. colic a. and plexus

L. common iliac a. and plexus

Sup. rectal a. and plexus

Superior hypogastric plexus (presacral n.)

Hypogastric nn. to r. and l. inferior hypogastric (pelvic) plexuses

L. sacral plexus

AUTONOMIC NERVES IN HEAD AND NECK

STRUCTURE	ANATOMIC NOTES	FUNCTIONAL SIGNIFICANCE
Superior cervical ganglion	Largest of paravertebral ganglia	Gives rise to 3rd-order fibers to lower 4 cranial and upper 4 cervical nerves, pharynx, external and internal carotid arteries
Middle cervical ganglion	Lies near C6 vertebra	Often absent
Inferior cervical ganglion	Lies near the lower border of C7 vertebra. Often fuses with 1st thoracic ganglion to form the stellate ganglion	Furnishes gray rami communicantes to C7-T1

Gray ramus communicans: Each spinal nerve receives a gray ramus communicans from the sympathetic trunk that consists of unmyelinated postganglionic fibers that innervate blood vessels, glands, and arrector pili muscles.

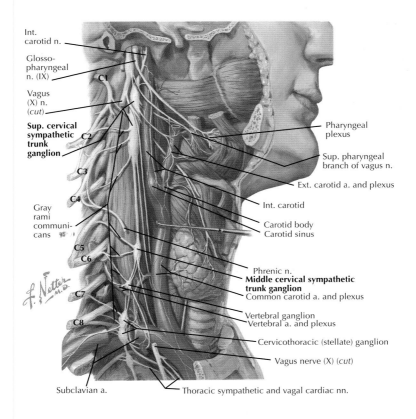

SCHEMATIC OF AUTONOMIC NERVES IN HEAD AND NECK

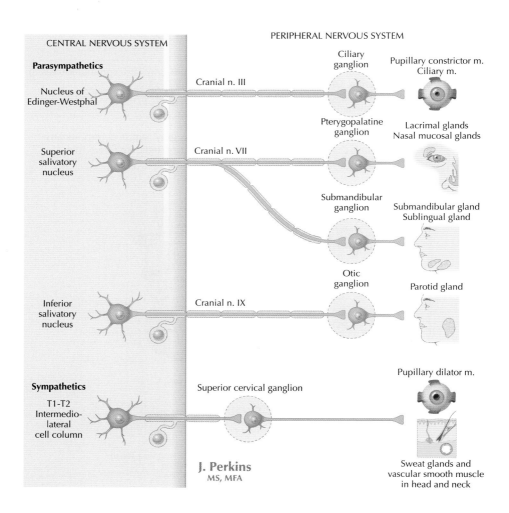

CENTRAL NERVOUS SYSTEM

PERIPHERAL NERVOUS SYSTEM

Parasympathetics

Nucleus of Edinger-Westphal

Cranial n. III

Ciliary ganglion

Pupillary constrictor m.
Ciliary m.

Superior salivatory nucleus

Cranial n. VII

Pterygopalatine ganglion

Lacrimal glands
Nasal mucosal glands

Submandibular ganglion

Submandibular gland
Sublingual gland

Otic ganglion

Parotid gland

Inferior salivatory nucleus

Cranial n. IX

Pupillary dilator m.

Sympathetics

T1-T2 Intermedio-lateral cell column

Superior cervical ganglion

J. Perkins
MS, MFA

Sweat glands and vascular smooth muscle in head and neck

AUTONOMIC INNERVATION OF LIMBS

STRUCTURE	ANATOMIC NOTES	FUNCTIONAL SIGNIFICANCE
T1-L2 intermediolateral cell column	Sends preganglionic fibers to sympathetic chain ganglia, which send postganglionic fibers into the peripheral nerves	Vascular smooth muscle: constriction Sweat glands: secretion Arrector pili: pilomotor contraction, goosebumps, or raise hair

Autonomic innervation of the limbs derives only from the sympathetic nervous system.

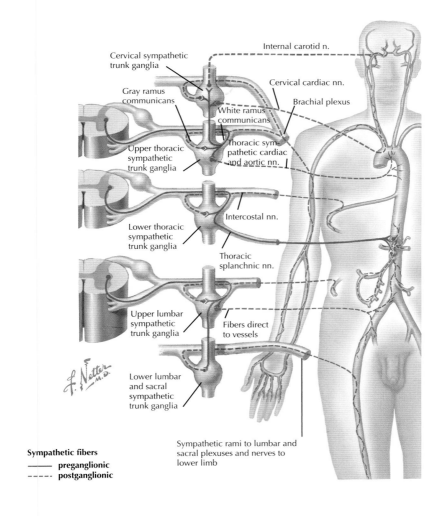

Cervical sympathetic trunk ganglia

Internal carotid n.

Cervical cardiac nn.

Gray ramus communicans

White ramus communicans

Brachial plexus

Upper thoracic sympathetic trunk ganglia

Thoracic sympathetic cardiac and aortic nn.

Lower thoracic sympathetic trunk ganglia

Intercostal nn.

Thoracic splanchnic nn.

Upper lumbar sympathetic trunk ganglia

Fibers direct to vessels

Lower lumbar and sacral sympathetic trunk ganglia

Sympathetic fibers
——— preganglionic
----- postganglionic

Sympathetic rami to lumbar and sacral plexuses and nerves to lower limb

AUTONOMIC INNERVATION OF STOMACH

STRUCTURE	ANATOMIC NOTES	FUNCTIONAL SIGNIFICANCE
Celiac and superior mesenteric ganglia (sympathetic)	Greater and lesser thoracic splanchnic nerves provide preganglionic input to ganglia	Decreases peristalsis and secretomotor (e.g., gastrin, HCl) activity
Celiac branches of vagus (parasympathetic)	Supply stomach and proximal duodenum	Increases peristalsis and secretomotor activity and relaxes associated sphincters

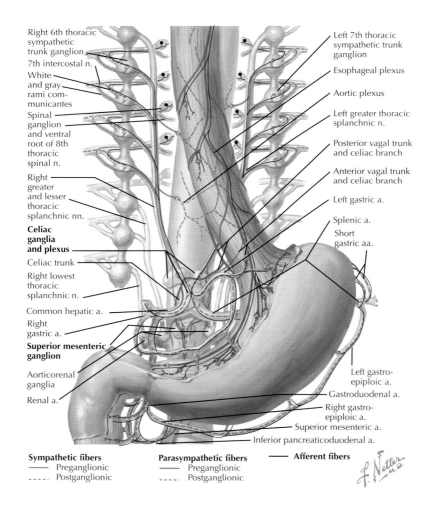

Right 6th thoracic sympathetic trunk ganglion

7th intercostal n.

White and gray rami communicantes

Spinal ganglion and ventral root of 8th thoracic spinal n.

Right greater and lesser thoracic splanchnic nn.

Celiac ganglia and plexus

Celiac trunk

Right lowest thoracic splanchnic n.

Common hepatic a.

Right gastric a.

Superior mesenteric ganglion

Aorticorenal ganglia

Renal a.

Left 7th thoracic sympathetic trunk ganglion

Esophageal plexus

Aortic plexus

Left greater thoracic splanchnic n.

Posterior vagal trunk and celiac branch

Anterior vagal trunk and celiac branch

Left gastric a.

Splenic a.

Short gastric aa.

Left gastro-epiploic a.

Gastroduodenal a.

Right gastro-epiploic a.

Superior mesenteric a.

Inferior pancreaticoduodenal a.

Sympathetic fibers
—— Preganglionic
- - - - Postganglionic

Parasympathetic fibers
—— Preganglionic
- - - - Postganglionic

—— **Afferent fibers**

F. Netter M.D.

AUTONOMIC INNERVATION OF INTESTINES

STRUCTURE	ANATOMIC NOTES	FUNCTIONAL SIGNIFICANCE
T5-11 intermediolateral cell column (sympathetic)	Distributes to the superior and inferior mesenteric and celiac ganglia	Decreases peristalsis and secretomotor (fluid secretion) activity
Vagus nerve, S2-4 intermediate gray (parasympathetic)	Distributes to the intramural ganglia	Increases peristalsis and secretomotor activity and relaxes involuntary sphincters

AUTONOMIC INNERVATION OF INTESTINES *continued*

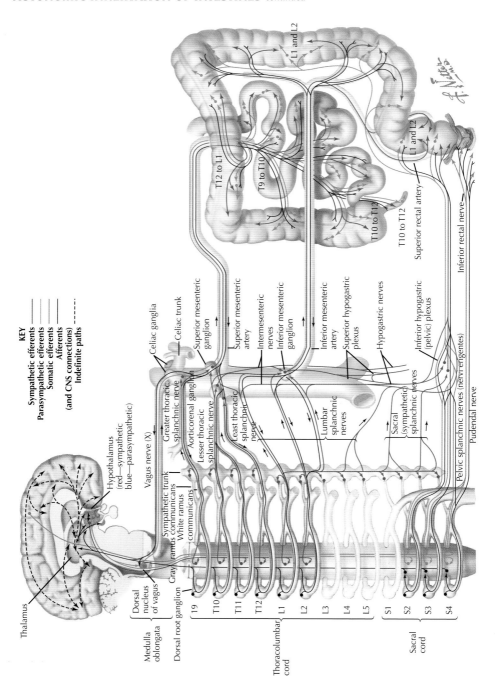

KEY

Sympathetic efferents
Parasympathetic efferents
Somatic efferents
Afferents
(and CNS connections)
Indefinite paths

Thalamus

Hypothalamus
(red—sympathetic
blue—parasympathetic)

Vagus nerve (X)

Dorsal nucleus of vagus

Medulla oblongata

Dorsal root ganglion

Sympathetic trunk
Gray ramus communicans
White ramus communicans

Thoracolumbar cord

Sacral cord

Greater thoracic splanchnic nerve
Lesser thoracic splanchnic nerve
Least thoracic splanchnic nerve
Aorticorenal ganglion
Celiac ganglia
Celiac trunk
Superior mesenteric ganglion
Superior mesenteric artery
Intermesenteric nerves
Inferior mesenteric ganglion
Inferior mesenteric artery
Superior hypogastric plexus
Hypogastric nerves
Lumbar splanchnic nerves
Sacral (sympathetic) splanchnic nerves
Inferior hypogastric (pelvic) plexus
Pelvic splanchnic nerves (nervi erigentes)
Superior rectal artery
Inferior rectal nerve
Pudendal nerve

T12 to L1
T9 to T10
L1 and L2
T10 to T12
L1 and L2

AUTONOMIC INNERVATION OF URINARY BLADDER

STRUCTURE	ANATOMIC NOTES	FUNCTIONAL SIGNIFICANCE
L1-2 intermediolateral cell column (sympathetic)	Through sacral splanchnic nerves to hypogastric plexus	Relax detrusor and contract trigone and internal sphincter
S2-4 intermediate gray (parasympathetic)	Through pelvic splanchnic nerves to intramural ganglia of bladder wall	Contract detrusor and relax trigone and internal sphincter to empty bladder

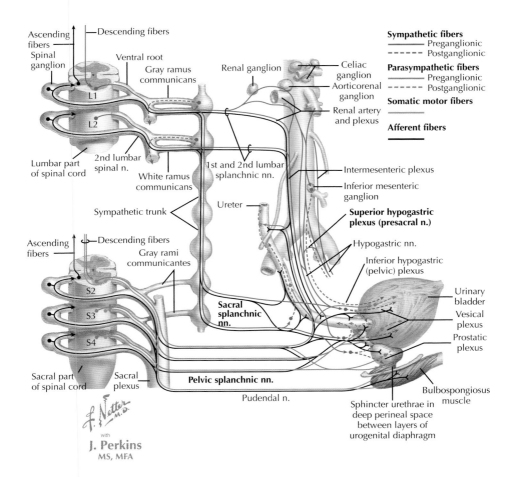

AUTONOMIC INNERVATION OF MALE REPRODUCTIVE ORGANS

STRUCTURE	ANATOMIC NOTES	FUNCTIONAL SIGNIFICANCE
T10-L2 intermediolateral cell column (sympathetic)	Via thoracic and upper lumbar splanchnic nerves to superior hypogastric plexus	Contraction of vas deferens and prostate capsule and contraction of the bladder sphincter to prevent retrograde ejaculation
S2-4 intermediate gray (parasympathetic)	Via pelvic splanchnic nerves to inferior hypogastric plexus	Vascular dilation to initiate and maintain erection

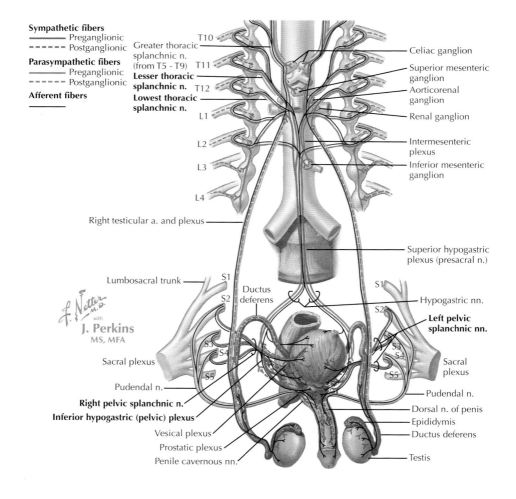

Sympathetic fibers
——— Preganglionic
– – – – Postganglionic
Parasympathetic fibers
——— Preganglionic
– – – – Postganglionic
Afferent fibers
———

Greater thoracic splanchnic n. (from T5 - T9)
Lesser thoracic splanchnic n.
Lowest thoracic splanchnic n.

T10
T11
T12
L1
L2
L3
L4

Celiac ganglion
Superior mesenteric ganglion
Aorticorenal ganglion
Renal ganglion
Intermesenteric plexus
Inferior mesenteric ganglion

Right testicular a. and plexus

Superior hypogastric plexus (presacral n.)

Lumbosacral trunk
S1
S2
Ductus deferens

S1
S2
Hypogastric nn.
Left pelvic splanchnic nn.

J. Perkins
MS, MFA

Sacral plexus
S3
S4
S5

S3
S4
S5
Sacral plexus

Pudendal n.
Right pelvic splanchnic n.
Inferior hypogastric (pelvic) plexus
Vesical plexus
Prostatic plexus
Penile cavernous nn.

Pudendal n.
Dorsal n. of penis
Epididymis
Ductus deferens
Testis

AUTONOMIC INNERVATION OF FEMALE REPRODUCTIVE ORGANS

STRUCTURE	ANATOMIC NOTES	FUNCTIONAL SIGNIFICANCE
T10-L2 intermediolateral cell column (sympathetic)	Via the thoracic and upper lumbar splanchnic nerves to the superior hypogastric plexus	Contraction of the uterus. Also supplies vaginal arteries, vestibular glands, and erectile tissue
S2-4 intermediate gray (parasympathetic)	Via pelvic splanchnic nerves to the inferior hypogastric plexus	Muscular and mucous coat of the vagina and urethra; stimulates erectile tissue of the vestibular bulb and clitoris and supplies vestibular glands

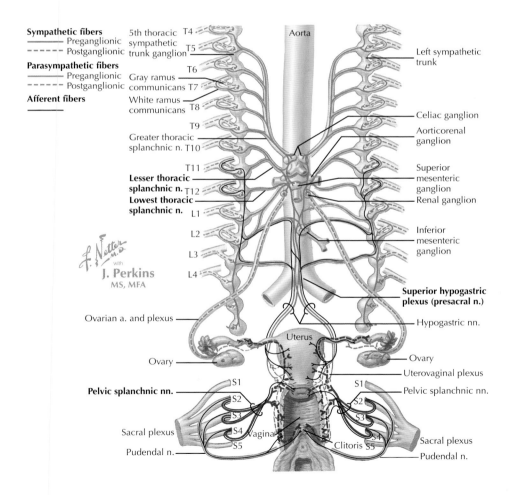

NETTER'S CONCISE NEUROANATOMY **391**

Index

Index

Index

Index

Index

Index